MW01029081

Dynamics of
Health and Disease

Dynamics of Health and Disease

CARTER L. MARSHALL, M.D.
University Dean for Health Affairs,
The City University of New York;
Associate Professor of Community Medicine,
Mount Sinai School of Medicine of
The City University of New York

DAVID PEARSON, Ph.D.
Assistant Professor,
Department of Epidemiology and Public Health,
Yale University School of Medicine

APPLETON-CENTURY-CROFTS
EDUCATIONAL DIVISION / MEREDITH CORPORATION
New York

Library of Congress Catalog Card Number: 72-78478

Second Printing

PRINTED IN THE UNITED STATES OF AMERICA
390-59893-3

Contributors

FRANK R. HARTMAN, M.D. *Clinical Instructor of Psychiatry, Albert Einstein College of Medicine; Consulting Psychiatrist, Time Incorporated*

EDWARD F. X. HUGHES, M.D., M.P.H. *Associate in Community Medicine, Mount Sinai School of Medicine of The City University of New York; Consultant to the Health Services Administration, New York City*

GEORGE W. JACKSON, M.D. *Epidemic Intelligence Service Officer, Center for Disease Control, Public Health Service; Department of Community Medicine, Mount Sinai School of Medicine of The City University of New York*

STANLEY MARINOFF, M.D., M.P.H. *Assistant Professor of Obstetrics and Gynecology, Mount Sinai School of Medicine of The City University of New York*

CAROL MARSHALL, M.P.H. *Coordinator for Program Planning and Development, Central Flushing Medical Center, Health Insurance Plan of Greater New York*

CARTER L. MARSHALL, M.D. *University Dean for Health Affairs, The City University of New York; Associate Professor of Community Medicine, Mount Sinai School of Medicine of The City University of New York*

DAVID PEARSON, Ph.D. *Assistant Professor, Department of Epidemiology and Public Health, Yale University School of Medicine*

ELIHU D. RICHTER, M.D., M.P.H. *Health Officer, Ministry of Labor, Government of Israel*

COURTNEY B. WOOD, M.D., M.P.H. *Associate Professor of Community Medicine, Mount Sinai School of Medicine of the City University of New York*

Preface

Dynamics of Health and Disease is an introductory text that has been written to meet the needs of students with little or no previous exposure to the health field. The objectives of this book are: (1) to provide a broad and general background which will enable the reader to read and to understand more advanced and specialized literature without undue difficulty; and (2) to make available a general reference text which consolidates and summarizes material from many sources.

Emphasis has been placed on the exposition of essential principles rather than on an exhaustive presentation of detailed information. Clarity has been a paramount concern. We have not hesitated to rely on secondary sources (such as newspapers and pamphlets) in preparing the material, and we wish to acknowledge a special debt to texts written primarily for medical students. Although such texts are more advanced than the present volume, they were of great value in organizing material and in suggesting alternative ways of presenting it.

The "vocabulary" or "jargon" of any specialized field universally presents a problem to the uninitiated, and the terminology of the health profession is no exception. Therefore, all newly encountered terms are defined either within the text itself or (if they appear in boldface) at the bottom of the page on which they occur. In addition, a list of essential word-roots is included in the first chapter. This should further assist the student in his efforts to understand the language of health.

Tabular material, photographs, and charts were developed or selected either because they helped to illustrate a principle discussed in the text, or because they added another dimension to the discussion. In all cases, their inclusion was approved by a college student who read the text specifically to identify the graphic material that would be most helpful to other students. Consequently, the various photographs, drawings, tables, figures, and so on should be considered an integral part of the text and their legends read as if they were part of the major body of the book.

Particular effort has gone into deciding what to include in this text, since it was obvious from the beginning that much would have to be omitted. In this necessarily arbitrary process of selection, we were guided principally by the desire to present material that would best exemplify basic concepts and principles. This book thus exposes the student to the representative tip of a vast and complex "iceberg" of knowledge. The essential nature of the iceberg is faithfully mirrored in the tip, even though the main body is larger, deeper, and less apparent. For this reason, the instructor can assign more specific and advanced reading which supplements and enlarges on the basic information offered in this text. In most introductory courses, this is difficult, if not impossible, because of problems with terminology or lack of exposure to basic principles.

The idea of writing this book grew out of several years' teaching experience in an introductory course for students of the allied health sciences at Hunter College. (Several of the contributors to the book have also taught in this course.) The allied health students at Hunter typically represent a wide and diverse range of experience, education, and interests. Some have had little or no previous exposure to any of the sciences. Others have good science backgrounds but no previous exposure to the health field. Still others have returned to school after years of work experience in one of the health occupations. We have therefore avoided any emphasis that might identify *Dynamics* as a book written for any specific group, such as nursing students, laboratory technologists, physical therapists, and so on.

The first and major part of the book deals with the nature of health and disease; the second part describes the ways in which society organizes itself to deliver medical care services. It is our hope that the broad scope of this book will enable it to be of value to a heterogeneous group of interested readers. In addition to students of the allied health sciences, *Dynamics* might also serve as a general introductory text for first-year medical students or for students in schools of public health. Moreover, at a time of growing interest in health and the delivery of medical care, this book could be helpful to lay people who want to know more about one or more aspects of a fascinating field.

Without the services of a good editor, books such as this one would be impossible to complete. We wish to acknowledge the untiring, imaginative, and thorough editing of Mrs. Marion Goodrich. Our thanks also go to Miss Ronnie Goldstein, a graduate student at The City University of New York, who developed and selected the illustrations and also told us when we were being obtuse. We also wish to thank The Mount Sinai Medical Arts Department for their cooperation. Needless to say, the contributors have fully earned a most profound acknowledgment; for without them, we would have only half a book.

C. L. Marshall
New York City
April 1972

Contents

Contributors   v

Preface   vii

List of Tables   xi

PART I: THE NATURE OF HEALTH AND DISEASE

1. SOME BASIC CONCEPTS OF HEALTH AND DISEASE   1
   Carter Marshall

2. SOME BACKGROUND DETERMINANTS OF HEALTH AND DISEASE   15
   Carter Marshall
   Carol Marshall

3. THE ANALYSIS AND MEASUREMENT OF DISEASE   62
   Carter Marshall

4. INFECTIOUS DISEASES   88
   Carter Marshall

5. CHRONIC DISEASES AND THEIR MANAGEMENT   127
   Carter Marshall

6. HEALTH PROBLEMS OF MOTHERS, CHILDREN, AND THE ELDERLY   163
   Carter Marshall

7. MENTAL ILLNESS   181
   Frank Hartman

8. THE SOCIAL ENVIRONMENT   222
    Carter Marshall
    Edward Hughes
    George Jackson
    Stanley Marinoff
    Elihu Richter

9. THE PHYSICAL ENVIRONMENT   281
    Carter Marshall
    Elihu Richter

PART II: THE DELIVERY OF HEALTH SERVICES

10. TRENDS AFFECTING HEALTH CARE   338
    David Pearson

11. RESOURCES FOR HEALTH CARE   356
    David Pearson

12. THE PROVISION OF MEDICAL CARE SERVICES:
    ORGANIZATION, FINANCING AND UTILIZATION   390
    Courtney Wood

    CONCLUDING NOTE   414
    David Pearson
    Carter Marshall

Appendix   417
Index   441

List of Tables

1-1	WORD ROOTS IN THE JARGON OF HEALTH	8
2-1	SALE OF THALIDOMIDE AND INCIDENCE OF THALIDOMIDE CASES	57
3-1	COMMONLY USED RATES	72
3-2	CRUDE AND AGE-SPECIFIC DEATH RATES IN TWO IMAGINARY TOWNS	73
3-3	RETROSPECTIVE VERSUS PROSPECTIVE STUDIES	80
3-4	ATTRIBUTABLE VERSUS RELATIVE RISK	80
3-5	SCREENING TESTS IN COMMON USE	84
3-6	IMPORTANT DISEASES AND EARLY DETECTION	85
4-1	DISEASE AGENTS AFFECTING COMMON SITES OF INFECTION	90
4-2	COMMONLY USED VACCINES	97
4-3	ANTIBIOTICS USEFUL AGAINST CERTAIN BACTERIAL AGENTS	108
4-4	TRANSMISSION AND CONTROL OF BACTERIAL DISEASES TRANSMITTED FROM MAN TO MAN	110
4-5	TRANSMISSION AND CONTROL OF VIRUSES TRANSMITTED FROM MAN TO MAN	111
4-6	INFECTIOUS VERSUS SERUM HEPATITIS	114
4-7	LEADING CAUSES OF DEATH, 1900 AND 1965, WITH SOME COMPARATIVE DEATH RATES	124
5-1	INFECTIOUS VERSUS CHRONIC DISEASE (A VERY GENERAL COMPARISON)	128
5-2	SOME FACTS ON CANCER— FIVE LEADING CAUSES OF CANCER DEATH	144
6-1	MATERNAL MORTALITY RATE (PER 100,000) BY RACE (UNITED STATES, 1915-1968)	164
6-2	LEADING CAUSES OF FETAL, NEONATAL, AND INFANT DEATHS 1960s, NEW YORK CITY AND GREAT BRITAIN	170
6-3	FIVE LEADING CAUSES OF DEATH BY AGE GROUPS IN UNITED STATES, 1967	173
6-4	FIVE LEADING CAUSES OF DEATH FOR THE AGED IN UNITED STATES, 1967	176
8-1	DRUG CLASSIFICATION	226
8-2	NARCOTIC-RELATED DEATHS IN NEW YORK CITY	230
8-3	ESTIMATED TOTAL SYPHILIS AND GONORRHEA CASES TREATED (FISCAL 1968)	252
8-4	CIGARETTE SMOKING AND MORTALITY RATIOS FOR SELECTED CAUSES OF DEATH	261
8-5	TYPES OF INJURIES ASSOCIATED WITH ACCIDENTS	266

8-6	SOME STATISTICS RELATED TO PRINCIPAL CLASSES OF ACCIDENT, 1970	268
8-7	TENEMENT PREVENTIVE MAINTENANCE AND ENVIRONMENTAL CONTROL—SELECTED HEALTH AND SAFETY BENEFITS	272
9-1	IMPORTANT ZOONOTIC DISEASES	285
9-2	A SUMMARY OF ZOONOTIC DISEASES WHICH DO NOT INVOLVE VECTOR TRANSMISSION	288
9-3	PRINCIPAL VECTOR-BORNE DISEASES	289
9-4	A SUMMARY OF SELECTED VECTOR-BORNE DISEASES	297
9-5	POLLUTANTS IN THE POST-WAR PERIOD	308
11-1	BEDS IN NURSING CARE AND RELATED HOMES: UNITED STATES, 1967	359
11-2	PERCENT DISTRIBUTION OF NURSING CARE AND RELATED HOMES BY BED SIZE: UNITED STATES, 1967	359
11-3	OWNERSHIP OF NURSING CARE AND RELATED HOMES: UNITED STATES, 1967	360
11-4	SELECTED HOSPITAL INFORMATION: UNITED STATES, 1960-69	362
11-5	HOSPITALS BY OWNERSHIP AND TYPE OF SERVICE: UNITED STATES, 1969	364
11-6	NONFEDERAL HOSPITAL OPERATING EXPENSE PER PATIENT DAY: UNITED STATES, SELECTED YEARS 1946-1969	370
11-7	EXPENSES INVOLVED IN AN AVERAGE HOSPITAL STAY IN COMMUNITY HOSPITALS: UNITED STATES, SELECTED YEARS 1946-1970	371
11-8	ESTIMATED EMPLOYMENT IN HEALTH OCCUPATIONS: 1900 AND 1967	378
11-9	CLASSIFICATION OF ALLIED HEALTH PERSONNEL	380
11-10	ESTIMATED EMPLOYMENT IN HEALTH FIELD BY OCCUPATION, 1965	381
11-11	HEALTH MANPOWER REQUIREMENTS: 1966 AND 1975 ESTIMATES	387
11-12	HOSPITAL MANPOWER REQUIREMENTS: 1966 ESTIMATES	388

Dynamics of
Health and Disease

CHAPTER

1

Some Basic Concepts of Health and Disease

The Question of Health

What is health? Its maintenance and preservation cost the American people about $60 billion a year, and health facilities employ more persons than any other industry except construction. And yet, health eludes exact definition. Suggested definitions are liable to change over time, always subjective, and never entirely satisfactory; moreover, they range from the over-simplified to the utopian. An example of the former is that health is the absence of disease. Most readers will find this definition unacceptable because it stresses not what health is but what health is not and because it raises the whole matter of what constitutes disease. The definition used in the constitution of the **World Health Organization** epitomizes the utopian view and equates health with a "state of complete physical, mental, and social well-being." While praiseworthy, this repre-

---

WORLD HEALTH ORGANIZATION: an agency within the United Nations concerned with
health

sents more a long-range goal than a definition and contributes little to a working understanding of health.

Most people seem to perceive health in terms of their own ability to function according to their own perception of what is normal. An individual seeks medical attention when pain or discomfort impedes function, or when he believes that medical care will prevent limitation of function at some future time. Accordingly, we can define health as that physical and mental state which maximizes the individual's ability to function in a normal manner, while disease may be defined as any condition which actually or potentially impedes individual function. There are problems here. For example, normal function differs from person to person. In addition, our definition of health implies that the individual is "healthy" so long as he is free of **symptoms and signs** that interfere with his ability to function; and this definition of disease includes potential conditions which may or may not produce symptoms. Thus, by our definitions a person can be ill and well simultaneously. This is in fact the case. Millions of Americans whose blood pressure is too high or whose blood sugar is abnormally elevated function without any difficulty whatever. Sooner or later, both of these conditions may seriously impede function, but at any given time the individual is likely to enjoy good health as we have defined it. This is an extremely important idea, for health and disease are not opposites—both may coexist in the same person. They tend to overlap and merge imperceptibly into one another. Is the asymptomatic man with an elevated blood pressure sick or well? This is much like asking whether a quart bottle containing a pint of milk is half empty or half full (Fig. 1-1). In each case the answer is neither one nor the other, but both. Throughout much of an individual's life, health and disease tend to counterbalance each other—with a slight tilt in favor of health. The fundamental task of those working in the health field is to maintain this balance in favor of the individual, i.e., to keep him healthy.

The activities that must be carried out to insure health are of three types: organizational, preventive, and restorative.

Health organization is both educative and administrative. The former primarily involves educating the public to the nature of health and disease in an effort to encourage behavior beneficial to health. Efforts directed toward reducing cigarette smoking, increasing safe-driving habits,

---

SYMPTOM: a functional change in the individual which is suggestive of disease, e.g., pain in the chest, or a sore throat

SIGN: an observable manifestation of disease, e.g., swelling of the ankles, or a body rash

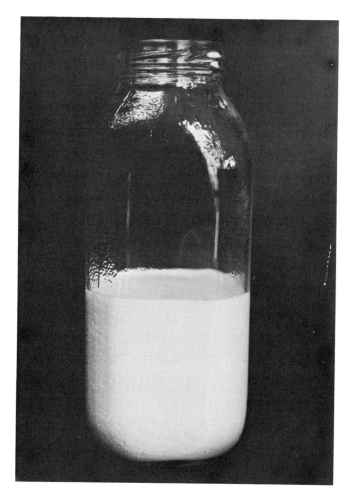

Fig. 1-1.   *Depending on your point of view, this bottle may be considered half empty or half full. In fact, it is both at the same time. So it is with health. People can be both sick and well simultaneously. (Courtesy of Dr. C. L. Marshall.)*

and disseminating sex information are examples of health education. Health organization at the administrative level is a responsibility of local, state, and federal governments. The ban of cigarette commercials from television and the requirement that the auto industry produce pollution-free vehicles by 1975 exemplify federal actions to promote health. Of equal if not greater importance are those governmental activities designed to assure the delivery of health services such as Medicare and Medicaid. The decision to seek legislation related to health is an administrative one, and the implementation of legislative mandates is an administrative task. With some major exceptions, health administration is general rather than restricted to specific disease entities. The objective is to remove barriers —such as polluted air or the inability to purchase medical care—which stand between people and good health.

Prevention is the classic function of the nation's health departments, and it can be approached in either or both of two ways: (1) manipulation of the environment to prevent contact between man and the agent of disease, and (2) manipulation of man to render contact with a disease agent harmless.

Environmental manipulation is known as primary prevention and almost always involves the applied science of engineering. Treatment of water supplies destroys **pathogenic bacteria** and keeps these harmful **organisms** out of human contact (Fig 1-2A). The manipulation of man himself is called secondary prevention, and the best example of this is the **immunization** of **infants** against diseases such as smallpox, diphtheria, tetanus, polio, and measles (Fig. 1-2B). Immunization does not prevent contact with the organisms responsible for these diseases, but it stimulates the body to create chemical defenses known as **antibodies** which destroy these disease agents if and when they are encountered again. In such cases, the disease agent serves as an **antigen.** Secondary prevention is the objective of programs initiated by health departments to control **communicable** diseases through direct patient care. The individual with **venereal** disease receives treatment for his own benefit, but essentially he is treated to prevent the transmission of the illness to others. For the same reason, tuberculosis and other diseases which spread directly or indirectly from man to man tend to be major concerns of public health agencies.

PATHOGENIC: that which is capable of producing disease

BACTERIA: a group of microscopic organisms, some of which produce disease; popularly referred to as "germs"

ORGANISM: a living entity, either animal or plant

IMMUNIZATION: the process of rendering an organism immune to a disease

INFANT: a child under one year of age

ANTIBODY: a protein produced by an organism in the presence of an antigen; the reaction of antibody with antigen inactivates the latter as a harmful agent

ANTIGEN: a protein-containing substance, such as a microorganism, which stimulates body-production of antibodies against it

COMMUNICABLE: capable of transmission from one person to another, either directly or indirectly

VENEREAL: caused or transmitted by sexual intercourse

CONCEPTUAL LEVELS OF DISEASE PREVENTION

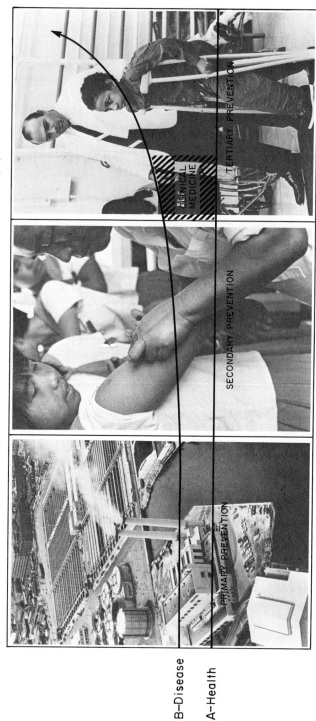

B–Disease

A–Health

PRIMARY PREVENTION

SECONDARY PREVENTION

CLINICAL MEDICINE

TERTIARY PREVENTION

Fig. 1-2A. *Water Treatment Plant (New York City). By treating water before people drink it, human exposure to waterborne pathogens is avoided. (Courtesy of Department of Water Resources.) B. BCG Vaccination (Okinawa). This vaccination protects the children against tuberculosis should they come into contact with the tubercle bacillus. (Courtesy of Dr. C. L. Marshall.) C. Learning to use crutches. Tertiary prevention does not prevent disease but attempts to minimize its effects. It is clinical medicine. (Courtesy of The Mount Sinai Hospital.)*

Restoration of health can be equated generally with the **diagnosis,** treatment, and **rehabilitation** of sick patients. Restoration is the province of **clinical medicine;** and most of the physicians, nurses, allied health workers, and hospital beds are devoted exclusively to it. Although they are less effective and more expensive than prevention, restorative services nevertheless monopolize public concern about health matters. The health programs undertaken by government usually arise in response to problems at the restorative level; and when people complain about the costs of medical care, the inability to find a doctor, or the need to wait a long time to see one, they are expressing dissatisfaction with some of the problems in this area. Restoration is occasionally referred to as tertiary prevention (Fig. 1-2C). Although in this case a disease is already present and cannot be prevented, it is often possible to minimize its disabling effects while maximizing the patient's ability to retain normal function. Thus, the treatment of cancer generally is most successful when the disease is detected early in its course. Similarly, the **aphasic** victim of a **cerebrovascular accident** stands a better chance of regaining normal speech if efforts to rehabilitate him begin as soon after the stroke as possible. Tertiary prevention thus refers not to prevention of disease, *per se,* but rather to prevention of its potential consequences.

We have chosen to understand health by defining it and examining its component activities; but it is of great importance that the reader fully appreciate that health is indeed the sum of its components, and all are of equal importance. We have seen that health and disease are not opposites but rather closely related and often coexist in the same person. It should be emphasized equally that the relationship between the preventive, organizational, and restorative aspects of health is also a close mutually interdependent one. Some diseases which cannot be treated successfully, e.g., polio, can nevertheless be prevented by im-

---

DIAGNOSIS: the differentiation of one disease from another
REHABILITATION: the restoration of normal function to a patient to the maximum extent possible
CLINICAL MEDICINE: the actual practice of medicine as opposed to theoretical or experimental medicine; the word clinical is derived from the Greek word for bed
APHASIC: loss of power of speech and/or the ability to understand verbal or written communication
CEREBROVASCULAR ACCIDENT: the unforeseen, usually sudden, interruption of the blood supply to the brain; commonly known as a "stroke"; "cerebro" refers to the brain itself, and "vascular" to the arteries and veins which transmit blood to and from **the brain**

munization. Others, like venereal disease, are very difficult to prevent. They can best be controlled through the treatment of individuals and the pursuit of their contacts. In order to be dealt with, all diseases, whether preventable or curable, require an adequate organizational base. The child who needs immunizations cannot get them without a system which assures the delivery of such health services. The poor person who delays seeking care because he lacks money is often deprived of medical attention when it would benefit him most.

The Jargon of Health

The preceding discussion on concepts of health and disease introduced many terms which may have been unfamiliar to the reader but which are common in the jargon of health. Table 1-1 lists and identifies a number of frequently encountered prefixes and suffixes; a knowledge of these will enable the reader to decipher the meaning of many technical words. Most of the terms used in medicine are derived from Greek or Latin, and once one gains a familiarity with these word roots the words themselves begin to make sense. A dash following the root identifies it as a prefix, a precedent dash identifies a suffix, and a root with dashes before and after shows that it usually falls in the middle of words.

Causality and Health

One of the thorniest problems in health care is that of distinguishing one disease from another. If you were to awaken one morning with a fever, a sore throat, a headache, and a stiff neck, you would probably diagnose your illness as a cold, "the flu," or "a bug." However, you might have an infection attributable to certain **streptococci,** and without treatment this could lead to troublesome **rheumatic fever.** It is also possible, though less probable, that you could have a lethal condition such as **leukemia,** or a potentially fatal one like **meningitis.** Each of these (and many other conditions) is capable of producing the indicated

---

STREPTOCOCCI: a group of round, pathogenic bacteria
RHEUMATIC FEVER: a disease associated with certain streptococci; rheumatic fever
    often results in serious damage to the heart
LEUKEMIA: cancer of the blood; characterized by uncontrolled proliferation of white
    blood cells
MENINGITIS: inflammation of the fibrous covering of the brain, i.e., the meninges

TABLE 1-1. Word Roots in the Jargon of Health

Root	Meaning	Example
a-, an-	no, not	*an*encephalic (no brain)
abdomin-	abdomen, belly	*abdomin*al (referring to the belly)
-alg-	pain	my*alg*ia (muscular pain)
angi-	vessel	*angi*na (pain related to the vascular system)
ant-, anti-	against, counter to	*anti*inflammatory
arter-	artery	*arter*iosclerosis (hardening of the arteries)
arthr-	joint	*arthr*itis (inflammation of the joints)
bacill- bacter-	a small rod	*bacill*i, *bacter*ia (microscopic rod-shaped organisms)
bi-	life	*bi*ology (the study of life)
bi-	two	*bi*sect (to divide into two parts)
bol-	ball	em*bol*ism (a ball of clotted blood that travels through the circulatory system)
bronch- trachi-	windpipe	*bronch*itis (inflammation of the windpipe)
canc- carcin-	crab	*canc*er and *carcin*oma (refer to the malignant disease which spreads from its center in much the same way as do the legs and claws of a crab)
cardi-, cor-	heart	*cor*onary (referring to the heart)
cephal- capit-	head	*capit*ation (counting heads)
cerebr-	brain	*cerebr*ovascular accident
cervi-	neck	*cervi*x (the neck of the uterus)
chron-	time	*chron*ic (lasting over time)
-cis, sect-	cut	in*cis*ion (a cut into something)
cocc-	seed or pill	gono*cocc*us (the round bacteria that causes gonorrhea)
col-, -colon	lower intestine	mega*colon* (enlargement of the lower intestine)
cort-	back or rind	*cort*ex (the outer layer of something)
cyst-	bladder	*cyst*itis (inflammation of the bladder)
dent-	tooth	*dent*ist
derm-	skin	*derm*atology (study of the skin)
dia-	apart	*dia*gnosis
dys-	bad	*dys*trophy (improper nutrition)
-ec-	out of	gastr*ec*tomy (removal of the stomach)
ede-	swell	*ede*ma (swelling)
em-, en-	in	*en*cephalon (that which is in the head, i.e., the brain)
-em-	blood	an*em*ia (deficiency of the blood)
-enter-	intestine	dys*enter*y (improper function of the intestine)
epi-	upon	*epi*demic (that which is upon the people)

TABLE 1-1. (Continued)

Root	Meaning	Example
-esthe-	feel	an*esthe*sia (absence of feeling)
gastr-	stomach	*gastr*itis (inflammation of the stomach)
gen-	originate or produce	carcino*gen*ic
gloss-, glott-, lingu-	tongue	macro*gloss*ia (an exceptionally large tongue)
-gno-	know, discern	pro*gno*sis (forecast of the outcome of a patient's disease)
-gram, -graph	write, record	electrocardio*gram* (an electrical recording of the heartbeat)
gyn-	woman	*gyn*ecology (the study of women's diseases)
hem-, haem-	blood	*hem*orrhage (loss of blood)
hemi-, demi-, semi-	half	*hemi*plegia (paralysis of one-half of the body)
hepat-	liver	*hepat*ic (of or pertaining to the liver)
hist-	web, tissue	*hist*ology (the study of living tissue)
hom-	same	*hom*osexual (one who prefers to have sexual relations with a member of the same sex)
hyper-, super-, ultra-	above, extreme	*hyper*tension (high blood pressure)
hypn-	sleep	*hypn*otic (medication to induce sleep)
hypo-, sub-	under, below	*hypo*thyroidism (deficient thyroid function)
hyster-	womb	*hyster*ectomy
iatr-	physician	*iatr*ogenic (physician-induced)
-itis	inflammation of	card*itis*, gastr*itis*
-ject	throw	in*ject*ion (literally, throwing something in)
lact-	milk	*lact*ate (to produce milk)
lymph-, hydro-	water	*lymph*oma (cancer of the lymph system)
macr-, mega-	large	*macr*oglossia
mal-	bad	*mal*function
-malac-	softening	osteo*malac*ia (softening of the bone)
mamm-, mast-	breast	*mast*ectomy (removal of the breast)
men-	month	dys*men*orrhea (disorder of *men*struation)
micr-	small	*micr*oorganism (a living thing of very small size)
my-	muscle	*my*algia
nephr-, ren-	kidney	*ren*al (of or pertaining to the kidneys)
neur-	nerve	*neur*ology (the study of the nervous system)
-nos-	disease	diag*nos*is, prog*nos*is
ocul- ophthalm-	eye	*ophthalm*ology (the study of the eye)

9

TABLE 1-1. (Continued)

Root	Meaning	Example
odont-	tooth	orth*odont*ia
-oma	tumor	hepat*oma*
orth-	right, straight	*orth*odontia
-osis	a disease process	brucell*osis* (a disease process caused by a bacterium known as *Brucella*)
path-, -pathy	sickness	*path*ogenic, lymphadeno*pathy*
ped-	child	*ped*iatrics
pha-	say, speak	a*pha*sia
pharyng-	throat	*pharyng*itis
phleb-	vein	*phleb*itis
plas-	to shape a form	rhino*plas*ty (reformation of the nose through surgical intervention)
-pne	breathing	dys*pne*a
pneumo- pulmo-	lung	*pneumo*nia
pro-	before	*pro*gnosis
proct-	anus	*proct*itis
py-	pus	*py*ogenic
rhag-	break, burst	hemor*rhag*e
rhin-	nose	*rhin*oplasty
scler-	hard	arterio*scler*osis
sep-	rot, decay	*sep*tic
ser-	watery	*ser*ous (watery)
sten-	narrow	aortic *sten*osis (the presence of an abnormal narrowing of the aortic valve, a part of the heart)
therap-	treatment	*therap*y
thorac-	chest	*thorac*otomy (surgery involving the chest)
thromb-	clot	*thromb*osis (the presence of a blood clot)
thyr-	shield	the *thyr*oid gland is shaped like a shield
-tomy	to cut	appendec*tomy*
tox-	poison	*tox*ic (of or pertaining to poison)
vas-	vessel	*vas*cular

symptoms; the process of pinpointing which disease is responsible for *your* fever, sore throat, headache, and stiff neck can be a real challenge. Yet such a distinction is basic because once we can identify and name

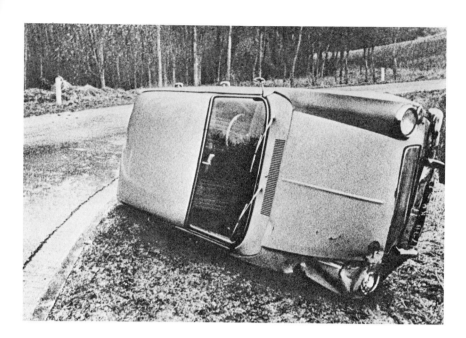

FIG. 1-3A. *Without automobiles, automobile accidents would be impossible.*

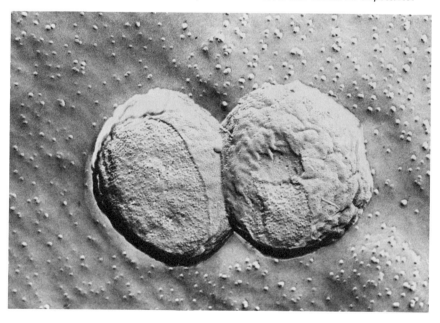

FIG. 1-3B. *Without these gonococci, there would be no gonorrhea. (Courtesy of Dr. J. Swanson.)*

the entity it becomes a known quantity; past experience enables us to predict its course with a high degree of accuracy. In other words, we know what to expect and can take steps to alter these expectations. The steps we take have been developed through accumulated experience with thousands and perhaps millions of previous cases.

A physician who considers your symptoms searches a kind of mental file from which, within the scope of his knowledge and skill, some or indeed most of the illnesses associated with your symptoms can be recalled. As he performs a physical examination and questions you on the history of your symptoms, he seeks to obtain information which, when added to what he already knows about you, will form a pattern of symptoms and signs that strongly suggest one or two diseases over all others. These patterns are known as **syndromes**. The information obtained by the physician not only suggests what you have but also what you do not have; symptoms which rule out something are just as valuable as those which rule in something. Laboratory tests and x-rays are simply extensions of this process of data collection. The most definitive information is the **pathognomonic** symptom, laboratory result, or x-ray finding.

The identification of the disease agent is also pathognomonic for the obvious reason that it is the recognized cause of the particular illness. Once identified, the cause, by definition, dictates the disease. The **spirochete**, *Treponema pallidum,* is the *cause* of syphilis, and the bacterium, *Mycobacterium tuberculosis,* is the cause of tuberculosis. Neither disease can exist in the absence of the causative organism (Figs. 1-3A, 1-3B). Note, however, that the reverse is not true because the organism which is causally necessary for a given disease to occur may not be sufficient unto itself to bring the disease into existence. Automobiles are the cause of automobile accidents in the sense that such accidents could not exist without motor vehicles; but not everyone who uses a car has an accident. Similarly, most people who are **infected** with polio **virus** or the **tubercle bacillus** do not develop paralysis or tuberculosis. In other words, A may be necessary for B to occur, but the mere existence of A does not dictate the existence of B. In this case A is a *sine qua non,* or a necessary cause. It is necessary but not invariably sufficient. The automobile "causes" the

---

SYNDROME: a group of symptoms and signs which together constitute a recognized clinical entity
PATHOGNOMONIC: that which is uniquely characteristic of a particular disease
SPIROCHETE: a coiled, corkscrew-shaped bacterium
Treponema pallidum: the spirochete causing syphilis
Mycobacterium tuberculosis: the bacillus (rod-shaped bacterium) causing tuberculosis

accident when, for example, the driver is drunk or the road is icy. Alcohol and ice thus become sufficient causes of our hypothetical accident, an accident which *could* not occur without the automobile itself and which *would* not occur without the inebriated driver or the poor road conditions. Some causes are necessary and some are sufficient; both are required for the effect to manifest itself.

It follows that any disease can be successfully attacked whose necessary cause is known and subject to human control. Medical science has been particularly successful in its efforts to control diseases caused by bacteria but far less so with still smaller microorganisms, the viruses. Unfortunately, the necessary cause of most **chronic** illnesses, such as heart disease, cancer, and cerebrovascular accidents, is elusive, and efforts to control these conditions are directed largely against sufficient causes.

A sufficient cause is essentially a **risk factor,** an entity whose presence increases the probability that a given disease will occur. Risk factors denote the existence of a **correlation**—or statistical association—between a particular disease and certain characteristics of potential groups of patients. Abnormal elevation of **serum cholesterol,** high blood pressure, obesity, lack of exercise, and cigarette smoking are all risk factors related to cardiovascular disease. In other words, the risk of this disease in smokers is greater than in nonsmokers, and if the smoker is also hypertensive the risk is greater still. At greatest risk is the individual who manifests all these characteristics. In the absence of firm knowledge as to the necessary causes of the disease, control measures are directed at the known risk factors. Dietary restrictions lower cholesterol; drugs and limited salt intake reduce blood pressure; people are encouraged to stop smoking, lose weight, and get more exercise. Each of these measures

---

INFECTION: the invasion by microorganisms of and their multiplication within a host (any animal, including man, which harbors and sustains a parasite); the infecting organisms are said to parasitize the host

VIRUS: a group of microorganisms which are smaller than bacteria and which exist only within susceptible host cells

TUBERCLE BACILLUS: *Mycobacterium tuberculosis*

CHRONIC: that which is long-lasting; in medical usage it refers to a large group of diseases which, with certain exceptions, are long-lasting, noninfectious, and not transmitted from man to man

RISK FACTOR: for our purposes, a characteristic associated with a particular disease or diseases

CORRELATION: an association between two things, such that a change in one implies a change in the other

SERUM: the liquid component of blood, i.e., that which remains when all cellular elements are removed

CHOLESTEROL: a chemical occurring naturally in all animal tissues

lowers the risk to the individual; but it should be noted that the presence of known risk factors does not guarantee the eventual appearance of the associated disease, nor does the absence of risk factors in an individual provide immunity to it.

The concepts of causality are important to an understanding of why certain general characteristics of some population groups tend to place their collective and individual health in particular jeopardy. Some groups live constantly exposed to a host of causal agents and risk factors rarely experienced by other groups, and the removal or neutralization of these factors is often more a social than a medical task. They constitute the field conditions with which the health worker must come to grips in order to prevent disease and to promote and restore health. In describing these field conditions it is useful and traditional to assign them such names as genetics, nutrition, poverty, population expansion, and pollution (the last of these is discussed separately in Chapter 9), but this categorization should not lead us to disregard their mutual interdependence.

References

Clark, D. W. A Vocabulary for Preventive Medicine. *In* Clark, D. W., and Mac-Mahon, B. Preventive Medicine. Boston, Little, Brown, 1967.

Dorland's Illustrated Medical Dictionary, 23rd ed. Philadelphia, W. B. Saunders, 1957.

Rice, D. P., and Cooper, B. S. National health expenditures, 1929–68. Soc. Sec. Bull. January, 1969.

Roenstock, I. M. Why people use health services. Milbank Memorial Fund Quarterly 44:3, part 2, July, 1966.

World Health Organization. The Constitution of the World Health Organization. W.H.O. Chronicle 1:29, 1947.

2

Some Background Determinants of Health and Disease

Genetic Inheritance

The health of every individual is partially determined before birth, for each of us is born with a unique genetic makeup which interacts with various environmental elements; the fate of the individual is largely determined by this interaction.

The cells of all the body organs contain 46 threadlike structures known as **chromosomes.** These 46 chromosomes are divided into 23 pairs, and the two chromosomes in each pair are identical to each other. The chromosomes carry on them smaller structures known as **genes,** which are arranged in a line like a string of beads. The principal chemical of the gene is a complex compound known as deoxyribonucleic acid (DNA). DNA has the ability to reproduce itself. It does this by transmitting in-

---

CHROMOSOME: the threadlike structure in cells which carries the genes
GENE: the basic unit of heredity

formation as to its makeup to a related cellular chemical known as ribonucleic acid (RNA). RNA, in turn, governs the intracellular production of proteins and thus acts as a messenger which mediates the replication of DNA. Just as the chromosomes exist as 23 matched pairs, each gene has a corresponding but not necessarily identical gene located in the same position on the second chromosome of that chromosome pair. Gene pairs are known as **alleles** or **allelomorphs**. In the immature reproductive cells of the male testicle and the female ovary the 23 chromosome pairs and the genes they contain undergo a process known as **meiosis**. Meiosis is also called reduction division; and, as a result of this process, the male sperm cell and the female ovum come to contain not 46 chromosomes but 23, half the normal number. This condition of having 23 rather than 46 is known as **haploid**. The haploid reproductive cells of each sex are called **gametes**. Now, it is elemental knowledge that human conception results from a fusion of male and female gametes (sperm and ovum). When this union occurs, the 23 male chromosomes plus the 23 female chromosomes restore the original chromosome number to 46 (the **diploid** condition), which results in 23 new chromosome pairs (Fig. 2-1). The process of meiosis redistributes genetic material in a manner which makes it most unlikely that any two individuals, even **siblings**, will have the same genetic makeup. Identical twins are the one exception to this. Such twins develop from the same fertilized ovum and consequently share an identical genetic composition. Although the total number of genes carried on all 46 chromosomes is not known, estimates range from 50,000 to 100,000. When one considers so large a number, it is not surprising that no two people except identical twins are exactly alike genetically. Failure of the meiotic process results in incomplete chromosome separation. This is called **nondisjunction** and results in an individual with an extra chromosome, a state known as **trisomy**. Trisomy, in turn, manifests itself as the familiar condition commonly called **mongolism**, which most often affects the offspring of older women and occurs in about 15

ALLELE; ALLELOMORPH: each of a gene pair; each gene located on the same site on the corresponding chromosome
MEIOSIS: cellular division which produces a reduction in the number of cellular chromosomes to one-half the normal number
HAPLOID: half the normal number of chromosomes
GAMETE: the haploid reproductive cell
DIPLOID: the full number of chromosomes
SIBLINGS: the brothers and sisters of an individual
NONDISJUNCTION: incomplete chromosome separation
TRISOMY: the condition of having 47 rather than 46 chromosomes
MONGOLISM: a condition characterized by arrested physical and mental development

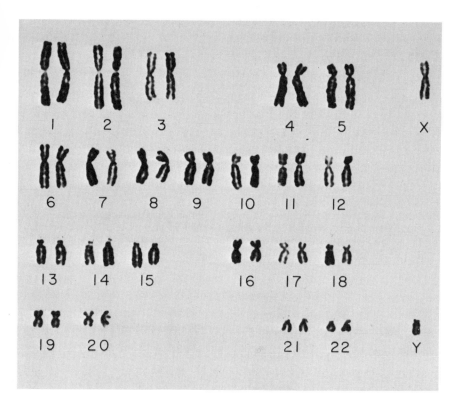

FIG. 2-1. *Normal karyotype. The word "Karyotype" refers to the specific chromo-somal constitution of the cell nucleus. This photograph depicts the karyo-type of a normal human male (one X and one Y chromosome). (Courtesy of Dr. K. Hirschhorn and Dr. L. Hsu, The Mount Sinai Hospital.)*

of every 1,000 births (Figs. 2-2, 2-3). Chromosome abnormalities are thought to account for about one-fifth of all spontaneous abortions.

The gene is known as the basic unit of heredity because it determines, either singly or in conjunction with other genes, the characteristics of each individual. Obvious characteristics such as eye color and hair texture are genetically determined, as are a host of more subtle traits, including a predilection for certain illnesses and the actual inheritance of others. We have seen that genes exist in pairs and that the two genes making up a pair need not be identical. To illustrate the importance of the gene pairs, let us consider the inherited malady known as sickle cell disease. This condition involves an abnormality of **hemoglobin**, the constituent of

HEMOGLOBIN: the oxygen-carrying constituent of red blood cells

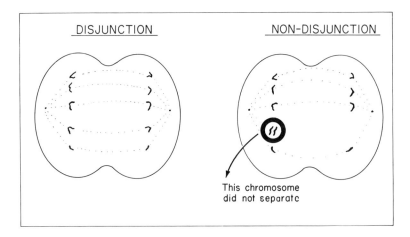

FIG. 2-2. *Chromosome separation. Normally, chromosome separation results in half the original number in the process known as meiosis. If a chromosome fails to separate, the resulting nondisjunction manifests itself phenotypically as mongolism. (Five chromosome pairs are shown in this illustration.)*

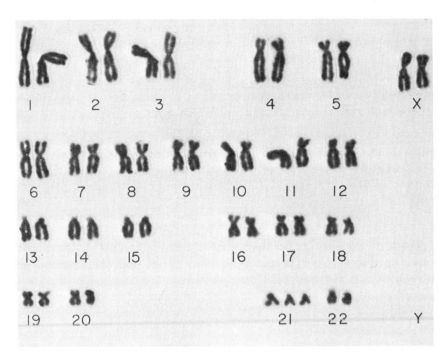

FIG. 2-3. *Abnormal karyotype: Trisomy. In this girl (note the two X chromosomes) there is an extra 21st chromosome; the condition known as trisomy. (Courtesy of Dr. K. Hirschhorn and Dr. L. Hsu, The Mount Sinai Hospital.)*

human red blood cells that transports oxygen. Normally the hemoglobin **molecule** is of the so-called A type. In sickle cell disease a large proportion of the hemoglobin is of the S type. Under certain conditions these abnormal red cells assume a sickle shape (they are normally shaped like a catcher's mitt) and are unable to transport oxygen (Figs. 2-4A, 2-4B). When this occurs the individual is said to experience a sickle cell crisis, an event characterized by severe muscle and joint pain, fever, and a tendency toward potentially fatal thrombosis.

To discover how this disease comes about, let us examine the makeup of the patient's parents (Fig. 2-5). The gene which dictates the production of normal hemoglobin A we shall simply call A, and that which leads to abnormal hemoglobin S we will call S. Since genes exist in pairs, a pair might be made up of two A genes (AA) or two S genes (SS) or one A gene and one S gene (AS). Let us assume that both parents' genes are of the AS type. In the process of meiosis the genes are separated, as are the chromosomes on which they sit. Thus, both parents produce one A gene and one S gene. The pregnancy of the female parent can produce an offspring whose gene pair for hemoglobin might be AA, in which case he receives one A gene from the father and one A gene from the mother; or AS, in which case the child receives the A from one and the S from the other; or SS, wherein the child receives the S gene from both parents. When the two genes of a pair are identical—i.e., AA or SS— the pair is called **homozygous;** when two genes are different (AS), they are termed **heterozygous.** Now, it so happens that only children who are homozygous (SS) manifest sickle cell disease. Heterozygotes are not so affected, although, as we have seen from the parents of our hypothetical child, two heterozygotes can transmit the disease to their offspring. The fact that heterozygotes contain the S gene but do not develop clinical disease is accounted for by the fact that the S gene is **recessive** and the A gene, which is also present in heterozygotes, is **dominant.** It is believed that diabetes is also a disease of this type. In other words, if we denote the gene for normal as A and that for diabetes as D, a person would be

---

MOLECULE: an aggregation of atoms which comprise the smallest unit of a compound having the characteristic of that compound
HOMOZYGOUS: possessing identical alleles in regard to a particular characteristic
HETEROZYGOUS: possessing different alleles in regard to a particular characteristic
RECESSIVE: referring to a characteristic which is manifested only in homozygotes
DOMINANT: referring to a characteristic which is manifested in both homozygotes and heterozygotes

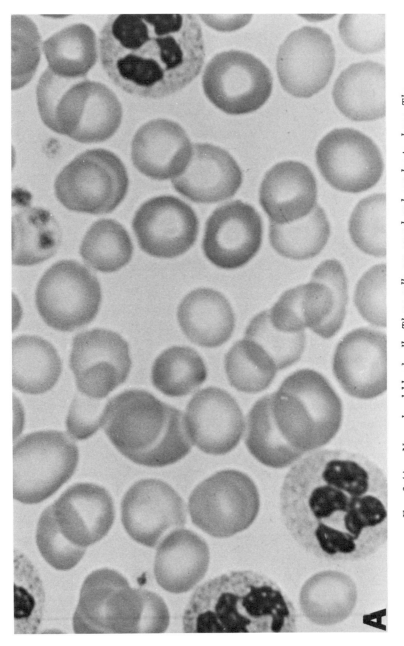

FIG. 2-4A. Normal red blood cells. These cells are round and regular in shape. The grainy cells with the dark lobulated nuclei are a normal type of white blood cell.

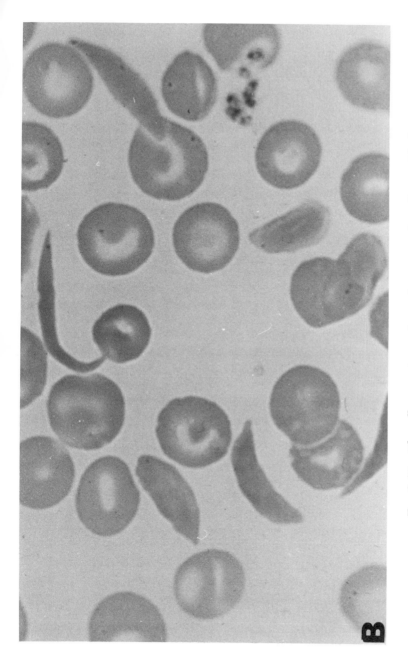

Fig. 2-4B. The cells appearing at the twelve, two, eight and nine o'clock positions are obviously sickled. They appear among a group of normal red blood cells. (Photographs courtesy of Dr. E. Davidson, Elmhurst Hospital.)

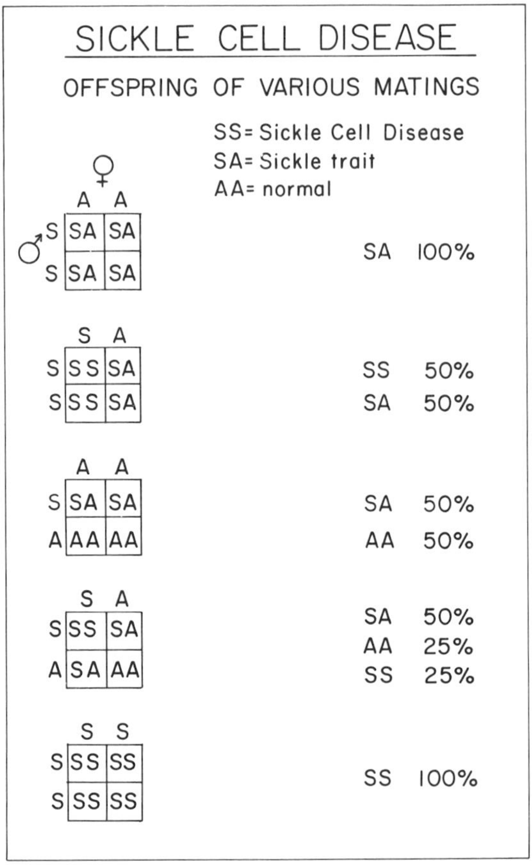

FIG. 2-5. *This chart depicts the possible offspring of various matings involving normal persons and those with sickle cell disease and sickle cell trait. It is important to realize that, for example, in a mating of two SA parents, the percentages represent the odds of each child being SA, AA, or SS. In other words, with each pregnancy the odds are 50% that the child will be SA, 25% that he will be SS and 25% that he will be AA.*

phenotypically diabetic (i.e., develop the disease) only if he were **genotypically** homozygous (DD).

Let us return to sickle cell disease to point out an important irony. For

---

PHENOTYPE: the actual physical representation of one's genetic makeup, i.e., eye color, height, and so on
GENOTYPE: the total genetic makeup of an individual

all practical purposes this disease is an exclusive affliction of black people, whose ancestral home, Africa, has for centuries been infested with malaria. Even today malaria is **endemic** to most of sub-Sahara Africa, where it remains an important cause of death and disability, especially in infancy. In the nineteenth century it was malaria which largely accounted for Africa's reputation as "the white man's grave." It is now widely accepted that malaria and sickle cell disease are related in that persons who are heterozygous for the sickle cell gene are resistant to the most lethal type of malaria. This heterozygous resistance may be regarded as a benefit bought at the cost of sickle cell disease in homozygotes. Obviously sickle cell disease is of no value whatever to individuals suffering from it. Nevertheless, it represents an indirect benefit in terms of the total population, for heterozygous resistance to malaria would cease to exist without the genetic contribution of the homozygote. In a real sense, the sickle cell phenomenon is an adaptive mechanism facilitating human existence in a variety of environmental circumstances. There are many types of hemoglobin, for example, although we have discussed only two. The ability of single genes to produce several phenotypic effects is known as **polymorphism.** The different blood types exemplify polymorphism, and although the original adaptive basis for the groups is unknown, some of the "cost" may be seen in the tendency of persons of blood group A to be particularly susceptible to stomach cancer and smallpox, while group O individuals seem to be more susceptible to plague. (See Chapters 4 and 5.)

Genetic inheritance is either **autosomal** or **sex-linked,** depending on the chromosomes involved. Autosomal inheritance refers to the 44 chromosomes not related to sex determination. The so-called sex chromosomes are somewhat different in that they vary according to sex. Females carry two identical chromosomes, designated XX; in males they are dissimilar and referred to as XY. Characteristics determined by the genes located on the sex chromosomes are considered sex-linked, or X-linked. Although autosomal characteristics may be either dominant or recessive, most X-linked ones are recessive, and, as such, they are expressed only in homozygotes. **Hemophilia** and color blindness are two of the best known X-linked recessive characteristics. Virtually all characteristics of any im-

---

ENDEMIC: referring to a disease normally present in a given population
POLYMORPHISM: the quality of occurring in many forms
AUTOSOMAL: refers to the 44 chromosomes not associated with sex determination
SEX-LINKED: refers to the two sex chromosomes
HEMOPHILIA: a hereditary disease, present in males and transmitted by females, which
     is characterized by a marked tendency to abnormal bleeding

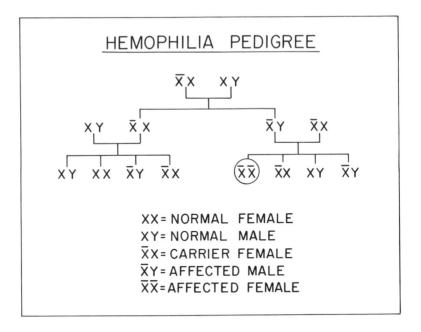

FIG. 2-6. *A carrier female (X̄X) mates with a normal male (XY) in the first generation. Two of the possible outcomes appear in the second generation. These same possibilities exist in the third generation if the female carrier mates with a normal male. Note, however, that in the unlikely event of an affected male mating with a carrier female, a female child with hemophilia may result. Thus, it is not true that females never have hemophilia. It is true, however, that female hemophiliacs are exceedingly rare.*

portance involve the X chromosome, and we have seen that all females have two of these, all males one X and one Y. Thus, the Y chromosome appears only in male offspring, while females receive one X from the father and one X from the mother. The point here is that the male lacks the second X chromosome of the female; in the absence of a countervailing X, the one X present in the male is, for all practical purposes, free to express itself. Thus, characteristics not expressed in the female, such as hemophilia, appear in the male, and the female can transmit the disease even though she herself may not suffer from it. (See Fig. 2-6.)

Generally speaking, human mating within defined population groups tends to be random; that is, any male is equally likely to mate with any female, or vice versa. There are obvious and important exceptions to this, however, for people tend to select mates of the same social class, educational background, nationality, religion, or race. Any or all of these factors can contribute to much inbreeding within relatively small sub-populations. This inbreeding, in turn, can produce situations in which certain genes are fixed, i.e., present in 100 percent of the population. Alternately, genes can disappear from a population altogether. The tendency of genes to become fixed or lost is known as genetic drift. Racial mixture in the United States is widespread, and about 30 percent of whites contain "black" genes, and vice versa. In the present climate of our society this statistic is no doubt regarded with distaste by both races.

Nutrition

In the public mind nutrition tends to be equated with **vitamins.** Important as these are, it is a consideration of proteins and calories that is most critical to an understanding of nutrition. Proteins are complex organic compounds made up of smaller molecules known as **amino acids.** Amino acids are the biochemical building blocks of all animal tissues. There are more than 20 such acids, 8 of which cannot be **synthesized** in the body and must be supplied by dietary intake. The body utilizes amino acids in maintaining its structural and functional integrity, but it depends on a dietary intake of **calories** to provide the energy needed in day-to-day living. (Appendix 2.) The calories supplied by food vary with the composition of that food. (Appendix 3.) **Carbohydrates** provide five calories per gram ingested, fats nine calories per gram, and proteins four calories. People on diets are thus steered away from foods high in fats and carbohydrates and are advised to eat those with a high protein content.

Health problems related to nutrition are peculiar in that malnutrition, in pronounced form often manifested as frank disease, deprives the body of the proteins and calories needed to resist other diseases, particularly infections. On the other hand, marginal nutritional status tends to lapse into gross malnutrition in the presence of infections and certain intestinal **infestations.** Thus, malnutrition and infection are intimately related—the one tends to promote the presence of the other in a circular pattern.

VITAMIN: an organic substance necessary to normal growth and function of the body
AMINO ACIDS: the structural constituents of proteins
SYNTHESIS: the creation of a chemical compound by a union of its elements
CALORIE: a unit of measurement of heat; specifically, the amount of heat necessary
to raise the temperature of one gram of water one degree centigrade
CARBOHYDRATE: a compound consisting of carbon, hydrogen, and oxygen, the latter
two in the same proportion as water, e.g., sugars, starches, cereals,
and so on
INFESTATION: establishment of parasitic organisms within or upon a host

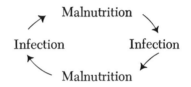

While insufficient nutrition is a constant reality for two-thirds of the world's population, the more common problem in the United States is over-sufficient nutrition, or **obesity.** Obesity does not enhance infectious processes as is the case with classic malnutrition, but it is a significant risk factor with respect to arteriosclerosis, diabetes mellitus, hypertension, hernia, and complications following surgery. About 12 percent of the people in the United States are overweight and about 4 percent are frankly obese, or more than 20 percent over desirable weight. (Appendix 4.) Among whites obesity is more common in men; the reverse is true of blacks, and no age group is exempt in either race. While overeating is the most common obvious reason for obesity, it is largely unknown why some people eat more than others or why some become fat and others do not. Overweight children are most commonly found in families where one or both parents are overweight, and the causes of obesity are probably both genetic and environmental. Regardless of the cause, the treatment of obesity has been generally unsatisfactory. Through special diets, appetite-suppressant drugs, and low-calorie foods, perhaps as many as 50 percent or more of those who try to reduce succeed in losing at least 20 pounds. (Appendix 5.) Unfortunately, only about half of these persons maintain their losses over a long period of time.

Like obesity, classic malnutrition is causally complex and is usually deeply rooted in the cultural, social, and economic characteristics of the population affected. While it is obvious that the necessary cause of malnutrition is a lack of essential food elements, there are many sufficient causes:

1. *Failure to ingest food.* Dietary restrictions traceable to customs, traditions, taboos, and poverty can result in reduced total food intake or in the exclusion of specific foods, such as eggs, milk, and certain meats, from the diet. Ingestion is also restricted in some psychiatric disorders, in diseases which produce loss of appetite, and those cases where a person has no teeth or cannot feed himself.

2. *Failure to utilize food.* Diarrhea, especially when it is prolonged,

---

OBESITY: an excessive accumulation of body fat

reduces the absorption of food in the gut. Since soluble vitamins (A, D, E, and K) are unavailable in such cases, the predictable deficiency disease develops. In addition, inadequate ingestion or absorption ultimately leads to a deficit in certain proteins and fats which transport vitamins and other necessary dietary components. When this happens these components cannot be utilized by the body even if they are ingested.

3. *Increased food requirements.* Basic nutritional requirements are increased in childhood and adolescence, during pregnancy and **lactation,** among people who do heavy physical labor, and in diseases which produce fever or increase the rate of body **metabolism.** Nutritional demands are greatest during adolescence, infancy, and pregnancy. The caloric requirement of adult females is about 70 percent of that for males, and in both sexes caloric needs decline with advancing age. A 22-year-old male normally requires 2,900 calories per day, compared to 2,600 at age 45 and 2,400 at age 65; the corresponding figures for women are 2,000, 1,850, and 1,700. In both cases the decline in caloric need between ages 25 and 65 is roughly 25 percent. (Appendix 6.)

Although malnutrition sometimes produces diseases which reflect a single dietary inadequacy, it is usual for several deficiencies to exist simultaneously. For this reason the following discussion of specific disease states is somewhat unrealistic. We have already noted the relationship between malnutrition, diet, and infection. An inadequate diet and a superimposed infection acts **synergistically** to produce either frank disease or an infinite variety of less serious conditions. The general term for these deficiency states is protein-calorie malnutrition.

Protein-calorie malnutrition signifies a deficiency in both these food elements, and its manifestations are most common in children living in developing countries. In milder forms the principal manifestation is retarded growth and development. This "mildness" is more apparent than real, however, for the affected child is not only smaller in stature but suffers as well from a number of biochemical abnormalities. In addition, evidence is mounting which suggests that protein-calorie malnutrition in infancy and early childhood results in permanent adverse effects on the ability to learn. Eighty percent of adult brain growth occurs before the

---

LACTATION: secretion of milk from the female breast
METABOLISM: the sum total of bodily physical and chemical processes by which energy is expended in converting simpler compounds to more complex ones, and by which energy is released through the breakdown of complex compounds to simpler ones
SYNERGISTIC: refers to cooperation among two entities, such that the effect they create is greater than that produced by either one alone

CLINICAL AND SUBCLINICAL MALNUTRITION

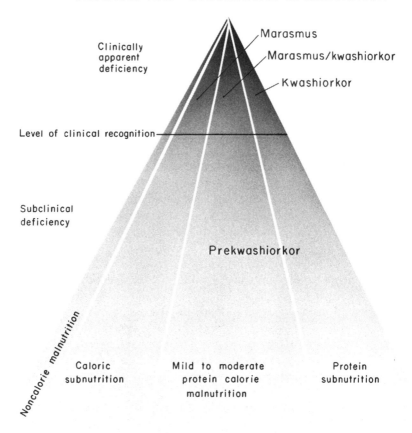

FIG. 2-7.   *While the diagram deals with nutrition, it illustrates a very important health principle: Regardless of the particular disease, subclinical cases which are inapparent vastly outnumber known clinical cases. In the next chapter we will identify this principle as "The Iceberg Effect." Here we have the subclinical precursors to marasmus and kwashiorkor. (Adapted from* Roche Image of Medicine and Research, Volume 13, No. 6, Septem-*ber, 1971.)*

age of three, and malnourished children have abnormally small head circumferences and perhaps a diminished number of brain cells. In addition, it has been suggested that the effects of malnutrition in one generation spill over into the next, in that poor nutrition in the infant female may influence the development of children born to her many years later.

In developing countries the ravages of poor nutrition are especially serious in the first three years of life. During the first months of life when the infant is at the mother's breast, nutrition tends to be adequate regardless of the nutritional status of the mother. However, the weaned child is too often the recipient of an inadequate diet and frequently goes into a nutritional tailspin which may prove fatal. In addition, the immunity to infections, which is passed on by the mother, declines toward the end of the first year of life, and the child is exposed to infectious diseases without the protection of adequate nutrition. For this reason the death rate of children between 2 and 3 years of age is the best single index of malnutrition in developing countries.

As we have indicated, malnutrition and infection are synergistic. In the presence of severe nutritional deficit common diseases of childhood become lethal, especially measles, whooping cough, and diarrhea. The most serious forms of protein-calorie malnutrition are known as marasmus and kwashiorkor. The former, most commonly associated with the weaning period, is frank starvation; it primarily reflects the ingestion of too few calories. Kwashiorkor develops somewhat later. It is usually preceded by infection and is caused by a lack of protein and essential amino acids. The word kwashiorkor is from the Swahili language and means "disease of the first son," referring to the health catastrophe which too often befalls the first child when the second occupies his place at the mother's breast (Fig. 2-8).

Vitamin and mineral deficiencies are the constant companions of protein-calorie malnutrition and cut across economic boundaries (Fig. 2-9). Vitamins, dietary constituents found in food, perform a specific function in the body, although some vitamins have been identified whose exact role in man is unclear. Vitamins are well known to the American people, who read about them on food wrappers and cereal boxes and guzzle them by the billions each year. Vitamin-A deficiency, most common where people subsist on a rice diet, causes softening and degeneration of the **cornea** of the eye and can lead to blindness. Vitamin A is present in leafy vegetables and is usually readily available. Vitamin D prevents a condition known as rickets, which is characterized by deformed bone structure and is seen most often in children. This vitamin is synthesized in the layers of the skin upon exposure to sunlight and is also present in human milk.

The eight important B vitamins are usually found together in a variety of foodstuffs and are of two types. Thiamin, niacin, riboflavin, pantothenic acid, pyridoxine, and biotin are involved in carbohydrate metabolism and are necessary to the release of body energy. In contrast, folic acid and vitamin B_{12} are involved in the production of red blood cells. Thiamine

---

CORNEA: the clear, most anterior portion of the eye, i.e., the part against which a contact lens rests

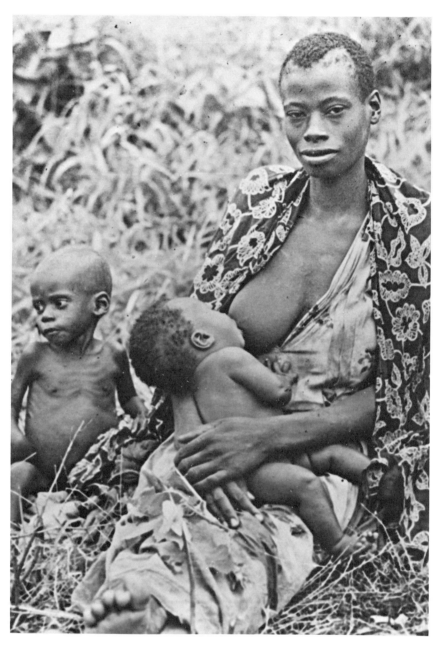

FIG. 2-8. *Kwashiorkor, "the disease of the first son." The child on the left has been taken from the mother's breast. The contrast between him and his younger sibling is striking. (Courtesy of Dr. F. J. Bennett.)*

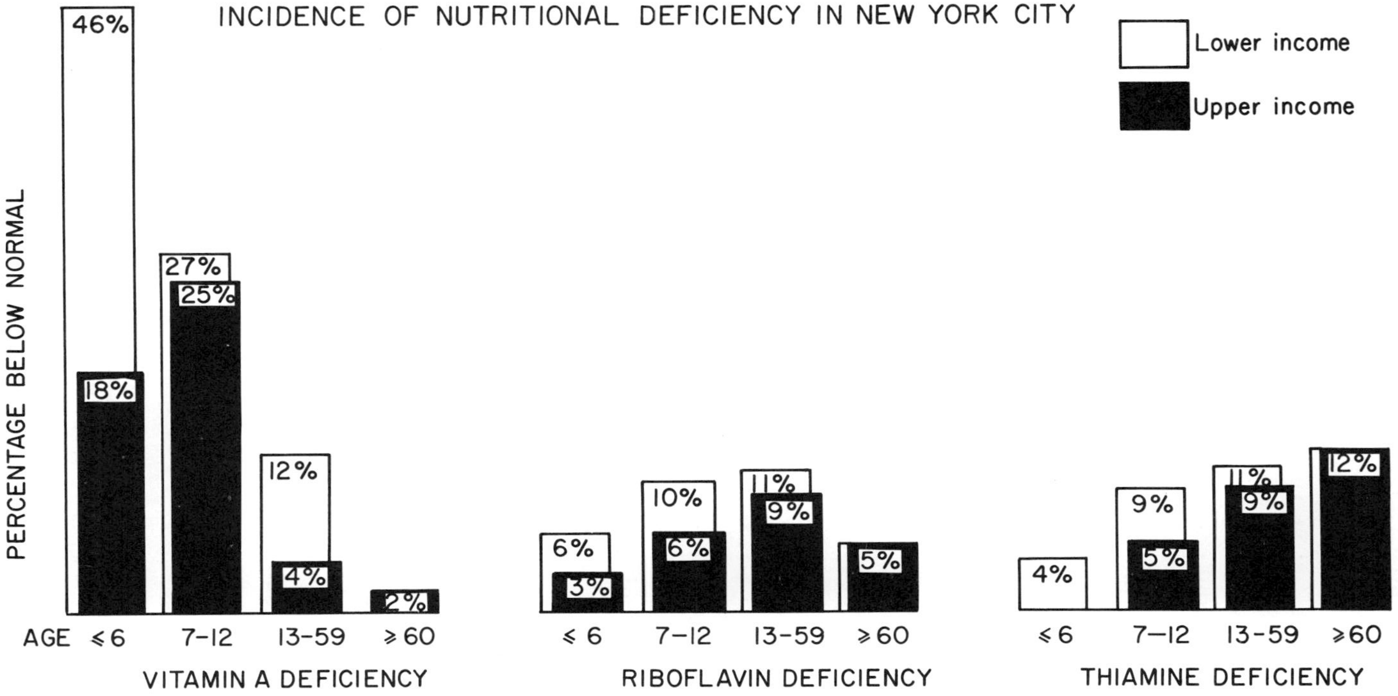

INCIDENCE OF NUTRITIONAL DEFICIENCY IN NEW YORK CITY

☐ Lower income
■ Upper income

PERCENTAGE BELOW NORMAL

VITAMIN A DEFICIENCY

AGE ≤6: 46% / 18%
7-12: 27% / 25%
13-59: 12% / 4%
≥60: 2%

RIBOFLAVIN DEFICIENCY

≤6: 6% / 3%
7-12: 10% / 6%
13-59: 11% / 9%
≥60: 5%

THIAMINE DEFICIENCY

≤6: 4%
7-12: 9% / 5%
13-59: 11% / 9%
≥60: 12%

FIG. 2-9. *Vitamin deficiencies vary with income but less than might be expected. In spite of the relatively high rate of Vitamin A deficiency shown here, the vast majority of Americans have no therapeutic need for vitamins. (Adapted from Roche Image of Medicine and Research, Volume 13, No. 6, September, 1971.)*

deficiency manifests itself in a condition known as beriberi. This disease affects the heart, **central nervous system,** and **gastrointestinal tract.** In infants it is rapidly fatal and commonly associated with thiamine-deficient mother's milk. Older children raised on a diet of polished rice are quite susceptible, as are adults who suffer from alcoholism. Niacin deficiency leads to pellagra, an illness characterized by **glossitis,** dermatitis, **dementia,** and a wide range of vague gastrointestinal complaints. Riboflavin deficiency is reflected in eye symptoms and the cracking and ulcerating of the corners of the mouth. This latter condition is called cheilosis and is virtually pathognomonic of riboflavin deficiency. Since they are widely distributed in nature and tend to be present or absent with other B vitamins, pyridoxine, pantothenic acid, and biotin are rarely associated with specific illnesses, although pyridoxine deficiency is sometimes implicated in pellagra. Low blood pressure, and a syndrome characterized by skin pallor, elevated serum cholesterol, and anemia, have been experimentally induced in humans fed diets deficient in pantothenic acid and biotin, respectively. Liver is the best single source of the B vitamins; but dairy products, vegetables, some cereals, and other meats are also acceptable sources.

Vitamin B_{12} and folic acid are necessary to the formation and metabolism of red blood cells. In B_{12} deficiency the red cell becomes abnormally large and the patient suffers from neurological symptoms brought on by degeneration of part of the spinal cord, a condition known as pernicious anemia. There is a high correlation between pernicious anemia and cancer of the stomach. The absorption of vitamin B_{12} depends on the presence of a so-called "intrinsic factor" normally found in the acid juices of the stomach. Persons who lack the intrinsic factor (a lack which tends to be **familial** and is probably genetically inherited) do not absorb the vitamin. Folic-acid deficiency leads to a similar type of anemia, but there is no accompanying neurological problem. Most commonly, this vitamin is lost in the presence of diseases which reduce or prevent its absorption from the gut. There are many such precursor diseases, and they tend to exist primarily in developing countries. Deficits in folic acid also arise when demands for it exceed intake, a situation which occurs most frequently in pregnancy.

Vitamin C (ascorbic acid) occupies an honored place in the history of

---

CENTRAL NERVOUS SYSTEM: brain and spinal cord
GASTROINTESTINAL TRACT: esophagus, stomach, small and large intestine, and rectum
GLOSSITIS: inflammation of the tongue
DEMENTIA: impairment of mental function
FAMILIAL: relating to or occurring in families

nutrition. A deficiency of ascorbic acid compromises the integrity of inter-cellular **connective tissues** and produces scurvy, a serious disease char-acterized by hemorrhage, anemia, delayed wound-healing, and greatly increased susceptibility to infection. Scurvy was largely a disease of sailors, and in 1753 an English naval physician, Joseph Lind, discovered that it could be prevented and cured by feeding lemon juice to the men (citrus fruits and leafy vegetables are particularly rich sources of vitamin C). Lind's discovery marked the beginning of the science of nutrition.

Vitamin K is found in most leafy vegetables and many other foods as well. After ingestion, it is extracted from food by bacteria normally present in the gut. From there it is transported to the liver, where it is converted into **prothrombin,** a compound which is essential to the blood-clotting process. Predictably, vitamin-K prothrombin levels decline in severe liver disease, in illnesses which prevent food absorption, in patients receiving **antibiotics** which destroy normal intestinal **flora,** and in **neonates** before the normal flora develops. Because of insufficient prothrombin and/or vitamin K, any of these situations may produce abnormal bleeding ten-dencies and hemorrhage.

In addition to its requirement for **organic** substances such as proteins, amino acids, and vitamins, the body needs a host of inorganic substances called **minerals.** These include sodium, calcium, chlorine, phosphorus, potassium, magnesium, sulphur, manganese, copper, cobalt, fluorine, iron, and iodine. Only the last two of these are commonly associated with deficiency states. Iron is an integral part of the hemoglobin molecule, and iron deficiency leads to a form of anemia characterized by small red cells which are relatively pale in color. Abundant in vegetables and legumes, iron is usually present in the human diet; by far the most fre-quent cause of iron-deficiency anemia is chronic blood loss. This is com-paratively rare in men, in whom it usually implies frank hemorrhage. In women, blood loss occurs with menstruation, and iron lost with the blood must be replaced by dietary intake; during pregnancy, iron requirements of the **fetus** must be met as well. Blood loss also occurs in hookworm

---

CONNECTIVE TISSUE: tissue whose function is that of binding together the various body-organs; the "glue" which holds us together
PROTHROMBIN: a protein, produced in the liver and essential to normal blood clotting
ANTIBIOTIC: a substance which destroys or prevents the growth of certain microor-ganisms
FLORA: a term used to denote bacteria normally present in the human body
NEONATE: a newborn child less than 30 days old
ORGANIC: carbon-containing compounds produced by living organisms or synthesized in the laboratory
MINERAL: a nonorganic substance of uniform composition
FETUS: the product of conception while still in the uterus

infestation. Hookworms are small worms which live in the gut, where they attach themselves to the intestinal wall and are nourished on a diet of blood. Hookworm is especially common in children, and the iron deficiency it promotes is compounded by the high iron requirements of childhood, a period of rapid growth. Hookworm eggs, which develop in soil, are passed in the **feces.** The use of human fecal matter as a fertilizer is widespread in developing countries; children, who rarely wear shoes, work alongside their parents and are thus constantly exposed to hookworm infestation through the skin of their bare feet. In its severest form iron-deficiency anemia leads to heart failure and, occasionally, death. The presence of anemia always dictates a search for a sufficient cause. The chronic blood loss which produces the anemia may also be the first clue to the existence of cancer, an ulcer, or disease of the respiratory or genitourinary system. It is estimated that in the United States iron-deficiency anemia, most common in the rural areas of the South, affects about 10 percent of the population.

Lack of dietary iodine leads to enlargement of the thyroid gland, a condition known as simple **goiter.** The thyroid gland regulates the rate of body metabolism and is important to growth, brain development, sexual maturity, and pregnancy. Iodine deficit is more related to the soil in which food grows than to the food itself, and goiter is therefore most common where the soil lacks iodine. The "goiter belts" of the United States were in the Great Lakes area and the Pacific Northwest. The main problem produced by goiter is usually a cosmetic one, an unsightly bulge in the neck. Occasionally, the enlarged thyroid presses against the **trachea** or **esophagus** and interferes with respiration or the swallowing of food. In areas where goiter has been endemic for years, some of the population suffer from hypothyroidism. These people are often apathetic, mentally retarded, and sometimes deaf. Today goiter is rare in the United States, and worldwide it is largely restricted to mountainous areas and islands where rainfall is heavy. In such areas 10 percent of the population may be affected. Goiter is more common in women than in men. Some foods, notably soy beans, rhubarb, and cabbage are goitrogenic in that they contain substances which prevent iodine uptake by the thyroid.

Both prevention and treatment of nutritional deficiencies are based on provision of the missing element. Goiter is effectively prevented by the

---

FECES: excrement discharged from the bowel; stools
GOITER: enlargement of the thyroid gland
TRACHEA: the windpipe
ESOPHAGUS: the tubular organ through which food passes from the throat to the
    stomach

addition of iodine to table salt. Rice can be enriched with thiamine, and vitamins A and D are added to bread, breakfast cereals, macaroni, and other foods. Fluorine added to drinking water reduces dental **caries.** A more recent innovation is the development of protein supplements in the form of bottled drinks and as a powder that is added to food. Malnutrition can be attacked indirectly as well. Education acquaints people with their own nutritional needs and, more importantly, the needs of their children. Education can also be expected to affect taboos against certain foods and eventually to eliminate such traditional customs, prevalent in parts of Africa, which dictate that the father eat first, the mother second, and the children get whatever scraps remain. Since infection and malnutrition are synergistic, efforts to control infectious diseases have a positive effect on nutrition. The best way to prevent hookworm is to insist that children wear shoes. However, the best means of coping with malnutrition is to grow more food and to provide a system that assures its adequate distribution. Food grown in one area is of no value elsewhere unless it can be transported, stored, and marketed. Malnutrition is more than a medical problem; its solution involves not only medicine but a range of other disciplines, including engineering, education, and soil science.

The importance of nutrition to health cannot be overemphasized. Simple measures to promote adequate nutrition are often remarkably effective. In Newfoundland, for example, enrichment of flour resulted in a 40-percent decline in infant mortality. In Guatemala, a food-supplement program for preschool children in one village proved as effective a health measure as a full-scale medical program for the entire population of a second village. The effect of the nutritional supplement was to reduce the incidence of disease so that fewer children became ill. The medical program, in contrast, failed to reduce the number of illnesses but was quite successful in reducing case fatalities.

The Population Problem [1]

The growth of human population has emerged as one of the greatest problems to challenge mankind, and the scope of this problem is such that it involves every field of human activity. There are several reasons why overpopulation is of particular concern to health professionals. Providing health care for the existing population is already extremely difficult even in a rich, industrialized country like the United States. The

---

caries: dental cavities; the erosion of the surface of a tooth

idea of organizing a system to assure the health of two or three times as many people is staggering. Secondly, the health professional has a significant role in defusing the population explosion through the mass use of contraceptives. Finally, it is a very common assertion that the primary cause of overpopulation has been the application of modern health techniques to the developing countries. We shall examine this idea presently.

The rate at which a population grows is a function of its **birth rate,** its **death rate,** and the prevailing pattern of migration into or out of the area under consideration. These rates are related as follows: Rate of population growth = birth rate − death rate ± **migration rate.** This formula shows that population will increase in any of the following circumstances: (1) a decreased death rate with no other changes; (2) an increased birth rate with no other changes; (3) increased in-migration; (4) a simultaneously increased birth rate, increased in-migration, and decreased death rate.

Obviously, the magnitude of the population increase depends on the magnitude of the change in the several components of the formula. The effects of a high birth rate may be cancelled by either a high death rate or a rise in out-migration, or both. Alternately, even with a decline in the birth rate, the population will grow if the death rate declines to a greater degree than the birth rate or if the population loses many people to out-migration. Usually migration is of secondary importance, but its effects depend to a large extent on who migrates. If the people leaving are young adults their departure will reduce the childbearing population and, if many such people leave, the birth rate will decrease. Also, since the departure of young people increases the proportion of the population that is of middle or old age, the death rate may increase. In this situation the rate of population growth will decline because the birth rate drops concurrent with a high rate of out-migration and a rise in the death rate. Actually, this very situation exists to a greater or lesser degree in many, if not most, rural areas of the United States and is particularly important in the plains states such as Kansas, Nebraska, and the Dakotas.

BIRTH RATE: the so-called "crude birth rate;" the total number of live births during the year divided by the total population as of the middle of the year: the result is multiplied by 1,000 to eliminate the fractional number

DEATH RATE: crude death rate $= \dfrac{\text{number of deaths in a year}}{\text{mid-year population}} \times 1{,}000$

MIGRATION RATE: may be positive or negative, depending on whether more people move in (positive) or out (negative); the rate is the $\dfrac{\text{net gain or loss of persons to migration in a year}}{\text{mid-year population}} \times 1{,}000$

The effects of migration show that both the birth rate and the death rate are affected by changes in the age distribution of the population under study. (The importance of age distribution is discussed in Chapter 3.) **Demographers** have attempted to get around this problem by the use of what is known as the **net reproductive rate** (NRR). The NRR is concerned with the average number of female children who will be born to a woman in her lifetime. Since women have about 35 years in which to bear children, the NRR deals with population changes over a generation rather than a single year. If during their childbearing years (roughly ages 15 to 44) 1,000 women bear 2,000 girl babies, the NRR is 2,000 ÷ 1,000, or 2.0. Because each woman replaces herself and adds a female as well, the population will ultimately rise (given no dramatic changes in death or migration rates). Thus, if 1,000 women bear 500 girl babies the NRR will be 0.5; if the same 1,000 women have just 1,000 female offspring the NRR will be 1.0. In the former case the population can be expected to decline, while in the latter it will tend to remain unchanged.

Obviously, if each adult couple has only two children, and no children die, the ultimate deaths of the parents would leave the population unchanged. In fact some children do die before they reach reproductive maturity, and not all of the female survivors will have children. In the United States approximately 20 percent of women have no children, and this fact coupled with the inevitable death of some children accounts for a replacement number, in this country, of not two children but about 2.5 children per family.[2] The fractional child compensates for infertility and for deaths in childhood. It needs to be appreciated that for most countries of the world childhood mortality is very high. In much of Latin America, for example, half of all deaths occur in children under age 5. In such places the replacement number is not 2.5 as in the United States, but a much higher number, perhaps 6, 8, or even 10.

For the past 300 years or so the growth of the world's population has been rapid, and the basic change which has produced this population expansion has been a general decline in death rates. (Fig. 2-10) Birth rates have remained more or less constant, and, in considering the entire world, migration can be ignored because those who move from one place must go to another; although their reproductive performance may differ from place to place, they are not lost to the total count. It is this expan-

DEMOGRAPHY: the study of human population
NET REPRODUCTIVE RATE: average number of female children born to a group of women in their lifetimes
_____
total number of women in the group

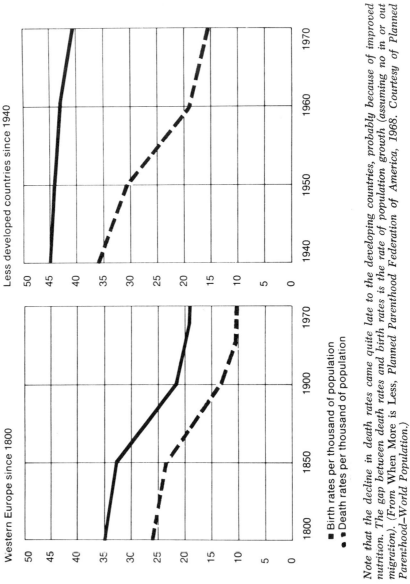

FIG. 2-10. *Note that the decline in death rates came quite late to the developing countries, probably because of improved nutrition. The gap between death rates and birth rates is the rate of population growth (assuming no in or out migration). (From When More is Less, Planned Parenthood Federation of America, 1968. Courtesy of Planned Parenthood–World Population.)*

sion that we now call the population explosion, and it is of interest to consider its cause before we discuss its effects.

The usual explanation is that, while birth rates remain unchanged, the universal application of modern medical techniques has radically reduced death rates. There is no denying the ability of health programs to lower death rates quickly and to alleviate human suffering with respect to most communicable diseases. However, this does not necessarily imply that operational programs have been applied on a scale so grand as to account for the global decline in death rates and the consequent expansion of population. Nevertheless, malaria eradication, particularly in Ceylon, is often cited as a prime example of this process. But the issue here is not malaria eradication *per se*. It is rather the dramatic decline in Ceylon's death rates, which coincided with and were attributed to this program. While mortality indeed dropped markedly in Ceylon, there is reason to doubt the impact of the malaria program as the sole major cause of Ceylon's population increase.

Only 38 percent of the population lived in malaria-endemic areas, and the program itself was confined to these areas. Therefore, if the malaria campaign were responsible for the nationwide decline in death rates, one would expect death rates in endemic areas to have dropped strikingly with respect to nonendemic areas. Yet, by 1948, when all of the endemic areas were included in the program, the death rates in endemic and non-endemic areas were 13.6 per 1,000 and 14.1 per 1,000, respectively. By 1953 these rates were 10.9 and 11.3. It is difficult to regard these small differences between endemic and nonendemic areas as significant. Moreover, a decline in Ceylon's death rates did not start with malaria eradication but began as early as 1905. Similarly, death rates in Africa have been declining for years, but as late as 1966 only Zanzibar and tiny Mauritius had programs to eradicate malaria. Ninety-two percent of the population of sub-Sahara Africa lives in malaria-endemic areas, and of these 158 million people only 3 percent are covered by any kind of malaria-eradication program. The global effort against malaria did not begin until the middle 1950s, and this comparatively recent development occurred after, not before, death rates began falling throughout the world.

In addition to malaria control, two other measures are often held responsible for declining death rates. These are the widespread use of antibiotics and improvements in sanitation. The use of antibiotics is in fact not at all "widespread" in developing countries. Although in many of these countries antibiotics are available without prescription, their use is greatly restricted by their cost and by lack of public knowledge about them. In any case, uncontrolled mass self-medication is unlikely to have much effect on the death rate. The effective use of these drugs depends heavily on the availability of personnel to supervise their administration, and none of the developing countries has anything close to adequate medical and paramedical personnel.

Finally, it should be noted that, as was the case with malaria, death rates began falling before the discovery of antibiotics. Between 1920 and 1949, for example, death rates in 18 representative developing areas fell about 35 percent. Penicillin was first used in 1944 and the **broad-spectrum antibiotics** did not become generally available until about 1948.

With regard to sanitation, there is little doubt that improved water supplies and adequate disposal are capable of preventing deaths. Moreover, these measures are most effective against waterborne pathogens so often responsible for the highly fatal diarrheal diseases of infancy and early childhood. It is also true that, worldwide, the greatest decline in deaths has probably occurred at the younger end of the pediatric age group. But it does not follow that these childhood deaths have been prevented by improvements in environmental sanitation. Like malaria eradication, drugs, and doctors, the availability of applied sanitation is insufficient to explain the global drop in death rates. In Latin America, death rates generally and infant mortality specifically have been falling since the beginning of this century, with some acceleration since the end of World War II. Yet, 80 percent of the rural areas of this region have no treated water, and the World Health Organization identifies the development of community water supplies as one of mankind's greatest needs, a need which is unmet for 90 percent of the population of developing countries. The global decline of death rates has been attributed to mass campaigns against malaria which are as yet inconclusive, to drugs which are largely inaccessible, to doctors who are unavailable, and to sanitation programs which do not exist.

What we now call the population explosion began in Europe around 1650 and was, until quite recently, a phenomenon generally restricted to Caucasians. (Figs. 2-11A, 2-11B) Caucasians accounted for about 19 percent of the world's population in 1650 and almost 27 percent some 300 years later. This remarkable increase occurred primarily in Europe and North America and is rivaled only by that of Latin America, which of course contains vast numbers of Caucasians and their mestizo descendants. Paradoxically, more than half of Europe's 300-year net gain took place between 1650 and 1800, a period when the physician's art was poorly developed and of dubious value. This period also preceded the advance

---

BROAD-SPECTRUM ANTIBIOTICS: antimicrobial drugs which are effective against a wide range of bacteria

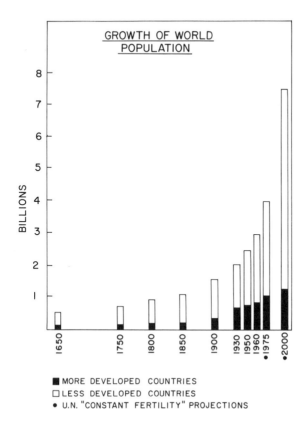

FIG. 2-11A.   *Man as we know him appeared for the first time about 40,000 years ago. It took 39,900 of those years for the human population to reach one billion (around 1850). However, just 50 years were required for the population to reach two billion (around 1900). Projections call for 7½ billion by 2000. Note that most of the increase is occurring in the poorer countries. (From* When More is Less, *Planned Parenthood Federation of America, 1968. Courtesy of Planned Parenthood–World Population.)*

in public health which began in the latter half of the nineteenth century with the development of water filtration systems. Similarly, the role of bacteria as disease agents was unknown until the 1870s, and the first effective antimicrobial drugs, the sulfas, came along in the 1930s. It is also of interest that in the last 300 years the proportionate numbers of both Africans and Asians have declined relative to whites and the mixed peoples of Latin America. Since 1930, however, both of these darker populations have been gaining ground, and cynics might wonder what role this most recent version of the "yellow peril" plays when westerners bemoan

World Population and Percentage Distribution by Continent, 1650–1965+

Continent	Year							% Change between 1650–1965
	1650	1800	1850	1900	1930	1950	1965	
Africa	100(18.3)	90(9.9)	95(8.1)	120(7.4)	154(7.6)	198(8.1)	310(9.4)	−8.9
Asia***	327(60.2)	597(65.7)	741(63.1)	915(57.8)	1,080(53.5)	1,320(53.8)	1,825(55.5)	−4.7
Latin America	12(2.2)	19(2.1)	33(2.8)	63(3.9)	109(5.4)	162(6.6)	243(7.3)	+5.1
North America	1(0.2)	6(0.7)	26(2.3)	81(5.1)	135(6.7)	168(6.8)	214(6.5)	+6.3
Europe	103(18.7)	192(21.4)	274(23.5)	423(25.4)	531(26.3)	593(24.2)	675(20.8)	+2.1
Oceania	2(0.4)	2(0.2)	2(0.2)	6(0.4)	10(0.5)	13(0.5)	17.5(0.5)	+0.1
Total	545(100)	906(100)	1,117(100)	1,608(100)	2,019(100)	2,454(100)	3,285(100)	

+ Population in millions.
*** "Asia" excludes all of the USSR, which is included in the Europe figures.

FIG. 2-11B. (From Marshall, et al. Improved Nutrition vs. Public Health Services as Major Determinants of World Population Growth. Clin. Pediat., 10 (No. 7) July, 1971.)

the population crisis. It would seem that a vital clue to the cause of population expansion may be found by identifying a factor or factors which became operative in Europe and North America relatively early and which have become operative in the developing world since around 1930.

While the positive relationship between adequate nutrition and resistance to disease is well established, the role of nutrition in maintaining health is nevertheless frequently considered secondary to medical care programs. We have already seen that this view is probably incorrect. Better nutrition, by promoting better health, lowers death rates without substantially affecting birth rates, and food changes have been historically associated with rapid population growth. The population of Ireland grew from 3 million in 1754 to 8 million about 100 years later, and the best available explanation is the introduction of the white potato in the middle of the eighteenth century. Likewise, the expanded use of corn, sweet potatoes, and peanuts seems to have been the prime factor in the Chinese population expansion which occurred in the sixteenth century. More recently, the introduction of enriched flour was followed by prompt decline in childhood mortality in Newfoundland and Scandinavia.

It is vital to recognize that there is more to nutrition than bushels of grain produced. What is crucial is what is consumed, how much, and by whom. For example, the 1965–66 grain famine in India seems to have reflected a distribution problem as well as an inadequate supply of food. Some of the Indian states had grain surpluses which were nevertheless unavailable to their less fortunate neighbors. Whether it involves political squabbles, lack of roads, or inadequate storage facilities, the matter of distribution is vital to any consideration of nutrition. The construction of a new road or the redrawing of political boundaries can be as potent a nutritional factor as a substantial increase in yearly crops or the introduction of a new food source. Insofar as improved transportation and communication tend to bring better means of marketing, better storage facilities, a greater variety of available goods, and the introduction of superior agricultural techniques, the nutritional benefits may be considerable. Presently, harvest losses in developing countries amount to as much as 75 percent and rarely less than 50 percent. Improved storage, distribution, and marketing of food could result in a food supply sufficient to feed millions of additional people.

Although thousands of children still suffer today from kwashiorkor and marasmus, it is entirely possible that in any given country the people are nevertheless somewhat better nourished than they were 20, 60, or 100 years ago. This is no "either/or situation," but rather a matter of a little bit more or a little bit less. A general improvement in global nutrition is probably the most significant single factor in explaining the recent decline of death rates in developing countries.

At the beginning of the Christian Era the world population was roughly 250 million. Sixteen hundred years elapsed before this figure doubled in size. At this point death rates began to drop, especially in Europe, and by 1850 world population had doubled again to 1 billion. By 1930, when population growth began to accelerate further, the world total had once more doubled to about 2 billion. At present, the population is about 3.5 billion and growing at a rate of 2 percent per year. Each year there are 102 people for every 100 who existed the year before. This may seem trivial but its import is clear when one considers that an annual increase of 1 percent will double the population in 70 years. A rate of 2 percent will thus double the population in 35 years ($70 \div 2 = 35$). Some countries grow at a rate of 3.5 to 4.0 percent per year, and their doubling time is only 18 years. The large cities in most developing countries grow even faster because of in-migration, often as high as 6 percent annually, in which case the doubling time is only 12 years. Asia and Latin America are growing most rapidly, Africa somewhat less rapidly, and the industrialized countries of Europe and North America least rapidly.

It is not difficult to envision the obvious implications of this kind of population expansion. For one thing, two-thirds of the present world population lives at a subsistence level (annual per capita income around $100), and the increasing number of people will strain governments which cannot provide adequately for their present populations. Human needs grow along with population. An obvious need is for enough food (Fig. 2-12). Even now the productivity of the labor force is often compromised by malnutrition. In addition to food, housing presents almost as critical a problem, not to mention schools, hospitals, and medical care. The implications for health can be appreciated if one considers that the United States is presently facing a physician shortage with one physician for every 700 people. Rural India's ratio at this time is one for every 23,000 people; nurses and other allied health personnel are in even shorter supply.

The basic problem is one of too many people for too few resources. It can be expressed in a simple formula: $PCI = SP - G$, where PCI is per capita income, or the total national income divided by the total population; S is the rate of investment, the amount of money spent yearly on capital goods;[3] P is productivity, i.e., the annual return on money invested;[4] G is the rate of population growth. In most developing countries S is about 10 percent of national income and P is roughly one-third. Referring to the formula, we have: $PCI = 10\% \times \frac{1}{3} - G$, or $PCI = 3.3 - G$. With a G of 2 percent, PCI will be 1.3 percent: $PCI = 3.3\% - 2.0\%$, or $PCI = 1.3\%$. In other words, the yearly per capita income will increase by 1.3 percent. If, on the other hand, G is 4.0 percent, the PCI will de-

U.S. availability of grain for food aid needs of 66 less developed countries 1965-1985

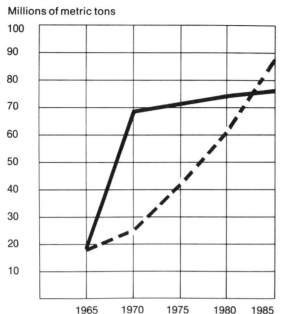

Millions of metric tons

1965   1970   1975   1980   1985

●● Food aid needs of less developed countries
■ Maximum U.S. grain production beyond
domestic and commercial need
Source: U.S. Department of Agriculture

FIG. 2-12. *Food production in developing countries is growing at the rate of only one percent a year while the population is increasing at 2.5 to 3 percent a year. As the grain deficit grows, massive U.S. aid cannot by itself avoid catastrophic famine in these countries. This kind of graph is very popular with advocates of population control. It shows what many of us have suspected all along, that the U.S. cannot feed the rest of the world. (From When More is Less, Planned Parenthood Federation of America, 1968. Courtesy of Planned Parenthood–World Population.)*

cline by 0.7 percent per year, and the people will be poorer than before. The most important thing about this equation is that economic growth depends on the product of S times P. As long as S times P exceeds G, PCI will rise. At present, there is no conclusive correlation between low per capita income and high rates of population growth among the developing countries. There is little evidence to support the oft-repeated idea that national poverty *must* accompany rapid population growth. Note well, however, that the PCI is a very gross measure which assumes an equal distribution of income. A high PCI is quite compatible with the most abject poverty if 10 percent of the people command 80 percent of the income, as is the case in many developing countries.

It is quite apparent that if the rate of population growth is to be controlled the birth rate must drop or the death rate must rise. Positive efforts clearly must be directed at the former. The most widespread method of birth control presently employed is induced abortion. Indeed, it is a philosophical question whether abortion represents a decrease in births or an increase in deaths; but it has been practiced for centuries and its use may be on the rise. It seems to be gaining favor in the United States, where several states have liberalized their abortion laws. Often opposed on moral grounds, its main disadvantage healthwise lies in the hazard it poses for the mother, particularly late in the pregnancy.

In addition to abortion, contraception seems to be an important key to the population problem. Several contraceptive methods can be mentioned simply to discard them. The rhythm method depends on sexual abstinence 48 hours before and 3 days after ovulation. It is not reliable because ovulation is often irregular, because its effective practice involves meticulous record-keeping and arithmetical calculation, and most of all because it involves abstinence, a utopian notion. Withdrawal before ejaculation, sometimes known as **coitus** interruptus, is ineffective in practice although more feasible in theory. The postcoital douche is ineffective in both theory and practice.

There are three superior methods of contraception: surgical intervention, drug therapy, and mechanical devices. Surgical intervention ties off the **fallopian tubes** in the female and severs the **vas deferens** in the male. Both operations are simple, especially that for males, and this method is 100 percent effective. Its disadvantages are its permanence and the reluctance of people to volunteer for surgery. Females seem more receptive than males, but male surgery is easier, quicker, and safer.

Drug therapy means "the pill," an agent which prevents ovulation. The pill is virtually 100 percent effective when taken as prescribed. Its advantages are its effectiveness, its easy use relative to other methods, and the fact that it is only slightly more expensive. Its disadvantages are its side effects and the fact that ultimately its effectiveness depends on the memory and motivation of the woman taking it. Motivation is of course a

---

COITUS: sexual intercourse
FALLOPIAN TUBES: a pair of muscular tubes which transport ova from the ovary to the uterus
VAS DEFERENS: the narrow tubes through which male sperm cells are carried to the penis from the testicles

problem with all methods and is not restricted to the pill. Only about 20 percent of American women of childbearing age have used oral contraceptives, although the publicity this method receives would suggest much wider usage. Side effects include vaginal bleeding, nausea, vomiting, breast tenderness, weight gain, and depression. Of greater importance is the increased risk of thromboembolism, especially in older women. In addition, the possibility cannot be ruled out that side effects might develop after years of use or years after use. Nevertheless, the lower dosage presently available does much to eliminate the less serious side effects, and the use of oral contraceptives is expected to increase.

Mechanical devices include the condom (probably the most commonly used device), the diaphragm, and the intrauterine device (IUD). Over 400 million condoms are sold in the United States each year. About 85 percent effective, the condom's major drawback as a means of contraception is that too often the male partner fails to put it on. The diaphragm, usually used with a spermicidal foam or jelly, presents a similar difficulty with respect to the female. The diaphragm-foam combination is about as effective as the condom. Neither diaphragm alone nor foam alone is recommended.

The IUD is the favorite of mass campaigns in developing countries. It is a small plastic loop or coil which is inserted into the uterus, where it is 95 percent effective in preventing conception. The IUD is inexpensive and, in addition, foolproof in that once in place it does not depend on further human cooperation. On the other hand, insertion involves an uncomfortable, often embarrassing procedure, and bleeding and abdominal cramps are frequent transient side effects. One unsolved problem with the IUD is that of spontaneous expulsion. Unfortunately, the woman is occasionally unaware of her loss, and when this happens she is of course unprotected. The IUD will probably remain the backbone of family planning in developing countries because of its low cost and the freedom it affords from continuous medical supervision.

It is sometimes proposed that living standards in developing countries would improve if health programs were downgraded in favor of family planning. Economists examining the effects of the malaria programs in Ceylon concluded that the costs of providing new housing, schools, hospitals, and the like for an expanded malaria-free population exceeded the value of increased productivity from healthier workers. For this reason malaria eradication has been widely regarded as an economic liability. It is further assumed that the death rate would stabilize if only the health people would stop meddling with it.

It is difficult to see how the results of this kind of thinking can avoid ultimate failure. The whole idea of birth control assumes that planning is possible. The family should therefore be able to plan with a high degree of probability that existing children will survive to adulthood. It seems unlikely that parents would be very enthusiastic about contraception in the presence of high infant and child mortality. A female population festooned with intrauterine contraceptive devices cuts into births but provides no insurance against disease problems compounded by inadequate nutrition. Much has been made of the economic role of children in developing areas. They help with the farming and, by supporting their parents when the latter grow old, provide a built-in social security program. What is more important, however, is that children are also desired for themselves, i.e., adults are fond of them, enjoy having them around, and do not like to be without them. For these reasons, it will probably be impossible to check population growth in the absence of better child care.

Although the long-range success of family planning programs remains to be seen, there is no question that the movement is gaining ground. In 1960, India and Pakistan were the only two developing countries with government-sponsored programs. A decade later 30 countries had official programs. That the United Nations endorsed worldwide family planning could be seen in the establishment of a Fund for Population Activities and the commitment of the United Nations Children's Relief Fund (UNICEF) to distribute birth control devices.

Health and Poverty

Poverty is the common denominator of malnutrition and population growth. There are some who see a genetic basis in domestic poverty, especially with regard to blacks and other minorities. There is little or no solid evidence to support this view, although the basic racism it represents may be genetically inherited. (Of course there is no evidence for this latter point of view either.) Indeed, the relationship between genetics and poverty is obscure except in genetically determined diseases which prevent gainful employment.

Like health, poverty is difficult to define. Most commonly it is described in terms of a predetermined income level. The income amount varies but usually reflects what is required to maintain only a minimum subsistence. A second means of defining poverty is based on the unemployment rate in a given area. The use of "negative risk" criteria is a third approach. This involves a combination of "risk characteristics," such as lack of education, old age, physical disability, or racial discrimination, which make it difficult to enter or remain in the labor force. Finally, poverty is sometimes defined in terms of a "culture" in which a distinctive set of values, behavior traits, and beliefs distinguish the poor from the affluent.

For our purposes we will define poverty as a set of circumstances which prevent employment at a wage sufficient to provide the necessities of life within the context of a particular economy, and a life style subject to resources so limited that human hopes and aspirations are destroyed. Poverty is relative, and even though a population group in the United States might be well off in other societies, its members could be considered poor by contemporary American standards because they live below the level enjoyed by the majority of citizens. Poverty, then, is far more than a simple lack of money. It is rather a state that involves a person's total life—his food, clothing, housing, education, health, job opportunities, family life, and aspirations. It is a vicious cycle in which each component relates to and reinforces the other. The total poverty population in the United States is 15 to 20 million—mostly farmers, the aged, children, and racial minority groups.

What are the medical needs of the poor, and what are their patterns of utilization of medical services? For one thing, the poor have higher rates of infant and perinatal mortality. Fatality rates from tuberculosis, many types of cancer, and other major diseases are higher than those of other socioeconomic groups. Tuberculosis, venereal disease, and disability resulting from heart disease, arthritis, and other chronic diseases are all more common among the poor. There are more episodes of psychosocial distress and clinical psychiatric disorders and a very high prevalence of untreated dental caries. In addition, the poor have generally higher fertility rates, higher illegitimacy rates, a greater incidence of premature births and larger family size (Figs. 2-13A and B). As might be expected, prenatal care, immunizations, and other aspects of preventive medicine are utilized less by this group than any other; and even the most acute problems, those which cause disability and great suffering, are often untended until late in their course.

Although the poor have great need for medical services, they utilize physicians less than any other socioeconomic group. Members of low-income groups are more likely to consult friends, pharmacists, or chiropractors about health problems and to seek the physician only when they are seriously ill. They remain longer when hospitalized, although fewer poor people are insured and less of the bill is covered for those who are. This disadvantaged population endures more days of restricted activity, more bed-disability days, and more days lost from work per person. When considered together, these patterns indicate that neither the health of the poor nor their utilization of health services is adequate.

One of the most obvious explanations for their poor health is the low priority assigned to illness among low-income groups. The poor often

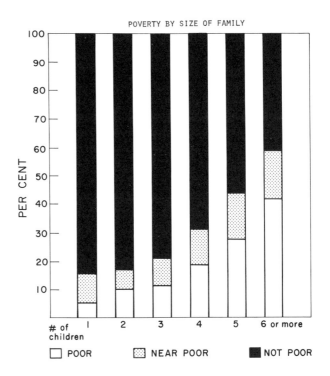

FIG. 2-13A. *While poverty is clearly associated with large family size, it is unclear whether poverty causes large families or whether large families cause poverty. In any case, many of the children in the larger families are unwanted. (See Fig. 14B.) (After* When More is Less, Planned Parenthood Federation of America, 1968. *Courtesy of Planned Parenthood–World Population.)*

proceed from one crisis to another, and this tendency to cope only with each immediate problem produces an outlook locked to the present. Expenditures for housing, clothing, food, and transportation are necessary and unavoidable; medical care, particularly any preventive measure, is too often postponed indefinitely. The poor rarely have the financial resources to purchase needed medical care, let alone to buy insurance against what might happen. They live in the present, and in many cases only when an individual becomes incapacitated does he consider himself ill. Emphasis on health is unrealistic in this context, and it is often easier to ignore symptoms than to do something about them.

In addition, disadvantaged populations have less contact with news media and agencies from which they might obtain health information. Poor people often have less general knowledge and more incorrect ideas about health-related matters and thus tend to defer medical care partly

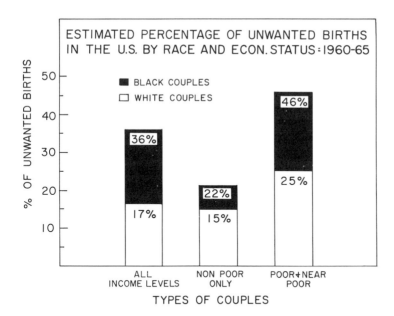

Fig. 2-13B.   *The percentage within the bars in the chart refer to the percentage of black and white couples within that income group who had unwanted children. Thus, 46 percent of black couples in the poor and near poor income group had unwanted children vs. only 25 percent of white couples. (Adapted from Westoff, 1968. From* Now to Zero. *Courtesy of Little, Brown and Company.)*

because they do not recognize the importance of symptoms. It is this lack of knowledge which leads them to consult friends, relatives, or the local druggist about medical problems, a process which usually results in delaying adequate care. All this is often compounded by fear of losing a day's work, a day's pay, and possibly a job if time is taken off for medical care.

Even when the importance of a symptom is recognized, it is usually difficult for low-income individuals to obtain medical care. Long distances, inadequate transportation, inability to hire a babysitter, inconvenient hours, complex eligibility requirements, lack of money, long waits, and rude personnel often make medical care inaccessible even when it is available. Low-income families are less skilled in the use of medical services and find it difficult to understand the health care system. The fragmentation, specialization, division of labor, and apparent impersonality of the modern medical institution can be both confusing and extremely frustrating. While the affluent patient often knows how to "beat the system" by seeking out key personnel, the poor rarely know who these people are.

The "professionalism" of health workers and the social distance perceived by both patient and medical staff lead to further gaps in communication and understanding. Seeking help in a large hospital often involves attendance at several specialty clinics and sometimes even referral to clinics in several different hospitals. The latter is especially disastrous in terms of continuity of care and follow-up, but good comprehensive care is difficult, if not impossible, in any large outpatient department. The patient is rarely seen more than once or twice by the same physician. In addition, the physician working in an institution far removed from the patient's environment is denied much of the information necessary to understand that patient's total life situation. This is extremely important because what goes on in the ghetto can and does have a direct influence on how effective the medical care will be. Indeed, it is often the patient's social and economic environment which contributes to the development of his illness.

Until very recently, medical care for the poor was based entirely on middle-class mores, was conceived by professional health planners, and was staffed largely by middle-class personnel. It was expected that the poor would understand, accept, and be grateful for this largesse. This approach has been ineffective because it ignores the manner in which poverty groups define illness, the barriers they must overcome to obtain care, and the frustrations of dealing with institutionalized medicine. Health planners have devoted years to the development of comprehensive care for the poor without realizing that the low priority of medicine in their lives makes treatment of the immediate need the prime necessity and the most pressing demand.

Like health, education is intimately related to the life situation of the individual and to his surrounding environment. Ill health, cultural deprivation, inadequate home-preparation for school, poor school facilities, less talented teachers, and racial discrimination make the learning process difficult and uninteresting for low-income children. The home environment of poor children does not provide the stimulation and range of experiences found in many affluent homes. Parents are less able to help their children with school work, to provide learning materials and supplies, and to arrange proper places for study. Frequently the child has an undetected hearing or visual problem. The results are poor academic performance, high drop-out rates, and marginal capabilities for employment. Financial resources to further the education of the student who does well in school are often unavailable, and he is forced to end his studies prematurely.

Unemployment and underemployment are closely related to education. Without the skills and education increasingly required to qualify for the better jobs, the individual is relegated to unskilled or semiskilled labor, which pays the least and offers minimal job security. The availability of simple, repetitive jobs has declined, while the demand for highly skilled personnel has increased. One result of this trend is that it is extremely difficult for dropouts and even some high school graduates to find work. If the individual is black his chances for employment are even worse. Blacks tend to be paid less than white workers with the same amount of education, and black college graduates earn less on average than whites who have only a high school diploma. Because of discrimination and exploitation blacks are disproportionately concentrated in the unskilled and semiskilled occupations. They lack the training required for skilled jobs and have no means of obtaining it. The prospect of constantly searching for one dead-end job after another offers little incentive to seek work, and in some cases welfare offers more financial security. Unskilled jobs usually provide only a subsistence wage, and even these jobs are hard to find and easy to lose. The unskilled wage earner is thus frozen in poverty, with little or no hope of advancement.

Although the poor are frequently accused of mismanaging their finances, excessive spending is often a function of exploitation. This is particularly true of food and durable goods. Stores within the ghetto tend to charge higher prices than those in other areas. This may be unavoidable where small shops must mark up goods to realize a profit, but frank exploitation is both common and well organized. Door-to-door peddlers, persuasive sales techniques, and ambiguous sales contracts lock people into purchases at exorbitant prices. The cost of credit is also usually far higher for the poor than for others, and a purchased article is promptly repossessed if payments are not maintained. In some cases wages are attached, and the family sinks further into poverty. Lack of knowledge about the legal aspects of such situations leaves the individual relatively helpless.

Because poor people have less money, they are rarely able to buy in quantity and are thus limited to a succession of small purchases which are more costly. Lack of money means difficulty in paying for proper food and housing, not to mention medical care when it is needed. Serious illness results in days lost from work as well as frequently large medical bills, both of which lead to further depletion of financial resources. Families who must worry about meeting everyday expenses rarely are able to save any substantial amount for emergencies. When an emergency does arise, the family is often unable to cope with it.

Environmental hazards are particularly prominent in low-income areas, largely because of poor housing. Not only are the buildings firetraps and generally unsafe for their occupants, but the lead-based paint so commonly found in these dwellings constitutes a special health hazard to young children. Infrequent garbage collection and improper disposal turn an area into a breeding place for rats and insects. Poorly lighted streets and lack of safe play areas for children are conducive to crime and accidents, both of which adversely affect health and welfare.

The effects of poverty are perhaps most devastating on family structure. Men not only have difficulty supporting a family but often hold jobs too low on the occupational scale to maintain self-respect. Their feelings of inadequacy are enhanced if the wife becomes, in effect, the breadwinner. If in addition the man is forced to stay at home because of unemployment or poor health, tensions frequently become so extreme that they lead to the breakup of the family. Often the male head leaves to escape his painful feelings, or because his absence would make his family eligible for welfare and thus more secure financially. This sequence of events places the total family burden on the female head, and it is estimated that 25 to 40 percent of the child-rearing units in urban slum areas are headed by a woman. She is sometimes assisted by older children, who often must leave school to care for younger ones or to find work. The absence or sporadic presence of a father is often detrimental to the social and emotional development of the children. Without support from a stable home environment they quickly become discouraged in school and drop out; and thus, with education interrupted in one way or another, the problem of low-income jobs comes to the forefront again. And poverty, like a hereditary disease, is transmitted from one generation to the next.

In this context it is not surprising to find the poor beset with feelings of helplessness. With little hope for future success, the individual comes to expect failure, and failure becomes a self-fulfilling prophecy. The son comes to experience the same failures as his father, and for the same reasons. The situation of women also remains unchanged. If change is to come, it is not sufficient to deal only with some components of the problem. The total life situation of the poor must be considered.

What does all this mean for the delivery of medical care to the poor? It means that simply treating acute medical problems will not substantially improve the health of persons from disadvantaged areas. The problem of lead poisoning, for example, will not be solved by medical care but by legislation and housing-code enforcement. Lead poisoning is, in other words, one of the many medical problems which require a nonmedical solution.

The idea is growing that such nonmedical solutions are the proper concern of health workers, whose fundamental responsibility is to maintain and improve the health of individuals. Treatment carried out in medical institutions meets only part of this responsibility. As we have previously suggested, if a physician knows only the medical history of a patient and nothing of the environmental conditions which contribute to making or keeping him sick, then the physician can relate only to symptoms, not causes. Yet the physician must be responsive to the total situation if he genuinely wants to help the patient. It is not necessarily the doctor's responsibility to go into the home to determine what problems might affect the health of his patient, but it is his responsibility to be concerned with and aware of those problems. It is meaningless to prescribe medication if the patient has no money to pay for it. Similarly, medical institutions must be aware of the situations that affect health within poverty areas in order to guard against implementing programs which have no meaning to the target population.

Working for better health is by no means the sole responsibility of medical institutions or medical personnel. Medical care is only one of a wide range of needs, including housing, jobs, and education. Community agencies, social workers, school personnel, health workers, housing administrators, neighborhood associations, and, above all, the people themselves must work together to complement each other's role. The treatment of disease is not an isolated activity, and it is not enough to identify a necessary bacterial cause. Attention must be paid to those sufficient causes in the social and economic environment that critically affect health. Only when the underlying sufficient causes are understood is it possible to deal effectively with the necessary cause. In other words, those who are concerned with health must also concern themselves with poverty. It would be supremely naive, however, to suppose that health care somehow offers a solution to the poverty problem. It is obvious that the poor need health care and that improved health is often the *sine qua non* of individual progress through the fetters of an impoverished background. On the other hand, health programs, *per se*, offer no solution to the basic challenge of poverty.

Better health palliates and potentiates, but it does not represent a cure. For example, no amount of medical care will give a man the education required for job security or remove the stigma of black skin. Fortunately, the health establishment has more to offer than medical care—at least in theory. As the nation's second largest employer, the health industry has a growing demand for manpower. The organization of training programs in health-related occupations and the recruitment of the poor into these programs are probably worth more than hordes of doctors, nurses, and technicians toward a cure for poverty. In addition, providing jobs is also a nonmedical approach to better health in that a better standard of living is one of the most effective ways to improve public health. The challenge of poverty is probably the best example of the seldom-recognized truth that good health does not invariably emerge from the end of a stethoscope.

Iatrogenic Disease

Up to now, this chapter has concerned itself with a group of general background risk factors which act on the individual and which, under certain conditions, tend to affect his health adversely. Genetics is a prime determinant of a person's ability to cope successfully with his environment. Malnutrition is both a disease in its own right and a potentiator of other diseases, while related problems of population and poverty promote ill health and act as effective barriers to health care.

Iatrogenic disease is more a foreground than a background factor. It is illness which results from the ministrations of a physician and thus enters the picture after the patient seeks medical attention. Iatrogenic disease is the hazard of health care.

Twenty percent of patients admitted to a hospital acquire an illness arising from their hospitalization experience. These illnesses are not those for which the patients were admitted to the hospital, but additional illnesses. Most of these are minor episodes related to drug therapy or diagnostic procedures, and subside spontaneously. Nevertheless, about 40 percent of them are serious enough to prolong the hospital stay, require special treatment, or actually threaten life. About 2 percent result in death. The chances that such an episode will occur rise with the length of hospitalization.

By far the most common cause of such untoward illnesses is drug therapy. This is true both in and out of the hospital. Adverse drug reactions are more common in women than men and more frequent in black women than white. Diseases arising from drugs come about both directly and indirectly. The best example of the former is the surprisingly high incidence of reactions to penicillin. Fever is the most common such reaction but rashes are not unusual, and occasionally sudden death occurs in **anaphylactic shock.** In the early 1960s, a drug known as **thalidomide** was widely promoted as a sedative in Europe and Canada, although it was not approved by the Food and Drug Administration for general use in the United States (Table 2-1). Several years passed before the birth

---

IATROGENIC: induced by a physician
ANAPHYLACTIC SHOCK: a highly fatal condition which develops rapidly and is due to hypersensitivity to a drug or toxin previously encountered by the individual
THALIDOMIDE: a drug used to induce sleep; when administered during the first trimester of pregnancy, thalidomide causes malformation of the fetus

TABLE 2-1. Sale of Thalidomide and Incidence of Thalidomide Cases*

Country	Sale, in Kg	Thalidomide Cases
Portugal	37	2
Norway	60	11
Netherlands	140	25
Belgium	258	26
Great Britain	5,769	349
West Germany	30,099	5,000

*Modified from Lenz, Malformations caused by drugs in pregnancy. Amer. J. Dis. Child., 112, 1966

of children with poorly formed arms and, less frequently, legs was associated with maternal use of thalidomide during the first **trimester** of pregnancy. Thalidomide then disappeared from the medical scene, although its effects live on in the thousands of deformed children whose chances for a normal life were obliterated within three months of conception. Other drugs remain in use even though their dangers are well known. Prominent in this group is chloramphenicol, an antibiotic developed in the late 1940s. Chloramphenicol is the drug of choice in **typhoid fever** and is occasionally indicated when other antibiotics of its type prove unsuccessful. Typhoid is a rare disease in the United States— only 395 cases were reported in 1968—and the occasions on which chloramphenicol's substitute cannot be used are also rare. The trouble with this drug is that it sometimes produces a highly fatal condition known as **aplastic anemia.** Reactions to chloramphenicol are usually milder, but why use the drug against diseases for which other drugs are safer and equally effective? This is a hard question with no clear answer. Chloramphenicol remains popular even though the government and the medical profession are fully aware of its hazards.

Thalidomide was removed from the market once its effects were apparent; chloramphenicol remains despite its effects. Unfortunately, years pass in many cases before the hazards of a particular drug emerge. The popular drug, phenacetin, was in use as one of the components of

TRIMESTER: a period of 3 months; commonly, the first 3 months of pregnancy
TYPHOID FEVER: an infectious disease due to the bacterium, *Salmonella typhosa;* symptoms are primarily intestinal, sometimes fatal
APLASTIC ANEMIA: an anemia characterized by cessation of formation of the cellular elements of blood

"A.P.C." tablets for 75 years before it was learned that this drug causes kidney damage. Ten years of use was required before it became clear that the widely used **tetracycline** family of antibiotics can adversely affect bone development. The time lag between the introduction of a drug and a true appreciation of its side effects guarantees the continuance of drug-related iatrogenic disease for the foreseeable future, and it is highly probable that some of today's more popular drugs will ultimately fail the test of time.

Some drug reactions are indirect in that they are genetically determined. Certain antimalarial drugs, sulfa drugs, and other compounds produce a **hemolytic anemia** in some people. These persons lack an enzyme present in normal red cells. The lack, also genetically determined, of another enzyme leads to abnormally slow deactivation of isoniazid, the front-line drug in tuberculosis therapy. Fortunately, this defect is not severe and usually offers no interference to effective tuberculosis therapy.

Finally, the development and use of antibiotics against those pathogenic microorganisms which have historically been man's most implacable adversaries encourages the emergence of new strains in bacterial species previously a minor threat to man. Most famous of these is the Staphylococcus. Before the "wonder drugs" came along, "Staph" was a mundane bacterial pathogen playing second fiddle to its more potent brethren, the pneumococcus and the Streptococcus. When these organisms proved vulnerable to penicillin, the Staphylococcus became a prime concern because it developed resistance to penicillin; and staphylococcal infections became the scourge of the hospitalized patient. When these infections finally succumbed to new antimicrobials, still more obscure organisms, the **gram-negatives** and the **fungi,** arose to take the place of the Staphylococcus. And so it seems that despite our best efforts we often wind up trading one disease for another in the process of seeking a cure for what ails us.

"A.P.C.": a combination of drugs (aspirin, phenacetin, and caffeine) used for pain, especially headache

TETRACYCLINE: the original "wonder drug"; a broad-spectrum antibiotic

HEMOLYTIC ANEMIA: an anemia in which red blood cells are destroyed

GRAM-NEGATIVE: a group of bacteria characterized by failure to take a commonly used laboratory stain known as Gram's stain; these organisms are usually less pathogenic than those which are gram-positive

FUNGI: a group of organisms belonging to the plant kingdom, some of which are pathogenic for man

Notes

1   Parts of this section appeared in somewhat different form in Marshall, C., Brown, R., and Goodrich, C. Improved nutrition vs. public health services as major determinants of world population growth. Clin. Pediat. July 10, 1971.
2   Do not confuse the replacement number with average family size. The former tells how many children a couple must have for the population to remain at the same size. The latter tells us simply the average number of children per family. It may be higher, lower, or identical to the replacement number, but the two are not related.
3   Capital goods refer to goods produced which can then be used to produce additional goods. Machines, buildings, roads, and electric power are all considered capital goods.
4   If a factory is built which costs $3 million and this factory produces $1 million worth of goods per year, productivity is 1 million ÷ 3 million, or one-third, or 0.33.

References

Albrink, M. Obesity. *In* Beeson, P., and McDermott, W. Textbook of Medicine. Philadelphia, W. B. Saunders, 1971.

Andreski, S. Parasitism and Subversion. London, Wiedenfeld and Nicolsen, 1966.

Bamberger, L. Project planning and development by official health agencies. Amer. J. Pub. Health **56**, April, 1966.

Bearn, A. G., and Kilbourne, E. D. Genetic determinants of health and disease. *In* Kilbourne, E. D., and Smillie, W. G., eds. Human Ecology and Public Health, 4th ed. New York, Macmillan, 1969.

Benson, R. Handbook of Obstetrics and Gynecology. Los Altos, Calif., Lange, 1971.

Berg, A. Malnutrition and national development. J. Tropical Pediat. September, 1966.

Bergner, L., and Yerby, A. Low income and barriers to the use of health services. New Eng. J. Med. **278**:10, 1968.

Bhagwati, J. The Economics of Underdeveloped Countries. New York, McGraw-Hill, 1966.

Breslow, L. New partnerships in the delivery of services—a public health view of the need. Amer. J. Pub. Health **57**, July, 1967.

Browne, J. H. Provision of suitable and sufficient nutrition. *In* Hilleboe, H., and Larimore, G., eds. Preventive Medicine, 2nd ed. Philadelphia, W. B. Saunders, 1965.

Burton, L. E., and Smith, H. H. Public Health and Community Medicine. Baltimore, Williams and Wilkins, 1970, pp. 264–270.

Cluff, L. Reactions to drugs. *In* Wintrobe, M. *et al.*, eds. Harrison's Principles of Internal Medicine, 6th ed. New York, McGraw-Hill, 1970.

Committee on Human Reproduction. The control of fertility. J.A.M.A. **194**, October, 1965.

Dorn, H. F. World population growth. *In* The Population Dilemma. The American Assembly. Englewood Cliffs, N.J., Prentice-Hall, 1963.

Dubos, R. Man Adapting. New Haven, Yale University Press, 1965.

Easterlin, R. Effects of population growth on the economic development of developing countries. Ann. Amer. Acad. Polit. Soc. Sci. **369**, January, 1967.

Eickhoff, T. C. Hospital-acquired staphylococcal infection. *In* Clark, D. W., and MacMahon, B., eds. Preventive Medicine. Boston, Little, Brown, 1967.

Geiger, H. J. The neighborhood health center. Arch. Env. Health **14**, June, 1967.

Gibson, C. The neighborhood health center: the primary unit of health care. Amer. J. Pub. Health **58**, July, 1968.

Goodman, L. S., and Gilman, A. The Pharmacological Basis of Therapeutics. New York, Macmillan, 1965.

Gordon, J. The politics of community medicine projects: a conflict analysis. Med. Care **7**, November–December, 1969.

Hauser, P. M. The social, economic, and technological problem of rapid urbanization. *In* Novack, D. and Lekach, R., eds. New York, St. Martin's, 1964.

Heilbroner, R. The Great Ascent. New York, Harper and Row, 1963.

Horowitz, A., and Burke, M. H. Health, population, and development. *In* Stycos, M. and Arias, J., eds. Population Dilemma in Latin America. Washington, D.C., Potomac Books, 1966.

Kaprio, L. A. World resources of medical personnel. *In* Walstenhomle, G. and O'Connor, M., eds. Health of Mankind. Boston, Little, Brown, 1967.

Kent, J., and Smith, C. H. Involving the urban poor in health services through accommodation—the employment of neighborhood representatives. Amer. J. Pub. Health **57**, June, 1967.

Kessner, D. M., and Lepper, M. H. Epidemiologic studies of gram-negative bacilli in the hospital and community. Amer. J. Epidemiology **85**, January, 1967.

Kiefer, D. M. Population, parts 1 and 2. Chem. Engineering News **46**, October 7 and 14, 1968.

King, M., ed. Medical Care in Developing Countries. Nairobi, Oxford University Press, 1966.

Latham, M. Human Nutrition in Tropical Africa. Food and Agricultural Organization of the United Nations. Rome, 1965.

Lenz, W. Malformations caused by drugs in pregnancy. Amer. J. Dis. Child. **112**, 1966.

Marshall, C. L., Brown, R., and Goodrich, C. H. Improved nutrition vs. public health services as major determinants of world population growth. Clin. Pediat. **10**, July, 1971.

Mayer, J. Some aspects of the problem of regulation of food intake and obesity. New Eng. J. Med. **274**, 1966.

Muller, C. Income and the receipt of medical care. Amer. J. Pub. Health **55**, April, 1965.

Oral Contraceptives. Medical Letter **10**, April 26, 1968.

Perkin, G. W. Intrauterine contraception. Can. Med. Ass. J. **94**, February 26, 1966.

Rosenstock, I. Why people use health services. Milbank Memorial Fund Quarterly **44**, part 1, July, 1966.

Schact, L. C. Human Genetics in Public Health. Minneapolis, University of Minnesota Press, 1964.

Scrimshaw, N. S., and Behar, M. Malnutrition. *In* Kilbourne, E. D. and Smillie, W. G., eds. Human Ecology and Public Health. New York, Macmillan, 1970.

Scrimshaw, N. S., Behar, M., and Gordon, E., eds. Malnutrition, Learning and Behavior. Cambridge, Massachusetts Institute of Technology Press, 1968.

Shimmel, E. M. The hazards of hospitalization. Ann. Int. Med. **60**, January, 1964.

Singer, W. H. The mechanics of economic development. *In* Agarwala, A. N. and Singh, S. P., eds. The Economics of Underdevelopment. New York, Oxford University Press, 1963.

Straus, A. Medical ghettos. Transaction, May, 1967.

Vogel, A. J. A new breed of specialist moves in. Medical Economics, July 8, 1968.

Walter, C. Antipoverty medicine. Medical Economics, November 14, 1966.

Wise, H. Montefiore Hospital, neighborhood medical care demonstration. Milbank Memorial Fund Quarterly **46**:3, part 1, July, 1968.

Wise, H. *et al.* Community development and health education: community organization as a health tactic. Milbank Memorial Fund Quarterly **46**:3, part 1, July, 1968.

Wrong, D. Population and Society. New York, Random House, 1967.

Yerby, A. The Disadvantaged and Health Care. White House Conference on Health, Washington, D.C., 1964.

3

The Analysis and Measurement of Disease

"One death is a tragedy," wrote Joseph Stalin, "one million is a statistic." The implications of this statement perhaps offend the humanistic reader and offer him immediate grounds for a negative attitude toward statistics. However, studying and recording what happens to many is one of our most valuable tools for ultimately helping one human being. Moreover, statistics are actually like pieces of puzzles, perhaps dull and meaningless out of context, but with each additional piece helping the solver to see more of the total picture. And the health worker, confronted with the puzzle of disease, needs to know something about the methods used to study disease distribution and the factors which affect this distribution. The examination, diagnosis, and treatment of the individual patient is the province of clinical medicine; but though the individual is of great importance, he is not a reliable mirror of health problems in his community. If we consider all the people in a community who have some disease or other, only a small percentage of these potential patients will have signs or symptoms of illness at any given time. The remainder will be totally free of any manifestations of their disease. Because some diseases produce symptoms more readily than others or produce more distressing symptoms, those who seek medical care, a part of our small

ICEBERG OF DISEASE

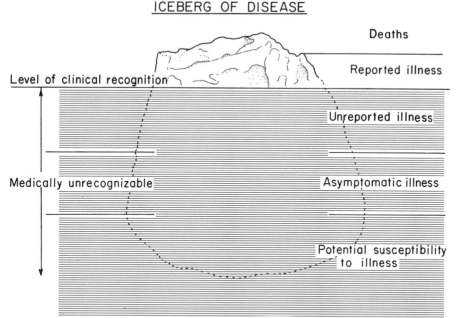

FIG. 3-1.   *Like the iceberg, most cases of disease are submerged below the "water-line" of clinical recognition. Other cases are unrecognized because the patient fails to report his symptoms to a physician. Notice that death is represented by the very top of the iceberg, i.e., the smallest portion of it.*

percentage, will be those who have the most symptomatology. The hinge that squeaks the loudest gets the most oil, but the need for oil at one hinge does not necessarily imply that all the hinges have the same need. The point is that the frequency with which people seek medical attention for diseases does not perforce reflect the frequency of those illnesses in the total population.

The existence of disease in the absence of symptoms or signs is illustrated by the so-called "iceberg effect" (Fig. 3-1). The "waterline" represents the division between apparent and inapparent disease, and, like the iceberg whose visible tip is but a small fraction of its total bulk, most diseases go through a latent phase before becoming apparent. In most cases hypertension usually produces no symptoms for 20 years or more, only to manifest itself without previous warning as a stroke or

MYOCARDIAL INFARCTION: death of a portion of the heart muscle; a "heart attack"

myocardial infarction. Other diseases, notably polio and hepatitis, only rarely produce distinctive symptoms. Most people who are infected with the polio virus recover without ever realizing that they had a potentially catastrophic disease. It is believed that there are 99 inapparent cases of polio for every clinical case. Inapparent cases are important because even though the individual escapes the obvious manifestations of disease himself, he is often capable of transmitting it to others who may not be as fortunate. In addition, it is generally easier to cope with diseases when they are detected early, and for conditions like hypertension early detection can be the difference between survival and death.

The logical approach to the study of diseases thus demands that all cases in a population be considered—the inapparent as well as the obvious. Among the benefits of this **epidemiological** approach to diseases are the following:

1. The *natural course of disease* can often be defined. The existence and importance of an asymptomatic phase can be clarified, as can the relationship between clinical and inapparent cases.

2. The *importance of a disease in the community* can be determined, and from this

3. The *effectiveness of control measures* and the *need for more or different types of health services* can be ascertained.

4. Contributory *risk factors* often come to light which provide clues to effective control, e.g., cigarette smoking and its association with lung cancer.

5. Often *new syndromes* are identified, or *new symptoms* suggestive of a known disease are uncovered.

6. Some of the time the *cause of the disease* in question can be determined.

Each item on the list provides information of value in the control of a particular disease, and it is the desire to control diseases that motivates us to study them in the first place.

The epidemiological approach basically is characterized by the process of comparing two or more groups of people. In this process the following question is asked: Are there any characteristics present in people who have this disease which are not present in people who do not have this disease? If positive, the answer to this question leads to a second: Is the existence of these characteristics in diseased individuals causally

---

EPIDEMIOLOGY: the study of disease distribution in populations and the factors which influence this distribution

related to the disease? The process of answering the first question is known as descriptive epidemiology because it describes the frequency and distribution of the disease and the characteristics with which it seems to be associated. The answer to the second question is ascertained through the technique of analytic epidemiology. From descriptive epidemiology we learn which characteristics are present in the disease group and absent in the group without the disease. This discovery suggests that certain characteristics may be causal, and from this observation the investigator derives an **hypothesis.** An hypothesis is essentially an unproved assumption which is used to explain certain observations and which acts as a basis for further study of a question. Hypotheses specify the causal factor, identify the effect derived from it, suggest how much cause is needed to produce the effect, and predict the time lag, if any, between the existence of the cause and the appearance of the effect. Most importantly, an hypothesis is formulated in a manner which suggests how it can be tested. For example, the statement that "cigarettes cause lung cancer" is an incomplete hypothesis. A correct formulation of this hypothesis might be stated as follows: The smoking of 30 to 40 cigarettes per day causes lung cancer in 12 percent of smokers after 20 years of exposure. This statement identifies cigarettes as the cause of lung cancer and it further specifies the amount of smoking required and the length of time one must smoke before lung cancer will appear. In addition, it clearly implies the kinds of data needed to test the hypothesis, i.e., numbers of cigarettes, years of exposure, and so on. Having stated the hypothesis, the investigator can proceed to design a study which will support or discredit it.

Before we examine the techniques of analytic epidemiology, let us consider the kinds of characteristics found through descriptive epidemiology. Characteristics may be related to time, place, or persons. All diseases must be studied in terms of time. Explosive outbreaks of disease produce a large number of cases in a few days, with subsequent cases appearing in lesser numbers until, after a period of weeks, no new cases occur. Such outbreaks usually suggest a common source through which the population comes into contact with the agent or agents of disease, e.g., bacterial contamination of a community's water supply, or the sudden exposure of a population to abnormally high levels of air pollution. Diseases which are transmitted from person to person reach a peak more gradually and tail off over a longer period of time (Fig. 3-2). Venereal disease is an example of this second type. Clustering refers to a tendency for events to occur within a relatively brief period after an antecedent

---

HYPOTHESIS: a supposition used to explain an event; an unproved theory

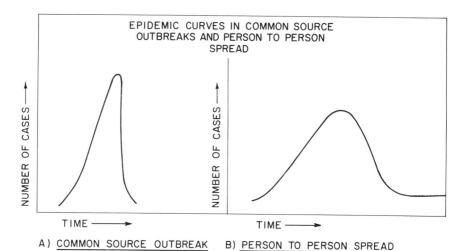

FIG. 3-2. *Epidemic curves in common source outbreaks and person to person spread.*

event. If a long period elapses between one event and another, the possible association between them is less clear and often overlooked altogether. When we speak of infectious diseases, the time lag between exposure to a disease agent and the appearance of the disease is called the **incubation period.** It is sometimes referred to as the latent period with respect to other diseases. In a second-grade class, cases of measles will cluster 10 to 14 days after the children are exposed to the first case in their class. The child who transmits the measles virus to his classmates is often called the **index case,** because all subsequent cases are discussed in relation to him.

Disease frequency also varies with the season of the year. Polio most commonly occurs in late summer and early fall, measles is at its height in early spring, and deaths due to accidents reach a peak in July. Sometimes disease occurrence varies over longer periods of time. These so-called secular trends may be a simple increase or decrease in the occurrence of a particular disease, i.e., lung or stomach cancer (Fig. 3-3). However, some secular trends are cyclical. Influenza tends to follow a cyclical pattern, with large outbreaks occurring between long periods of low

---

INCUBATION PERIOD: the time lag between exposure to an infectious disease-agent and the appearance of clinical disease

INDEX CASE: the reference case from which the disease is transmitted to others and to which other cases are related

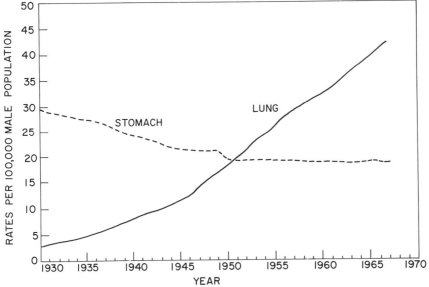

MALE CANCER DEATH RATES BY SITE
UNITED STATES, 1930–1967

FIG. 3-3.   *The dramatic rise of lung cancer deaths since 1930 has been matched by a more gradual decline in deaths from stomach cancer. (After Cancer Statistics, 1971, American Cancer Society, Inc., 1971. Courtesy of American Cancer Society, Inc.)*

incidence that are several years in duration. Some experts feel that infectious hepatitis is inclined to follow a seven-year cycle.

Characteristics of place involve several levels. First, disease patterns vary from country to country. **Schistosomiasis**, one of the world's most important diseases in terms of both **morbidity** and **mortality**, does not occur in the United States and most other temperate-zone countries. Other diseases may occur in all countries but with very different frequency. Stomach cancer is on the wane in the United States, even though it is very prevalent in Japan. On the other hand, cancer of the breast is

---

SCHISTOSOMIASIS: a chronic parasitic disease involving many organ systems; it is caused by a kind of worm and transmitted from person to person by several species of freshwater snails; it is usually debilitating and often fatal
MORBIDITY: illness
MORTALITY: death

far more common in American women than in Japanese. Disease frequency also varies from region to region within the same country. Urban disease-patterns often differ from those in rural areas. The reason for a particular regional difference is often an important clue to disease causation. Malaria does not occur in the absence of the anopheline mosquito which transmits it.[1] Similarly, schistosomiasis is transmitted by certain species of freshwater snails and cannot exist where temperature or other factors prove lethal to snails. Goiter depends on soil deficient in iodine, and the distribution of this disease is therefore limited to such areas.

Characteristics of persons are many, but perhaps the most important is age. This is because disease frequency varies more consistently with age than with any other characteristic, and generally the prevalence of chronic disease increases with advancing age. If a 40-year-old man is told that he has measles, this diagnosis is immediately suspect because measles is usually a disease of childhood. Similarly, the child who complains of chest pain almost certainly does not have arteriosclerotic heart disease because the age and the disease do not match.

Disease frequency also varies with sex. Males are more likely to have a "heart attack," but rheumatoid arthritis is more common in females. With the exception of those illnesses specifically related to the sexual organs themselves, chronic disease tends to be more common in males. Ethnic group is also an important **variable**. We know that sickle cell disease is virtually restricted to blacks. Conversely, skin cancer, **ulcerative colitis**, and **multiple sclerosis** are more common in whites. Religion is often used to subclassify whites, and, as one might expect, disease frequency does vary with religion. Other personal characteristics of importance in descriptive epidemiology include socioeconomic group, occupation, place of birth, size of family, marital status, and blood group. This list could be extended further, but these examples are sufficient for our purpose.

Disease Rates

Washington, D.C. is said to have about 17,000 narcotics addicts, and in New York City the figure is put at 200,000. Does this mean

---

VARIABLE: having no fixed numerical value; a characteristic or attribute
ULCERATIVE COLITIS: a chronic inflammation of the large bowel, with ulceration of the bowel wall
MULTIPLE SCLEROSIS: a swelling and hypertrophy (overgrowth) of connective tissues of the brain and spinal cord

that addiction is more common in New York than it is in Washington? It would certainly seem so, since New York has more than ten times as many addicts. However, things are often not what they seem to be. In fact, if the available information is correct, the magnitude of the problem in the two cities is approximately equal. Why? For one thing, the data we have tell us how many addicts there are in each city, but it does not tell us how many people in each place might become addicts. In other words, we know nothing about the population at risk. With regard to drug addiction, virtually every person in the population is at risk: from the newborn baby who becomes addicted in the uterus of an addicted mother, to the oldest citizens. Washington, D.C. has about 700,000 people, while New York's population is almost 8 million. It is illogical to comment on the prevalence of addiction in the two cities without considering the **population at risk.** This is done by noting that out of 700,000 potential addicts (population at risk) Washington has 17,000 actually addicted. Obviously, only a fraction of the people are addicted:

$$\text{number addicted} = 17,000$$
$$\text{population at risk} = 700,000$$

$$\text{addicted fraction} = \frac{17,000}{700,000} = 0.024$$

For New York:

$$\text{number addicted} = 200,000$$
$$\text{population at risk} = 8,000,000$$

$$\text{addicted fraction} = \frac{200,000}{8,000,000} = 0.025$$

Now, it so happens that the world is full of people who break out in a cold sweat when they see a number as hostile and incomprehensible as 0.025 or 0.024. Fortunately for those of us who feel this way, there is an easy way out. That 0.025 really means that for every single person at risk in New York City there is 0.025 person addicted. But it is hard to visualize 0.025 person, let alone to sympathize with him. Yet, if there are 0.025 addicts for each single individual at risk, there must be 0.25 for every 10 persons at risk, or 2.5 addicts for every 100 New Yorkers, or

---

POPULATION AT RISK: all the people who might contract an illness; usually the entire population of a neighborhood, city, state, or nation

25 addicts for every 1,000. Note how reassuring it is to be rid of that decimal point. It is also easy. You simply multiply your fractional number by 10, 100, 1,000, or 100,000 until it vanishes, only to emerge in a respectable form such as 25 or 24 per 1,000 persons at risk.

In our example we multiplied Washington's 0.024 and New York's 0.025 by 1,000 to produce a pair of rates by which the addiction problem in the two cities can be compared. Even though the actual number of addicts in Washington is less than one-tenth the number in New York, the rates of addiction are 24 per 1,000 population at risk and 25 per 1,000 population at risk, respectively. In other words, the proportion of the population addicted to drugs in each city is virtually identical. The use of a rate enables us to compare disease frequency in different populations because the size of the population being compared is automatically taken into consideration.

Rates are used to compare not only disease frequency (morbidity), but also births (natality) and deaths (mortality). Regardless of what they are used to measure, all rates are fractions derived from a numerator and a denominator. The numerator counts the number of times that a particular event occurs, i.e., babies born, persons dying, or individuals becoming addicted. The denominator counts the population at risk, i.e., the number of individuals in whom or to whom the same event *might have* occurred during the time interval in question. As we have seen, most rates are small fractional numbers. To avoid the confusion generated by decimal points and zeros, these fractions are generally expressed in terms of large numbers of persons, e.g., 2.5 per 100, 25 per 1,000, 250 per 10,000, and so on.

The two most important rates in epidemiology are incidence and prevalence. These rates are measures of morbidity in that they both deal with the frequency with which a disease occurs. Incidence is defined as the number of new cases of a particular disease during a specified time interval (usually one year), divided by the estimated population at risk at the midpoint of the time interval (usually midyear). Prevalence is defined as the number of cases (new and old) existing at a given point in time divided by the estimated population at risk at that same point in time. For most diseases both incidence and prevalence are expressed in terms of cases per 100,000, although very common diseases such as dental caries are better expressed as cases per 100 (percent). The term frequency is a general one which should be avoided because it is nonspecific and imprecise.

Incidence and prevalence are related to each other by the factor of time. Specifically: prevalence = incidence × duration of disease. To clarify this relationship, let us consider two diseases: staphylococcal food poisoning and tuberculosis. The former is an acute, mild, brief illness caused by ingestion of food containing an **enterotoxin** produced by the staphylococcus. Most important for our present purpose is that staphylococcal food poisoning rarely lasts more than a couple of days. Tuberculosis, on the other hand, is a disease of long duration, usually several years. The prevalence of food poisoning is also its incidence, because it consists only of the new cases that occur at a given point in time. The disease is so short-lived that there are no "old" cases. The same is true of conditions which are rapidly fatal, such as homicide or electrocution. Strictly speaking, these events have no prevalence. The equation shows that prevalence equals the *product* of incidence and duration. This means that the longer the duration of the disease the greater its prevalence and the lesser its incidence, and vice versa. Tuberculosis, unlike food poisoning, has a relatively high prevalence, because not only do new cases occur each year but the old ones persist year in and year out. The equation is a useful aid in understanding the relationship between incidence and prevalence. However, it has little practical value because the duration of a particular disease usually varies over a great range of time, and it is often difficult, if not impossible, to determine the precise time of the onset of the disease. Also, it will be remembered that diseases are subject to seasonal variation. There is, for example, little or no measles in September. For these reasons duration is hard to measure, and incidence and prevalence often depend on what disease we study and when we study it.

In spite of their importance, incidence and prevalence are only two of the rates in common use. The others are defined in Table 3-1. Note that many use a midyear population as a denominator. This is done because populations change over a year's time, and the midyear population represents the best single figure to describe the population during any given year. It should also be noted that the crude death rate is influenced by sex, race, environmental factors, and other variables as well. Although this rate is often misleading, as the hypothetical data in Table 3-2 demonstrate, it is commonly used because the data from which it is derived are readily available. The table reveals two towns, A and B. They are of equal size and their populations are divided into four age groups. Town A has a crude death rate of 10.5 per 1,000, while that of town B is 10.8 per 1,000. Yet, even though the crude death rate in town B is slightly higher than that in town A, town A has higher age-specific death rates for every age group except the 65+ group. This apparent paradox is ex-

---

ENTEROTOXIN: a poison produced by staphylococci; it affects the intestines and causes vomiting and diarrhea

TABLE 3-1. Commonly Used Rates[a]

Name	Numerator	Denominator	Rate Usually Expressed per
Crude birth rate	No. of live births in 1 year	Midyear population	1,000
Fertility rate	No. of live births in 1 year	No. of women of childbearing age (15–44) at midyear	1,000
Crude death rate	No. of deaths in 1 year	Midyear population	1,000
Age-specific death rate	No. of persons dying in 1 year at a specific age	No. of persons of that age in the midyear population	1,000
Infant mortality rate	No. of deaths in children under 1 year of age	No. of live births during that year	1,000
Maternal mortality rate	No. of deaths related to pregnancy in 1 year	No. of live births during that year	10,000
Case fatality rate	No. of deaths from a specified disease	No. of cases of the same disease	100
Proportional mortality rate	No. of deaths due to a specified cause during 1 year	Total deaths from all causes reported in the same year	100
Neonatal death rate	No. of deaths in children under 28 days of age in 1 year	No. of live births during that year	1,000
Fetal death rate	No. of fetal deaths during the year	No. of live births plus fetal deaths in that year	1,000
Perinatal mortality rate	No. of fetal deaths plus infant deaths under 7 days of age in 1 year	No. of live births plus fetal deaths in that year	1,000
Incidence	No. of new cases of a disease occurring in a time interval, usually 1 year	Population at the middle of the time period, e.g., midyear	1,000; 10,000; or 100,000
Prevalence	No. of cases, new and old, on a given date	Population on that date	1,000; 10,000; or 100,000
Five-year survival rate	No. of cases of a particular cancer which survive 5 years	No. of cases of that cancer at the beginning of the 5-year period	100

[a]To determine the rate, divide the denominator into the numerator and multiply the result by the number in the last column.

TABLE 3-2. Crude and Age-Specific Death Rates in Two Imaginary Towns

Age Group	Population (in percent)	Deaths	Population	Age-Specific Death Rate
		Town A		
0–20	10	60	2,000	30.0
21–44	20	20	4,000	5.0
45–64	50	70	10,000	7.0
65+	20	60	4,000	15.0
	100	210	20,000	10.5 = crude death rate[a]
		Town B		
0–20	12.5	50	2,500	20.0
21–44	22.5	20	4,500	4.4
45–64	35.0	45	7,000	6.4
65+	30.0	100	6,000	16.7
	100	215	20,000	10.8 = crude death rate

[a]*Note that the crude death rate is not the average of the four age-specific groups.*

plained by the differences in the sizes of the population groups in the two towns. Town B has more elderly people, among whom death rates are highest, and fewer middle-aged persons, in whom death rates are somewhat lower. Similar differences in crude death rates exist in populations with marked variances in income levels.

Two other rates deserve mention. The accuracy of the fetal death rate is compromised by the fact that although all 50 states collect data on fetal deaths, there is disagreement as to when an embryo is entitled to the designation "fetus." In some states a fetus comes into being after the twentieth week of gestation. In others it is 24 or 28 weeks, and, unless you know which designation is being used, it is hazardous to compare fetal death rates from state to state. Also, fetal deaths are often the result of induced abortion and thus tend to be underrepresented except in those states which have legalized abortions.

Perinatal mortality is of special interest because it measures the deaths of children just before and just after birth. It is estimated that the number of deaths during this period equals the total number who die during the next 40 years of life.

Rates are very useful in the study of disease distribution. They enable us to compare groups of people and, in so doing, to define groups who are at high risk for certain diseases. This knowledge, in turn, can often be used to prevent disease insofar as we are able to remove or neutralize the risk. Finally as we shall see, the association of a particular disease with a specific set of characteristics frequently provides insight as to the cause of the disease.

Analytic Epidemiology

Once it has been determined that a disease seems to be associated with certain characteristics—and our hypothesis has been developed to explain this association—the task remains of designing a study to support or discredit the hypothesis. There are two basic ways to do this. The first begins with a population at risk, e.g., the people of the New York City metropolitan area; from this large population a smaller population, or **sample**, is selected. The sample is then divided into two groups of people as alike as possible in all respects, except that one group manifests the suspected characteristics while the other does not. Both groups are followed over time, often a decade or more, to see if there is a difference between them in the incidence of disease. If we were interested in air pollution and **emphysema**, for example, we might select an urban group which is constantly exposed to polluted air and compare it with a second group which is not thus exposed. Ideally, we should use a group of urban dwellers who live in a city with clean air. Since cities like this are hard to find, we would probably have to settle for a more rural group. This is the kind of compromise which must often be made with reality, and it creates problems because it introduces a **bias** into the study. By this we mean that the two groups, whose only difference optimally should be exposure or nonexposure to air pollution, differ in at least one other important respect: One group is urban, the other rural. Quite apart from pollution exposure, life styles differ markedly in the two areas and even if the two groups were alike as to age, sex, race, income, housing, smoking habits, education, occupation, and so on, the rural-urban problem would still limit the credibility of our results.

SAMPLE: a selected portion of the population used to represent the whole

EMPHYSEMA: a respiratory disease in which the lung loses its elasticity, thus making breathing difficult; thought to be causally related to air pollution and smoking

BIAS: that which influences the outcome of a study, often to a degree sufficient to render the results useless

If this problem cannot be avoided, we must decide whether it is worthwhile to proceed. To do so we must answer a couple of questions. First, does the condition (emphysema) occur more often in the group with the characteristic (exposure to air pollution) than it does in those without the characteristic? Let us answer affirmatively by assuming that we find a higher incidence of emphysema among the exposed group. The second question might be stated as follows: Are these results generally true in that we can expect emphysema to occur more often in *all* persons exposed to air pollution than in unexposed persons? It is in the consideration of this question that there are some other ways in which bias can sneak into our study. For example, we did not study *everyone* exposed to air pollution or *everyone* not exposed to air pollution. We only studied some of the people. The problem is that the people we studied may not be like the people we did not study. In other words, the study group may not be representative of the population at risk. Maybe the study group consists of bankers who are fat, rich, and well educated, while the general population at risk is less fat, less rich, and less well educated. In this case it is not possible to draw conclusions about the general population from the results of the study. Ideally, the study group should be selected in such a way that every individual in the population from which it is drawn has an equal chance of being included in the study. Like most ideals this one is often sought but seldom achieved. Nevertheless, accuracy demands that we design a study as free as possible from bias.

The type of study we have just examined, in which we follow an exposed group and an unexposed group over time and compare the incidence of disease in each, is called a **prospective** or **cohort study.** Strictly speaking, the exposed group is the study group and the nonexposed group, which serves as the basis of comparison, is known as the **control group.**

The prospective study is diagrammatically represented in Figure 3-4. Obviously, some of the exposed (study) group developed emphysema and some did not. The rate at which the former developed the disease, i.e., the incidence of emphysema, is given by $(a) \div (a) + (b)$. Similarly, the incidence of emphysema among the nonexposed (control) group is $(c) \div (c) + (d)$. In drawing conclusions from the study, what we are doing is comparing these incidence rates. If the rate in the exposed group is significantly higher than the rate in the nonexposed group, and if our

---

PROSPECTIVE or COHORT STUDY: one in which a group of people are followed over time to determine the existence of an association between a characteristic and a disease

CONTROL GROUP: a group which is identical to the study group in all characteristics except the one under study

DIAGRAMMATIC REPRESENTATION OF A PROSPECTIVE STUDY

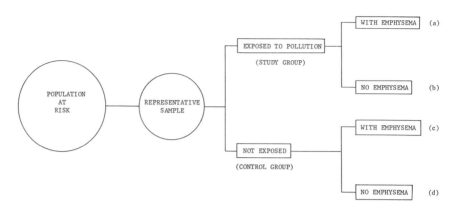

FIG. 3-4.   *Diagrammatic representation of a prospective study.*

study design is not riddled with biases, we can cautiously advance the view that air pollution and emphysema are related as to cause and effect. How do we know what is "significant?" The best we can do in this regard is to determine the likelihood of a difference of this magnitude turning up by chance alone. Let us assume that the incidence of emphysema in the exposed group is 50:100,000, and that of the nonexposed group is 10:100,000. Usually, if the probability that a difference of this size would occur purely by chance is less than 1 in 20 (sometimes 1 in 100), the investigator will accept the results as indeed related to air pollution rather than chance variation. The calculation of this probability lies in the realm of biostatistics and will not be discussed here. However, you need not be confused if, when reading an article, you run across a statement like this hypothetical one: "Our study shows that the incidence of venereal disease is related to military service. Males in the military have twice as much venereal disease as males of the same age who are civilians ($p < 0.05$)." Do not let that peculiar "$p < 0.05$" throw you. It may also appear as $p < 0.01$ or $p < 0.001$. It means only that according to a statistical test run by the investigators, the probability (p) of a twofold difference in rates occurring by chance alone is less than ($<$) 1 in 20, or 5 percent expressed as 0.05, in 100 ($p < 0.01$), or 1 in 1,000 ($p < 0.001$).

It has been mentioned that there are two ways to conduct an analytic study. The prospective method is one. The second type is called a **retro-**

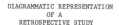

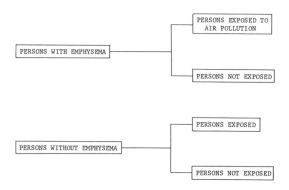

FIG. 3-5. *Diagrammatic representation of a retrospective study.*

spective or **case history study.** The prospective method begins with two groups of people and looks forward in time to see how many develop disease in each group. The retrospective study also starts with two groups, but the study group has the disease in question rather than a characteristic thought to be associated with the disease, as in prospective studies. Retrospective studies also differ from prospective studies in that they look *backward* in time to see if the characteristic (e.g., exposure to air pollution) was more common in the study (emphysema) group than in the control (nonemphysema) group. A diagrammatic view of the retrospective study is seen in Figure 3-5.

Notice that the retrospective study differs from the prospective study in an additional and very important respect: the retrospective study lacks a reference population. Instead of drawing an exposed study group and a nonexposed control group from a common population, we begin with cases of disease and compare them with a control consisting of non-cases. We then seek to examine the past histories of the persons in the study and control groups to see if those in the study group possess a characteristic more often than those in the nondiseases control group. In

---

RETROSPECTIVE or CASE HISTORY STUDY: one in which the past histories of a group of people are examined to determine the existence of an association between a disease and a characteristic

terms of the diagram, we compare $(a) \div (a) + (b)$ and $(b) \div (b) + (d)$. What we learn from retrospective studies is whether or not a certain characteristic is more common in diseased persons than it is in nondiseased persons. For example, let us assume we find that a majority of those with emphysema were exposed to polluted air and that those without emphysema were not so exposed. We still have not answered the question we really want to answer, i.e., to what extent does exposure to air pollution lead to emphysema? This question is answered in a prospective study, but a retrospective study tells us something else: that a majority of emphysema patients were exposed to air pollution. This does not mean that a majority of those exposed developed emphysema. To use another example, it is interesting to learn that many people who have diabetes (disease) are or were obese (characteristic), but it is illogical to conclude from this that many obese people become diabetic. Similarly, the fact that about 85 percent of those who develop lung cancer are smokers does not mean that 85 percent of smokers develop lung cancer.

The retrospective study does not answer the right question because the results this type of study provides cannot be related to a reference population. There is no assurance that the cases and the associated characteristic represent the true extent of the characteristic in the population. Another way of looking at this problem is to consider that there is always doubt about the cause-and-effect relationship in retrospective studies because we begin with effect and search the past for cause. In prospective studies we begin with a supposed cause and discover if the expected effect materializes. If in a retrospective study it is discovered that heroin addiction is most common in the poor, we would probably conclude that poverty is a cause of such addiction; but from our retrospective study we can never be certain that heroin addiction is not a cause of poverty. Finally, retrospective studies deal only with *survivors* of a disease; those who died of it before we decided to do our study are excluded. If we find that smoking is associated with lung cancer, it may be that all nonsmoking patients with cancer of the lung died of their disease and that smoking actually protects the cancer victim against death.

In view of the problems associated with them, the reader is probably curious to know at this point why retrospective studies are used at all. The answer is that there are advantages and disadvantages to both types of studies. Retrospective studies are essentially case histories, and we do not have to wait for the disease to occur as we must in prospective studies. For this reason retrospective studies can be done at relatively low cost and in a relatively brief period of time. After all, it often requires 20 years or more for a smoker to develop lung cancer. Studies conducted over this period of time are costly and subject to a high rate of attrition, since people move away, die of another disease, or lose interest and refuse to cooperate further. The attrition/cost problem is enhanced if we study a rare disease. In this case a huge sample is needed to get a few cases, and both the cost and the attrition rate become major obstacles to a successful study. The attrition problem is sometimes partially solved by the use of life tables and the person-years approach. These are biostatistical methods used to maximize the value and extend the applicability of the available data.

As we have seen, a major drawback of retrospective studies lies in the problems this method raises with respect to interpretation of the results. A second drawback is that neither incidence nor prevalence can be calculated from a retrospective study because there is no population at risk. Incidence rates can be derived from prospective studies because these studies specifically look for the emergence of new cases. Retrospective studies suffer also because it is often hard to get the accurate historical information needed to document the characteristic and because the control group is often unlike the study group. Commonly, control groups in retrospective studies are a sample of the general population from which the study cases come, e.g., they might be relatives of individuals in the study group or patients who have a different disease but are in the same hospital as members of the study group. With none of these controls can we be certain of having a sample which adequately reflects the actual population at risk. Since the study group is not drawn from the general population in the first place, we do not know to what extent, if any, the two are alike. Patients and relatives also present problems in that both are special groups unto themselves and may or may not be representative. Nevertheless, because of low cost and relative ease of data collection, retrospective studies are usually carried out first. If they suggest an association between the disease and a characteristic, they are followed by the more costly and time-consuming prospective approach. A partial summary of the differences between retrospective and prospective studies can be seen in Table 3-3.

Prospective studies are particularly suitable for estimating risk. To illustrate this, let us consider the hypothetical data in Table 3-4. The incidence of disease is 100 in persons with the characteristic and 20 in persons without the characteristic. Two risk measures can be calculated: relative risk and attributable risk. Relative risk relates the disease rate in those with the characteristic to the disease rate in those without the characteristic, i.e., $100 \div 20 = 5$. In other words, persons with the characteristic are five times as likely to develop the disease. This ratio depends on the size of the difference between the rates in the characteristic group and the noncharacteristic one. It also depends on the size of the rate in

TABLE 3-3. Retrospective versus Prospective Studies

	Disease Present	Disease Absent	Total
Characteristic present	*a*	*b*	*a+b*
Characteristic absent	*c*	*d*	*c+d*
	a+c	*b+d*	*a+b+c+d*

1. Retrospective begins with disease and searches for an associated characteristic. In the table you therefore read *down* in that you compare *a÷a+c* with *b÷b+d*.

2. Prospective begins with the characteristic and follows the sample over time to record the appearance of the disease. In the table, therefore, you read *across* in that you compare *a÷a+b* with *c÷c+d*.

3. Retrospective studies are inexpensive and quickly carried out, but they are more difficult to interpret because of the absence of a reference population, inadequate control groups, and the inclusion of survivors only.

4. Prospective studies are expensive, time-consuming, and plagued by the problem of attrition. Yet they produce incidence rates and better estimates of risk.

TABLE 3-4. Attributable versus Relative Risk

Characteristic Present	Incidence (per 100,000)
Yes	100
No	20

noncharacteristic persons. These persons get sick without exposure to the characteristic we are studying, but one we are *not* studying and about which we know nothing might be responsible for this. Although we thus cannot predict from relative risk the effects of a control measure aimed at the studied characteristic, what we do gain is an estimation of causal relationships. The higher the value of the relative risk, the stronger the case for a causal relationship between characteristic studied and disease.

To predict the effect of a control measure, attributable risk is used. It is simply the rate of disease in those with the characteristic, minus the rate of disease in those without it, i.e., 100 − 20 = 80. This means that 80 of the 100 cases in the group exposed to the characteristic can be *attributed* to it, while 20 cases of the disease would have occurred without it. Thus, if the characteristic were eliminated, the disease would decline by 80 percent (80/100).

Prevalence Studies and Mass Screening

Prevalence studies, sometimes called **cross-sectional studies,** produce prevalence rates and are surveys done over brief periods of time. They yield information on the number of cases of one or more diseases in a defined population at risk, e.g., the number of drug addicts in the population of Washington, D.C. Because they deal with the present, prevalence studies are neither retrospective nor prospective but sort of midway between the two. Like the latter, they are based on a representative sample of a reference population at risk; but unfortunately, like the former, they count survivors only, and cause-and-effect relationships are often blurred. Specifically, if we select two samples from our population at risk, one representative of the rich and one representative of the poor, and if we find that the prevalence of hypertension is greater among the poor, we still are faced with determining what this finding means. What we have is a prevalence rate, and we know that prevalence equals incidence times duration of disease. Therefore, the higher prevalence rate among the poor could be explained by higher incidence *or* longer duration. It is impossible to tell which is the case from a prevalence survey, and for this reason we can draw no causal conclusions about the association between poverty and hypertension. Causal inferences can be made from incidence rates but they are more difficult to come by than prevalence rates because two sets of observations are required, one at the beginning of the time interval in question and one at the end of the interval. This is necessary because incidence is concerned with *new* cases only.

Prevalence rates are useful for identifying cases of disease and thus enabling a community to assess its needs for health facilities, additional manpower, new programs, and so on. Mass screening programs are prevalence surveys intended to identify individuals with various diseases so that the required medical care for cure or control can be obtained. Screening is thus directed at finding cases of treatable or manageable diseases. A good screening program should be aimed at a high-risk target population. There is no point in looking for tuberculosis in a group of affluent suburban teen-agers, but there is good reason to look for this

---

PREVALENCE or CROSS-SECTIONAL STUDY: a survey designed to identify the prevalence of a disease in a defined population

disease among the inmates of a mental institution. Screening programs are sometimes aimed at a single disease, but more often multiple illnesses are sought. Surveys which screen for more than one disease are known as multiphasic screening programs. To be worthwhile a proposed screening program should be designed to meet the following criteria:

1. The diseases sought should be prevalent ones. Screening for rare diseases is extremely expensive.
2. The diseases sought should be the causes of a significant amount of discomfort, disability, or death. Screening for dandruff is a waste of time and money.
3. The diseases sought should be susceptible to medical intervention.
4. All cases uncovered should be assured follow-up care. There is no point in getting people anxious about an illness unless you are prepared to do something about it.
5. The diseases sought should be detectable through the use of a diagnostic screening test which is precise, valid, safe, inexpensive, easy to administer, and acceptable to the patient.

Few, if any, screening programs approach this ideal standard. Follow-up is by far the greatest problem. Either the patient is not referred to a medical resource, or he is referred but fails to show up. A major problem with most screening programs is that usually the middle class, the well educated, the white, and the affluent appear, while the poor, the poorly educated, and the minorities stay away in droves. A common reason for this is that screening tends to be carried on away from low-income areas, but even programs conducted in the ghetto do not produce a good turnout. Thus, for one reason or another, the people who in theory should benefit most from screening are those who in practice are rarely screened.

No screening program is any better than the tests it employs to identify possible disease. These tests are almost never completely satisfactory, and generally they suffer from defects in their precision or reliability, and/or in their validity. The person who administers the tests is called an observor; **precision,** or **reliability** (also known as **repeatability** or **reproducibility**), is the extent to which the results of a test would be the same if it were carried out by a different observor or by the same observor at a different time.

PRECISION, RELIABILITY, REPEATABILITY, REPRODUCIBILITY: the extent to which the same diagnostic-test result would be obtained if the test were repeated by a different observor or by the same observor at a different time

Validity is the extent to which a test actually detects the disease being sought. Validity is determined by a test's **sensitivity** and **specificity**. The former is the ability of a test to identify as positive those people who actually have the disease. The latter is the ability of a test to call negative those who do not have the disease. An insensitive test produces **false negative** results; a nonspecific test produces **false positive** results. This is a very confusing concept which may be clarified by thinking of it as follows: disease present + test negative = false negative = insensitivity; disease absent + test positive = false positive = nonspecificity.

In screening programs false positive results are preferable to those that are falsely negative. With adequate follow-up care, the former will be picked up at a later, more thorough examination; false negatives, in contrast, receive no further attention.

Table 3-5 lists the tests most commonly used in screening programs. Table 3-6 summarizes important diseases and the value of early detection in their control.

Sources of Health Data

It is obvious that our knowledge of health and disease is no better than the data from which this knowledge is obtained. The quality of health data varies as to completeness and accuracy. Death registration is required by law and is virtually complete throughout the United States. Although each state designs its own, all death certificates are similar and all require that the cause of death be listed. Since the listed cause reflects the opinion of the physician completing the certificate, data on the causes of death vary in accuracy and depend on the physician's concept of cause, his diagnostic skill, and the manner in which diseases are classified. Birth records are less complete than death statistics, but in the United States more than 95 percent of births are recorded. (Problems encountered in relation to fetal deaths were mentioned earlier.) Figures on births, deaths, marriages, and divorces are collectively referred to as vital statistics. (See Appendix 11.)

VALIDITY: the ability of a diagnostic test to detect the disease it is intended to diagnose
SENSITIVITY: the ability of a diagnostic test to identify as positive those who have the disease being sought
SPECIFICITY: the ability of a diagnostic test to identify as negative those who do not have the disease being sought
FALSE NEGATIVE: a person with a disease whose test result is negative
FALSE POSITIVE: a person without a disease whose test result is positive

TABLE 3-5. Screening Tests in Common Use

Test	Comment
Serologic test for syphilis	Precise, sensitive; some false positives; often avoided by patient
Chest x-ray	Primarily for heart disease, tuberculosis, lung cancer; errors of precision; good validity
Blood pressure	Imprecise; high validity, but depends on the blood-pressure range defined as normal
Self-administered medical history	Imprecise; marginal validity due to poorly worded questions, patient ignorance, etc.
Height and weight	Imprecise; high validity
Blood sugar	For diabetes mellitus; precise, but many false positives; rare problem of patient acceptance
Visual acuity	Precision and validity depend on method used
Hearing acuity	Precision and validity depend on method used
Tonometry	For glaucoma; measures the pressure of the fluid in the anterior chamber of the eye; fairly precise; good validity, but depends on the range accepted as normal
Hemoglobin determination	For anemia; precise and valid
Tuberculin testing	A skin test to determine past or present infection with the tubercle bacillus; imprecise in the hands of the inexperienced; results depend on a second contact with the patient after a 48- to 72-hour interval to classify skin reaction
Electrocardiogram	Precision often a problem; often invalid due to false negatives
Urinalysis	Tests mainly for renal disease and diabetes; precision and validity depend on what is being sought; sugar in urine as a screen for diabetes lacks validity due to false positives and false negatives
Pap smear	A test for cancer of the cervix; precise and valid in experienced hands; patient acceptance often a problem
Serum cholesterol	Precise and valid; problem of patient acceptance is rare
Female breast examination	Depends on method used; palpation most reliable; patient acceptance is a rare problem

As we have indicated, mortality data is complete even though questions can be raised as to the accuracy of information on the causes of death. Morbidity data presents far greater problems. A prime difficulty is that only some infectious diseases must be reported, and the reporting of these is far from complete. Nevertheless, general trends in infectious diseases can be inferred from the available reports. No chronic diseases are

TABLE 3-6. Important Diseases and Early Detection

Disease	Comment
Cervical cancer	Pap smear is an excellent test, credited with reducing mortality for this disease
Breast cancer	Most common cause of cancer deaths in women; early detection can improve 5-year survival rate substantially
Cancer of the colon (large intestine)	In men this cancer ranks second only to lung cancer; most large gut cancers are located within range of the sigmoidoscope (a tube with a small light on the end, which is inserted into the rectum); early detection can cure about two-thirds of the cases, but sigmoidoscopy is unpopular with patients
Lung cancer	Five-year survival rate is not affected by early detection through chest x-ray
Prostatic cancer	Accounts for 10 percent of male cancer deaths; with early diagnosis, more than 90 percent survive 5 years; early detection depends on a complete physical examination
Lymphomas	Cancer of the lymphatic system; early detection is of great value in some lymphomas, especially Hodgkin's disease; there is no substitute for the physical examination here
Skin cancer	Most common cancer; also most obvious and most curable
Stomach cancer	No adequate screening test; most cases detected late; poor prognosis
Hypertension	Easy to identify, but the value of early treatment is controversial except in very severe cases
Arteriosclerotic heart disease	No test available; electrocardiogram of little predictive value; look for associated risk factors such as obesity, high blood pressure, high serum cholesterol, inactivity, smoking, family history
Diabetes	Most common in persons over age 40 with a family history of diabetes; about 2 million Americans remain undiagnosed
Glaucoma	About 1 million undetected cases; early detection of great value in preventing blindness
Phenylketonuria	Detected by a simple test performed on the urine of infants; early detection can reduce mental retardation if follow-up is adequate; sometimes damage is done prior to birth, incidence is no greater than 1:10,000, so yield is low; testing required by law in most states
Tuberculosis	Chest films and skin testing are of greatest value among groups known to be highest TB risks—i.e., contacts of TB patients, institutionalized populations, alcoholics, immigrants, people living in very close quarters (e.g., naval personnel), the poor, and medical personnel

so reported, except in the few states that have cancer registries. The value of these registries depends on the extent to which physicians voluntarily report, but cooperation is usually of a high order.

In order to generate data on disease occurrence the United States National Health Survey was established in 1956. The survey consists of three parts:

1. Health interviews (of about 40,000 families per year). The interviews collect information about illnesses, injuries and resulting disability, absences from work and school, and so on. No attempt is made to corroborate the information provided by the individuals interviewed.

2. Health examinations. These constitute a series of prevalence surveys aimed at different groups at different times. To date, adults aged 18 to 79, children 6 to 11, and, most recently, adolescents aged 12 to 17 have been covered.

3. Health records survey. Record samples are drawn from hospitals, nursing homes, and other sources and are used as a supplement to the interviews and examinations.

In addition to the National Health Survey there are a number of other sources of health data. All of them are basically inadequate for public purposes because they are intended for other uses and because none is representative of the general population. Insurance companies compile client data based on claims against the company. The number of claims and what they say depend largely on the way they are administered by the company. Tax funds cover the cost of medical care for certain groups of people, including the military, American Indians, and merchant seamen. But these groups are not representative, a problem they share with records of hospital patients. Hospital records also lack a denominator, and numerator data is simply a count which cannot be converted into a rate. Absenteeism records from schools and industry are unreliable because of faked reports of illness to excuse absences. Routine physical examinations and screening programs are not only often remiss with regard to follow-up care, but share the problem of uncertainty about how well the few participants represent the enormous number of nonparticipants.

In spite of these and other numerous problems, the general quality of health data in the United States is good. What is important is that the student of health should never take quality for granted. An attitude of cautious skepticism about data sources and data accuracy is always wise policy.

Notes

1   One exception to this is the transmission of malaria through blood containing malaria parasites, e.g., blood transfusions and the sharing of a common needle by drug addicts.

References

Benenson, A. S., ed. Control of Communicable Diseases in Man, 11th ed. American Public Health Association, 1970.

Blum, H., and Keranen, G., eds. Control of Chronic Diseases in Man. American Public Health Association, 1966.

Cassel, J. Lectures in epidemiology. Unpublished.

Johnson, K. Epidemiology. In Kilbourne, E. D., and Smillie, W. G., eds. Human Ecology and Public Health. New York, Macmillan, 1969.

Larimore, G. Accident hazards. In Hilleboe, H., and Larimore, G., eds. Preventive Medicine. Philadelphia, W. B. Saunders, 1965.

Lewis, C. E., and Sisk, C. Lectures in epidemiology. Unpublished.

Linder, F. Sources of data on health in the United States. In Clark, D. W., and MacMahon, B., eds. Preventive Medicine. Boston, Little, Brown, 1967.

MacMahon, B. Epidemiologic methods. In Clark, D. W., and MacMahon, B. Preventive Medicine. Boston, Little, Brown, 1967.

MacMahon, B., and Pugh, T. F., eds. Epidemiology: Principles and Methods. Boston, Little, Brown, 1970.

Morris, J. N. Uses of Epidemiology, 2nd ed. Baltimore, Williams and Wilkins, 1964.

Sartwell, P. E. Epidemiology. In Sartwell, P. E., ed. Maxcy-Rosenau Preventive Medicine and Public Health, 9th ed. New York, Appleton-Century-Crofts, 1965.

Schor, S. Fundamentals of Biostatistics. New York, G. P. Putnam's Sons, 1968.

Schulman, J. Screening and mass surveys. In Kilbourne, E. D., and Smillie, W. G., eds. Human Ecology and Public Health. New York, Macmillan, 1969.

Siegel, M. Indices of community health. In Clark, D. W., and MacMahon, B., eds. Preventive Medicine. Boston, Little, Brown, 1967.

CHAPTER

4

Infectious Diseases

Coexistence with microorganisms and the infections they generate is the natural state of man. Indeed, mankind generally thrives on a variety of microbes which, in turn, thrive on him. For example, it has been mentioned that the normal presence of certain bacteria in the human gut is essential to the utilization of vitamin K. Man returns this favor by providing harborage and nurture for these and other microbes. A relationship between host and parasite wherein each benefit is known as **symbiosis**. The development of disease in a parasitized host is an expression of an inadequate adaptation of host and parasite to each other. It is the opposite of symbiosis.

The development of microbial disease follows a general pattern regardless of the particular organism involved. The organism gains entry into the host through the nose, throat, respiratory passages, gut, urethra, or skin. Once having entered, the agent begins to multiply and thus initiates a primary lesion which is restricted to the immediate area of entry. This

---

SYMBIOSIS: an association of different organisms in which each benefits from the presence of the other

localized infection becomes the site of an inflammatory response through which the host resists the invader. The blood vessels serving the area dilate, allowing increased blood flow. Certain types of white blood cells engulf invading bacteria while antibodies inactivate or destroy these disease agents or their products. Some pathogenic bacteria produce toxins which destroy **phagocytes,** while others produce **enzymes** which break down intercellular connective tissue or muscle. Viruses, in contrast, invade host cells and from this intracellular base proceed to replicate themselves and release new virus when the cell wall ruptures.

If the issue is not decided locally, the agent spreads to the bloodstream by way of the lymphatic system. Once access is gained to the bloodstream, which is an open channel to distant areas of the body, the agent usually produces distant, or secondary, lesions. Infectious diseases produce characteristic symptoms and signs which are, however, doubly nonspecific in that they tend to occur in some noninfectious conditions as well as in most infectious diseases. Fever, chills, abrupt onset, muscular aches and pains, sore throat, swelling and tenderness of lymph nodes, nausea, vomiting, diarrhea, an elevated or (less commonly) depressed white-cell count, and occasionally an enlarged spleen are cardinal manifestations of an infectious process. Often these and other disease indicators do not appear until the agent has successfully established a secondary lesion. In meningococcal infections, for example, the primary lesion is in the nose and throat, and rarely produces symptoms. The secondary lesion is meningitis, and it is at this stage that the patient becomes ill—not only with the symptoms listed above but with the stiff neck and other more specific manifestations of meningitis. The principal target organ of a particular agent can be either a primary or secondary site, and which one it is depends primarily on where the disease manifestations occur. Generally, the vast majority of human infections are asymptomatic; this is especially true of viral infections. In the United States and in most industrialized countries the important agents of infectious disease are bacteria and viruses; Table 4-1 lists the invading agents and the body sites most commonly involved. Of all infectious diseases, viral infections affecting the upper respiratory tract have by far the highest incidence. These are the ubiquitous colds, sore throats, and runny noses that harass mankind, especially in the winter. Other commonly affected body sites include the skin, gastrointestinal tract, and ear. The other infections listed in Table 4-1 tend to be less common but often more serious.

PHAGOCYTES: cells which engulf and destroy invading bacteria
ENZYME: a material which causes or enhances a chemical reaction

TABLE 4-1. Disease Agents Affecting Common Sites of Infection[a]

Site	Disease Agent	
	Common	Less Common or Rare
Bones	*Staphylococcus aureus*	Salmonella: Streptococcus
Joints	*S. aureus*; gonococcus	Other bacteria
Skin	*S. aureus*; Streptococcus	Various gram-negative bacteria
Throat, upper respiratory tract	Respiratory viruses; Streptococcus	Various bacteria
G.I. tract	Enteroviruses; Salmonella	Shigella
Lung	Pneumococcus; tubercle bacillus	Other bacteria and viruses
Ear	Pneumococcus; *Hemophilus influenza*	*S. aureus*; Streptococcus
Urinary tract	*Escherichia coli*	*Klebsiella aureus*; enterococcus
Brain	Arbovirus	. . .
Meninges	Pneumococcus; meningococcus	*H. influenza*

[a]*Modified after Bennet, J., and Petersdorf, R. An approach to infectious diseases. In Wintrobe, M., et al., eds. Harrison's Principles of Internal Medicine, 6th ed. New York, McGraw-Hill, 1970.*

Bacteria, Viruses, and Immunity

Bacteria are single-celled organisms belonging to the plant kingdom. Though small, they are larger than viruses, and when properly treated with a stain are easily identified under a microscope (Fig. 4-1A, Fig. 4-1B). Gram's stain is the one most commonly used, and organisms which take this stain are called gram-positive. The gram-positive bacteria listed in Table 4-1 are the Staphylococci, Streptococci, and pneumococci. The remainder are gram-negative, except the tubercle bacillus which has unusual staining characteristics. Traditionally, the gram-positive group has been the biggest problem for man, and it is against these organisms that antibiotic drugs like the penicillins are most effective. Ironically, the success of antibiotics against the gram-positive group has favored the emergence of gram-negative pathogens as very troublesome sources of infection, especially in debilitated patients. Unlike the gram-negatives in Table 4-1 which usually respond to antibiotics, many of these organisms are often resistant to antibiotics and not particularly pathogenic. Some were not even considered pathogens in the pre-antibiotic era. They bear unfamiliar names like Proteus, Aerobacter, Klebsiella, and Pseudomonas;

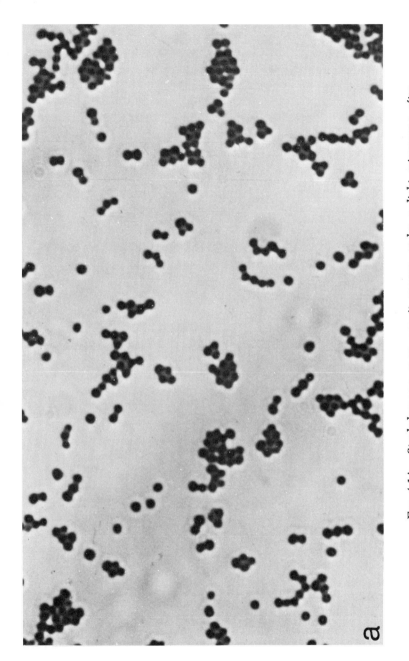

FIG. 4-1A. *Staphylococcus aureus as it appears under a light microscope after staining. Viruses, in contrast, are not visible under ordinary microscope. (Courtesy of Dr. S. Schneirson, The Mount Sinai Hospital.)*

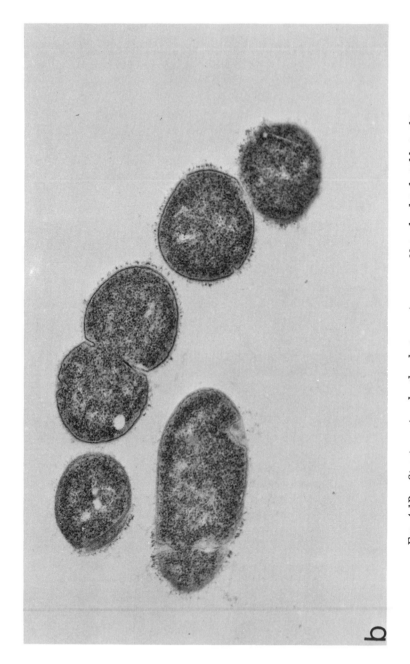

b

Fɪɢ. 4-1B.   *Streptococci under the electron microscope. Note the detail visible in this photo compared to the staphylococci photographed from a light microscope. (Courtesy of Dr. J. Swanson.)*

and their favorite targets are unfortunate people already weakened by a severe burn or a chronic illness such as cancer. In effect, it is medical progress itself which has produced new infectious diseases in that these disease agents rose from relative obscurity only after a previously important group of organisms were brought under more effective control.

Viruses are characterized by extremely small size and by the fact that they multiply only within living cells. Bacteria are rod-shaped, round, or spiral organisms (bacilli, cocci, and spirochetes, respectively) and, as has been indicated, are visible under the microscope. Viruses, on the other hand, come in a variety of shapes and sizes and all are too small to visualize under a normal optical microscope, although many can be studied with an electron microscope (Fig. 4-2). Viruses are so small that they often parasitize bacteria, just as bacteria parasitize humans. In some cases bacteria are pathogenic only when parasitized by the appropriate virus. Those viruses which invade and multiply within bacteria are known as bacteriophage. Because viruses can reproduce themselves only in living cells, their survival outside of an appropriate host is limited. Nevertheless, a few important viruses can survive for a time in the external environment. Smallpox virus persists briefly in the air and dust particles near a smallpox patient. Thus virus also survives on dishes, silverware, and other articles used by the patient. The viruses of infectious hepatitis and polio can be transmitted through water and food. However, smallpox, hepatitis, and a large group of viruses transmitted by insects are exceptions to the generality that common viral diseases are transmitted only by direct person-to-person contact.

The concept of immunity is vital to an understanding of the infectious disease process. Immunity refers to the resistance of a host to the effects of a pathogenic agent. Immunity can be complete or incomplete and is either natural (hereditary) or acquired. Natural immunity is probably dependent on genetic factors and relates primarily to racial groups and entire animal species. Each species of animal tends to have its own group of important infectious diseases, and by and large the diseases of one species do not occur in others. If cross-occurrence does occur, the form taken by the disease often may be so different that it is overlooked. Similarly, particular racial groups tend to resist certain infectious diseases to a greater extent than others. However, since it is extremely rare to find two races living under the same conditions even in the same country or city, racial immunity is often difficult to prove. Population groups living in relative isolation are catastrophically affected by the introduction of diseases with which they have had no previous experience. Measles proved devastating when introduced into previously unexposed peoples in Fiji and the Faroe Islands. Instead of being a mild disease of childhood,

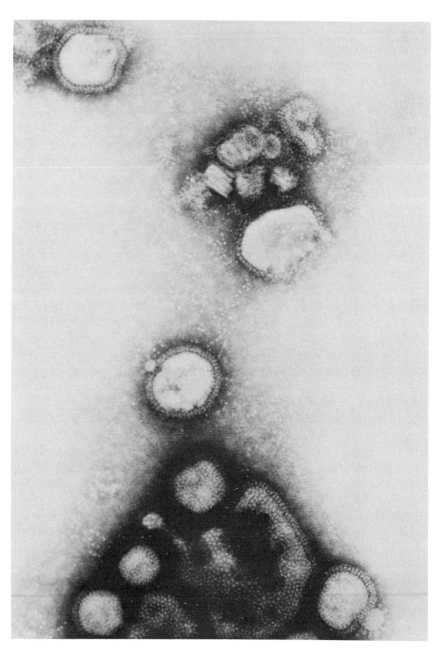

FIG. 4-2.   *Influenza virus. This photograph was made with the aid of an electron microscope. (Courtesy of Dr. J. Swanson.)*

measles among these peoples revealed a darker, more sinister face. It swept through the population in **epidemic** fashion and produced a very high case-fatality rate. This devastation was based primarily on generations of isolation from measles virus and a consequent gradual disappearance of antibodies, rather than a primary racial difference in susceptibility.

Disease agents stimulate the development of host antibodies. The agent itself, or a particular part of it, represents a foreign protein which the host attempts to destroy by manufacturing a chemical specifically aimed at the foreign protein, or antigen. This chemical is called an antibody. Antibodies are derived from a type of protein known as gamma globulin. On rare occasion individuals are born without the ability to produce gamma globulin. These people are generally susceptible to repeated infections, but they seem to have little difficulty with some diseases, including measles and chickenpox. This suggests that other protective mechanisms may be at work quite independent of antibody production. Human resistance to infection is decreased in many chronic disease states. We have previously noted the synergistic relationship between infection and malnutrition. Conditions which promote malnutrition, such as alcoholism and drug addiction, also favor the development of infectious diseases. Blood disorders, diabetes, and any condition which obstructs the **bronchus, ureters, urethra,** or other hollow body tube increases susceptibility to infection. Certain drugs also have this effect. Most notable are **cortisone** and cortisone-like preparations and the anti-cancer drugs, most of which have the unfortunate effect of suppressing the body's ability to produce antibodies.

Acquired immunity is that which results from the presence of antibodies in response to a specific pathogenic organism. Such immunity can be either active or passive. Active immunity results from exposure to the disease agent, in which case the body produces its own antibodies against the agent. Passive immunity is acquired when the host is inoculated with antibodies from an outside source.

Active immunity is perhaps best exemplified in the commonly encountered diseases of childhood. In these infections (measles, mumps, chicken-

---

EPIDEMIC: an abnormally high number of cases of a disease in a population over a brief period of time

BRONCHUS: a highly branched hollow structure through which air is transmitted from lung tissue; the lower end of the trachea, or windpipe

URETER: the tubular structure connecting kidney to bladder

URETHRA: the tubular structure through which urine is discharged from the bladder

CORTISONE: a drug of the steroid family which suppresses the inflammatory process and lowers host resistance to infection

pox, whooping cough, and so on) host antibodies are produced in response to the invading microorganism. If the individual is exposed to the same microorganism at a later time, the level of antibodies circulating in his bloodstream rises, and he is protected against the disease. The immunity acquired from subclinical, inapparent disease is usually just as effective as that from severe illness. Active immunity can also be induced artificially. Through the familiar process of vaccination, or immunization, the host is inoculated with **attenuated** but live bacteria or viral organisms. These attenuaced agents are too weakened to produce anything but mild disease, but the host nonetheless produces antibodies against them. Inoculation of inactivated organisms also stimulates antibody production, but vaccines derived from killed organisms are less effective than those from living agents. Some bacteria owe their disease-producing ability to toxins which act as body poisons. The disease agents of diphtheria and tetanus are important ones of this kind. To produce active immunity against these agents the important element is the toxin, not the organism. Toxin is modified chemically in such a way that it loses its **virulence** but retains its ability to act as an antigen. The preparation which results from this process is known as toxoid. The inoculation of toxoids stimulates antibody production in the host and renders him immune.

Passive immunity can be provided naturally or artificially. Newborn infants are resistant to those diseases against which the mother has antibodies. Maternal antibody passes to the child before birth and provides protection during the critical first six months of life. This mechanism buys time for the infant and gives him the opportunity to develop his own antibodies while still protected by the passive transfer of antibodies from the mother. Passive immunity is a very useful way to provide temporary protection against diseases. Immune gamma globulin is administered to protect contacts of patients with infectious hepatitis, measles, and polio. Live vaccines exist for the latter two conditions; their use is preferable because passive immunity provides only short-lived protection, usually six weeks or less. Passive immunity against tetanus and diphtheria is obtained by the use of antitoxins. Unlike toxoid, which is essentially a weakened version of the toxin itself, antitoxin is antibody against the toxin. Antitoxins are therapeutically useful in treating persons who have no active immunity. Before antibiotics, serum from horses and other animals was used to produce antiserum, i.e., serum containing antibody against a particular agent. Indeed, antiserum was long the key therapeutic agent against

---

ATTENUATED: thinned out, made less virulent
VIRULENCE: the ability of a disease agent actually to produce disease

TABLE 4-2. Commonly Used Vaccines

Disease	Agent	Vaccine	Immunity	Repeat Every[a]
Cholera	bacterium	killed	active	6 months
Diphtheria	bacterium	toxoid antitoxin	active passive	5 years
Tetanus	bacterium	toxoid antitoxin	active passive	5 years
Pertussis	bacterium	toxoid	active	b
Typhoid	bacterium	killed	active	3 years
Tuberculosis	bacterium	live	active	c
Influenza	virus	killed	active	d
Infectious hepatitis	virus	γ globulin	passive	6 months
Measles	virus	live γ globulin	active passive	c
Polio	virus	live killed γ globulin	active active passive	2–4 years
Rabies	virus	live killed γ globulin	active active passive	e
Rubella (German measles)	virus	live γ globulin	active passive	c
Smallpox	virus	live	active	3 years
Yellow fever	virus	live	active	10 years
Typhus	Rickettsia	killed	active	6–12 months
Plague	bacterium	killed live	active active	6 months
Mumps	virus	live	active	unknown

[a]*Passive immunity is short-lived and used primarily when a previously nonimmunized person is exposed to the disease in question.*

[b]*During the first, third, sixth, and twelfth years of life only.*

[c]*Does not need repeating.*

[d]*Influenza virus changes over time, and immunization must be repeated with each new variant of the virus, i.e, a separate immunization with an appropriately modified vaccine must be given with each outbreak of influenza.*

[e]*Every six months, but if the immunized person is bitten by a rabid animal vaccination should be repeated immediately.*

pneumococcal pneumonia. Table 4-2 summarizes vaccines now in common use.

Sometimes recovery from infection is more apparent than real. In these cases the patient enjoys a total recovery but continues to harbor the agent. This situation is known as latent infection because the agent can become active again and reproduces the same illness years later. Tuberculosis represents a classic example of latency. The patient can be free of all illness for years, only to have his TB reactivate as a result of physiological or emotional stress. Chickenpox often recurs in adult life as a similar condition known as herpes zoster. Typhus reappears as a milder condition called Brill's disease. In typhoid fever the disease itself may not occur again, but the patient can be a **carrier** who sheds typhoid bacilli and thus transmits the disease to others. For this reason, persons with a history of typhoid are usually forbidden by law to work as handlers of food. Millions of well people harbor staphylococci in the nose and throat, although these organisms can suddenly produce serious illness if the host's defenses are lowered. Staphylococcal infection among hospital patients is a major problem because such infections are often resistant to antibiotics. Latent infections are especially prone to activity in the presence of malnutrition and other conditions which lower host resistance.

Transmission and Control of Infectious Diseases

To the individual suffering with an infectious disease the cure of that disease is of paramount importance. To the community in which he lives, however, the prime consideration is how to prevent his case from spreading to others. Spread obviously cannot be prevented unless its mechanism is understood. It would certainly help to cure the individual case and thus eliminate a potential source of infection. But remember that most infections are asymptomatic, and many of those that produce symptoms are communicable before the symptoms appear. Consequently, curing the individual case is ineffective control, just as closing the proverbial barn door is of little help once the horse has galloped off.

An infectious agent must have access to a reservoir to sustain itself. A reservoir is a base of operations in which the agent normally lives and multiplies and on which it depends for survival. This reservoir can be a human, an animal or insect, a plant, soil, or nonliving organic matter; it is from the reservoir that the agent is transmitted to the human host.

Depending on their mode of transmission (Fig. 4-3), all human infections can be divided into two broad categories. In the first category are

---

CARRIER: an asymptomatic person infected with a disease agent which can be transmitted to others

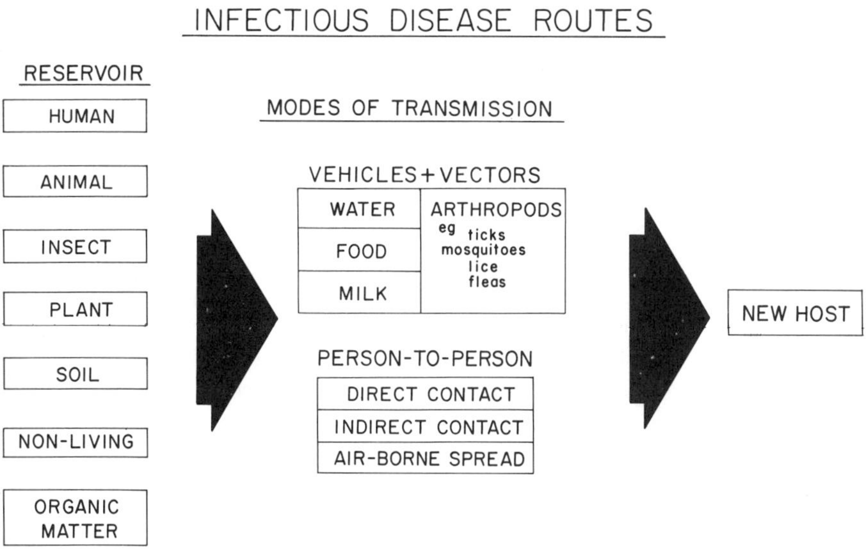

INFECTIOUS DISEASE ROUTES

RESERVOIR

| HUMAN |

MODES OF TRANSMISSION

| ANIMAL |

VEHICLES+VECTORS

| INSECT |

WATER	ARTHROPODS
FOOD	eg ticks mosquitoes lice fleas
MILK	

| PLANT |

NEW HOST

| SOIL |

PERSON-TO-PERSON

| DIRECT CONTACT |
| INDIRECT CONTACT |
| AIR-BORNE SPREAD |

| NON-LIVING |

| ORGANIC MATTER |

Fig. 4-3. *Infectious disease routes.*

those infections whose agents are transmitted to man from reservoirs in the external environment. Basically, these agents require a vehicle or a vector and sometimes both. A vehicle is any inanimate material by means of which the agent is transmitted from the reservoir and introduced into the host. Classic vehicles are water, food, and milk. Typhoid fever is a prime example of a disease transmitted in this way, the vehicle being water. Recently, blood and blood products have emerged as significant vehicles of serum hepatitis. This disease is a major hazard for patients receiving transfusions and for drug addicts who share a common needle. A vector is an **arthropod** which transmits disease by carrying the agent from an infected host to a new, noninfected host. The agent enters the new host as a result of a bite or inoculation, or through the absorption of infective materials deposited on the skin. Malaria is transmitted through the bite of an infected anopheline mosquito which inoculates the parasite into the host. Some diseases in this category are known as zoonoses. These are infectious diseases which primarily affect animals but which, under certain conditions, are transmitted to man. Perhaps the best example of a zoonotic disease is plague, the notorious "Black Death" of the Middle

ARTHROPOD: an insect

Ages. Epidemics of this disease are infrequent, but when they occur their scope is truly gargantuan. The fourteenth-century epidemic wiped out one quarter of the population of Europe and is presumed to be the basis of a still-popular nursery rhyme.[1] The irony of plague is that it is primarily a disease of rodents, especially rats. Plague is transmitted to the human host when a flea which has fed on an infected rat feeds on man. Plague is endemic in the wild rodent population of the western United States, and cases in humans occur sporadically. The most common infectious diseases transmitted from the external environment are less exotic than plague. Because their control is achieved through the engineering techniques of primary prevention, these diseases are discussed in Chapter 9, in which we consider man and his environment.

The second broad category consists of those diseases whose agents are transmitted from person to person. Transmission occurs in three ways: (1) direct contact, (2) indirect contact, and (3) airborne spread. In the first, there is actual physical contact between infected and noninfected persons. The second involves physical contact with an object contaminated by an infected person or with the waste products of an infected person. In airborne spread, the infected person propels infective droplets into the air when he sneezes, coughs, or talks. These droplets, which usually travel no more than a few feet from the source, often settle on objects such as furniture, where their water content evaporates. Droplet nuclei, small but infective residues of dust, are thus left behind. These particles may remain suspended in air for long periods and can be carried quite some distance via air currents.

As might be expected, the mode of transmission is the main determinant of the route the agent takes to enter the host. Airborne spread tends to produce respiratory tract infections. Direct contact means skin-to-skin contact, contact between skin and **mucous membrane**, or contact between mucous membranes. Venereal disease, some infections of the skin, and the feared disease known as leprosy, all result from such contact. Indirect contact usually involves contact with feces of an infected person, particularly the inadvertent ingestion of contaminated feces by the new host. Agents transmitted in this way tend to produce gastrointestinal symptoms, but the clinical manifestations of these **enteric** diseases are often those arising from a secondary lesion.

Enteric infections can be either bacterial or viral. The bacterial diseases are all subject to vehicular transmission; cholera, dysentery, and typhoid

---

MUCOUS MEMBRANE: the moist red tissue which lines certain bodily orifices, such as the nose, mouth, and vagina
ENTERIC: related to the intestine

fever are most commonly spread this way. Infections by the fecal-oral route are less common but do occur, and these diseases are primarily producers of diarrhea. Cholera is highly fatal primarily because the diarrhea is so massive that it depletes the body of fluids and leads to dehydration, **shock,** and death. In typhoid, constipation is as likely as diarrhea, which can be severe enough to produce an ulceration of the gut wall. This leads to gastrointestinal hemorrhage; perforation of the ulcer can produce a fatal **peritonitis.** Dysentery is caused by bacteria of the Shigella group. Usually it is a relatively mild diarrheal disease which is more common and more severe in childhood. Infantile diarrhea is a syndrome due to a number of bacteria, either singly or in combination. Children tolerate prolonged diarrhea poorly because they become dehydrated rapidly, and for this reason it is a leading cause of infant death, especially in the developing countries.

Enteric disease is also produced by a family of viruses known as enteroviruses. While the intestine is the site of primary infection, most of these viruses produce important secondary lesions. Enteroviruses include the following:

1. Coxsackie. These viruses are divided into groups A and B. Both groups can cause meningitis and both persist in the stool for as long as 30 days after the acute illness. Group A causes herpangina, a mild childhood disease whose main characteristic is sore throat. Group B causes pleurodynia, a syndrome characterized by fever and chest pain, as well as **pericarditis** in adults and **myocarditis** in infants.

2. Echo. These viruses produce a mild meningitis and skin rash.

3. Polio. Paralysis is a secondary lesion. Enteric symptoms are mild. Polio virus is shed in the feces for as long as four months after infection.

4. Reovirus. This virus produces mild enteric and respiratory illnesses.

5. Viral gastroenteritis. A pair of unidentified viruses produce this mild gastroenteritis.

6. Infectious hepatitis. Disease results from the effects of the virus on the liver.

Taken as a whole, viruses cause far more diseases of the gastrointestinal tract than bacteria. With the exception of polio and infectious hepatitis,

---

SHOCK: the general depression of body function brought about by a greatly lowered blood pressure
PERITONITIS: inflammation of the membranous lining of the abdomen
PERICARDITIS: inflammation of the pericardium, a membranous sac housing the heart
MYOCARDITIS: inflammation of the heart muscle

these diseases tend to be mild; with all of them, including the more serious, the ratio of inapparent to apparent infection is very high.

Respiratory diseases are transmitted primarily by the airborne route, usually through droplets and droplet nuclei. These diseases are caused by a number of agents, the more important of which are summarized in the outline that follows.

1. *Corynebacterium diphtheriae.* Diphtheria is primarily an upper respiratory infection (URI). The bacteria remain in the throat and produce a toxin which affects the nerves and heart muscles. The goal of immunization is to develop antibodies against the toxin.

2. *Hemophilus influenza.* This virulent organism produces a variety of syndromes, including pneumonia, sore throat, **otitis media,** and **septicemia.** Meningitis is a special problem in young children. The bacterium gets its name from its occasional occurrence in patients with influenza. In these cases *H. influenza* produces a pneumonia which was often fatal in the pre-antibiotic era.

3. *Hemophilus pertussis.* A highly contagious bacterial disease which is especially dangerous to children under 1 year of age; pertussis (whooping cough) is a leading cause of infant mortality.

4. *Meningococci.* These bacteria are harbored in the nose and throat of millions of people. Clinical cases represent only a tiny fraction of the total number infected. The most serious disease caused by these bacteria is meningitis, which is highly fatal in children and, for some reason, military recruits. Most commonly manifested by a sore throat, this disease also often produces a syndrome characterized by fever, rash, **polyarthritis,** and mild septicemia.

5. *Pneumococcus.* This bacterium is responsible for more than 90 percent of primary pneumonias, which are especially common in young adult males.

6. *Staphylococci.* Thirty to 50 percent of the population harbor these bacteria on the skin and in the nose. Staphylococci produce boils, **osteomyelitis, impetigo,** and septicemia. Infection is most common in infants and young children. Infections acquired in the hospital tend to be resistant to most antibiotics.

OTITIS MEDIA: inflammation of the bonelike structure of the middle ear, which transmits sound to the brain
SEPTICEMIA: the presence and multiplication of bacteria in the bloodstream
POLYARTHRITIS: inflammation of several or many joints
OSTEOMYELITIS: inflammation of the bone
IMPETIGO: a skin infection usually due to staphylococci

7. *Streptococcus.* This bacterium is a frequent cause of sore throat; in children a common syndrome consisting of sore throat and a skin rash is known as scarlet fever. Erysipelas is the name given to streptococcal skin infections. Postinfection sequelae include rheumatic fever and glomerulonephritis. Morbidity and mortality from rheumatic fever have dropped drastically in recent years.

8. *Adenovirus.* The incidence of adenoviral URI is very high among military recruits. In civilians the most common illnesses are mild sore throat and **conjunctivitis** ("pink eye").

9. *Rhinovirus.* This agent produces 25 percent of colds and is the most important cause of this very common syndrome.

10. *Influenza.* There are three distinct viral variants, known as A, B, and C. Type A is responsible for most epidemic diseases. Worldwide epidemics (pandemics) occurred in 1918, 1957, and 1968. This disease is a significant threat to life in cardiac patients, persons with chronic respiratory disease, and the elderly. Superimposed bacterial infection (pneumococcus, *H. influenza*) is a frequent complication. Viral types change over time and vaccines must be continually updated to be effective.

11. *Mumps.* This is a childhood disease which involves salivary glands. In adult males testicular involvement is a serious complication and sometimes leads to sterility if the involvement is bilateral.

12. *Varicella, herpes zoster.* In children this causes chickenpox, a mild disease characterized by an itchy body rash. Varicella sometimes reappears in adult life as herpes zoster in a disease called "shingles." Shingles is characterized by inflammation of nerves serving the skin and by a skin rash along the course of the involved nerves. Both chickenpox and shingles are self-limiting.

13. *Smallpox.* This virus can survive outside the human host for long periods of time. Smallpox is a very serious disease, with a fatality rate as high as 30 percent. The last individual case in the United States appeared in 1968, and the most recent outbreak occurred in 1949.

14. *Measles.* Epidemic cycles of measles occur every two to three years. Usually a mild childhood disease, measles is nevertheless capable of serious complications, including otitis media, pneumonia, and encephalitis.

15. *Rubella* is a very mild illness commonly known as German measles. Its main importance lies in the fact that women contracting the disease in

---

CONJUNCTIVITIS: inflammation of the protective membrane lining the inner eyelids and eyeball

the first three months of pregnancy have a 20-percent chance of bearing a dead or deformed child.

The skin infections, erysipelas and impetigo, are important diseases transmitted by direct contact. The transmission of leprosy is thought to be by direct contact also. This disease is perhaps more feared than any other because it mutilates and disfigures (Fig. 4-4). Children are most susceptible to leprosy, which is a common disease in the tropics and particularly prevalent in China and India. In the United States it is very rare and largely confined to Louisiana and southeast Texas. Perhaps the most important illnesses transmitted by direct contact are the venereal diseases, principally syphilis and gonorrhea. (They are discussed in detail in Chapter 8.)

Primary prevention (see Chapter 9) is rarely possible for diseases transmitted by direct contact, indirect contact, or airborne sperad. For these illnesses, secondary prevention implies the availability of vaccine (see Table 4-2); in the absence of a vaccine, tertiary prevention (restoration) is the rule. Tertiary prevention relies on the identification and treatment of clinical and inapparent cases. The latter are often very difficult to find because the carrier is unaware of his infection. Practically, a carrier can be identified only when he is a known contact of an index case. Subclinical cases of typhoid, meningococcal, and staphylococcal infections can often be detected by **cultures** of the organism obtained from stool (typhoid), the nose, or the throat. Past or present infection with the tubercle bacillus can be determined by a simple skin test. Culture is sometimes used to detect gonorrhea in contacts, who are often treated to abort the development of clinical disease and to eliminate a source of infection. Prophylaxis, as such treatment is called, is useful in cases of tuberculosis and gonorrhea and is sometimes employed, with mixed results, against meningococcal infection.

As we have already noted, the identification of clinical cases is not a very effective means of controlling most infectious diseases because of the problems presented both by inapparent infections and the fact that the patient is often capable of transmitting the disease before he becomes sick. Nevertheless, it is of some value to eliminate obvious cases and investigate their contacts to reduce the available sources of infection. The simplest way to deal with clinical cases is to cure them. When this is not possible, two other measures are used: isolation and quarantine.

CULTURE: the growth of bacteria and other microorganisms in an artificial environment

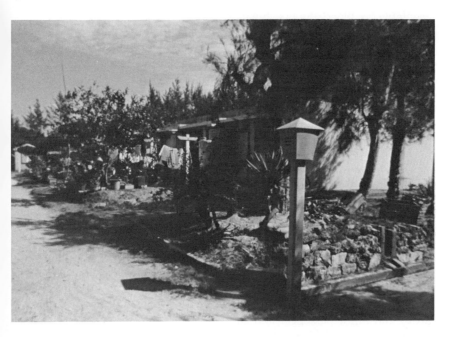

Fig. 4-4.   *This photo shows a small section of a leprosy hospital in Okinawa. The small box on the pole in the foreground contains a loudspeaker which broadcasts a signal. Blind leprosy patients can walk about the hospital grounds by moving from one audio box to another. (Courtesy of Dr. C. L. Marshall.)*

Isolation is the separation of the patient from other persons during the communicable period of his disease. It is seldom used today and is unnecessary if the disease can be successfully treated. Moreover, it is of little value if the **communicable period** begins prior to the onset of symptoms. Smallpox is the only disease for which isolation is commonly recommended. Drugs for the treatment of smallpox do not exist, and its communicable period begins only with the appearance of symptoms. Certain diseases which are difficult or impossible to treat are dealt with through modifications of the isolation idea. Leprosy patients are often isolated for life, while the blood of patients with serum hepatitis, a disease transmitted by blood, is isolated in the sense that such patients are not

---

COMMUNICABLE PERIOD: the time during which a communicable disease is transmittable from man to man; it usually begins during the incubation period and extends into the disease itself

acceptable as blood donors. Smallpox and measles are not curable, but clinical cases usually lead to contacts who can be protected by vaccination.

Quarantine involves restricting the movement of contacts of a known case for a time period equal to the longest usual incubation period of the disease in question. Quarantine is obviously difficult to enforce because rarely are all contacts known, and those who remain undetected are free to move about at will. Quarantine is applicable mainly to international travel. When most persons travelled by sea, quarantine was practical because, in the event of a case aboard ship, all the possible contacts were immediately known. In such cases, a ship was required to sit out the incubation period before its passengers were allowed into the country. The jet age of air travel has made quarantine increasingly irrelevant, but six diseases are quarantinable under international agreement: yellow fever, cholera, typhus, relapsing fever, plague, and smallpox. In practice, quarantine is rarely invoked against any of these but cholera, and it is rare even against this disease. As for the others, the population into which the potential case seeks entry is better protected by requiring that the individual be vaccinated (yellow fever, smallpox) or by killing the fleas, lice, mosquitoes, or rats which transmit disease (plague, typhus, relapsing fever) and infest passenger and ship alike.

Cure of disease is obviously preferable to both isolation and quarantine. The mainstays of infectious disease therapy are the antibiotics. Despite the value of this family of drugs, they are not without drawbacks. They are not effective against viral diseases, although the notion is widespread among the public that penicillin is good for colds. The organisms against which antibiotics are used often become resistant to them, and allergic reactions and other often serious side effects are not uncommon in patients for whom these drugs are prescribed. Prolonged administration can alter the normal flora of the body and result in the overgrowth of resistant organisms. Following is a summary of the major antibiotics:

1. Penicillin is the standard against which other antibiotics are measured; it is probably the most valuable drug ever introduced into medicine. Allergic reactions to penicillin are fairly common, and the drug is limited in effectiveness to gram-positive organisms, some of which (notably staphylococci) develop resistance to it. To get around the resistance problem and to deal with gram-negative organisms, variants of penicillin have been developed—the two most important being ampicillin and methicillin. Unlike most antibiotics, which prevent bacterial multiplication, the penicillins kill the organisms outright.

2. Erythromycin, cephalothin, and *lincomycin* are essentially penicillin substitutes, useful when the patient is allergic to penicillin or when the organism is resistant. Organisms rapidly develop resistance to erythromycin. Like the penicillins, these drugs are effective against gram-positive bacteria.

3. *Sulfonamides* are drugs of particular value in dysentery and meningococcal infections. They are effective against both gram-positive and gram-negative organisms, but primarily the sulfas are back-up drugs. One group of variants of the sulfa drugs, called sulfones, are the drugs of choice against leprosy. Resistance to sulfas is common, as are side effects.

4. *Tetracyclines* are commonly identified commercially by the suffix, "mycin." These were the original "wonder drugs." Although resistance is a problem, they are effective against both gram-positive and gram-negative bacteria and tend to produce fewer and less serious side effects than most antibiotics.

5. *Chloramphenicol* is a highly toxic and dangerous drug, which is effective against gram-negative and gram-positive bacteria and is the drug of choice against typhoid and typhus.

6. *Isoniazid* (*INH*), *para-aminosalicylic acid* (*PAS*), and *streptomycin* are the front-line drugs against tuberculosis. They are usually used in combination, but isoniazid is used alone for TB prophylaxis. While PAS is used only against tuberculosis, streptomycin is effective against many gram-negative organisms and is the drug of choice against plague. Its major fault as an antibiotic is the extreme rapidity with which resistant organisms appear.

7. *Kanamycin* and *polymycin* exemplify a number of strictly secondary drugs whose use is confined to organisms like *Klebsiella, Aerobacter, Proteus,* and *Pseudomonas.* These are resistant to most drugs and present special problems in debilitated patients. Kanamycin is of some value in urinary tract infections due to *E. coli.*

Table 4-3 shows the use of antibiotics against common bacterial disease agents. Tables 4-4 and 4-5 summarize the transmission and control of the infectious diseases covered in this chapter.

Less Important Types of Disease Agents

A variety of organisms, including Rickettsiae, fungi, Protozoa, and helminths are "less important" only in the parochial sense that they are not major problems in the United States. In much of the developing world they are very important sources of death and disability. Typhus is the classic rickettsial disease, and it is transmitted from man to man via the body louse. Untreated typhus produces a fatality rate which often

TABLE 4-3. Antibiotics Useful Against Certain Bacterial Agents[a]

Agent	Disease	Best Drug	Secondary Drugs
Corynebacterium diphtheriae	diphtheria	erythromycin	penicillin, tetracyclines
Diplococcus pneumoniae	pneumonia, otitis, meningitis	penicillin	erythromycin, ampicillin
Mycobacterium leprae	leprosy	sulfones	⋯
Mycobacterium tuberculosis	tuberculosis	INH, PAS, streptomycin	various drugs
Staphylococcus	skin infections, pneumonia, osteomyelitis, meningitis, septicemia, lung abscess, brain abscess, infection of surgical wounds	penicillin, methicillin	ampicillin, streptomycin
Enterococcus	urinary tract infection, diarrhea	penicillin plus streptomycin	ampicillin plus streptomycin
Aerobacter aerogenes	secondary infections	kanamycin	chloramphenicol, polymycin
Borrelia recurrentis	relapsing fever	tetracycline	penicillin
Escherichia coli	urinary tract infection, diarrhea	ampicillin	tetracycline, kanamycin
Hemophilus influenza	pneumonia, sore throat, otitis, meningitis	ampicillin	chloramphenicol
Klebsiella pneumoniae	secondary infections	cephalothin	ampicillin, tetracycline
Neisseria gonorrhoeae	gonorrhea	penicillin	ampicillin, tetracycline
Neisseria meningtidis	meningitis, arthritis, otitis, sore throat	penicillin	ampicillin, tetracycline
Pasteurella pestis	plague	streptomycin	tetracycline, chloramphenicol
Pseudomonas aeruginosa	secondary infections, urinary tract infections	polymycin	tetracycline
Proteus vulgaris	secondary infections, urinary tract infections	kanamycin	chloramphenicol
Rickettsiae	typhus	chloramphenicol	tetracycline

TABLE 4-3. (Continued)

Agent	Disease	Best Drug	Secondary Drugs
Salmonella typhosa	typhoid	chloramphenicol	ampicillin
other *Salmonella*	diarrhea	chloramphenicol	ampicillin
Shigella	dysentery	sulfonamides	tetracycline
Treponema pallidum	syphilis	penicillin	erythromycin, tetracycline

[a]*Modified after Jawek, E., Melnick, J. L., and Adelberg, E. A. Review of Medical Microbiology, 8th ed. Los Altos, Calif., Lange, 1968.*

TABLE 4-4. Transmission and Control of Bacterial Diseases Transmitted from Man to Man

Disease	Spread	IP[a]	CP[b]	Prevention
Bacterial cholera	vehicular, indirect contact	2–3D	O–14D	primary
Dysentery	vehicular, indirect	4D	O–14D	primary, tertiary
Infantile diarrhea	indirect	1–4D	O–variable	tertiary
Typhoid	direct, indirect	14D	O–30+D	primary, secondary tertiary
Staphylococcal	direct, airborne	4–10D	O–duration	tertiary
Streptococcal	direct, airborne	1–3D	3D–3D	tertiary
Tuberculosis	indirect, airborne	4–6W	varies	secondary, tertiary
Diphtheria	direct, indirect	2–5D	O–2W	secondary, tertiary
H. influenza	airborne	1–3D	unknown	
Pertussis	direct, indirect, airborne	7D	O–3W	secondary, tertiary
Meningococcal	direct, airborne	3–4D	varies	tertiary
Pneumococcal	airborne, direct, indirect	1D–3D	indefinite	tertiary
Gonorrhea	direct	3D–4D	indefinite	tertiary
Syphilis	direct	3W	indefinite	tertiary

[a]IP = incubation period: D = days; W = weeks

[b]CP = communicable period: D = days; W = weeks; O = onset of disease. The first number stands for onset (O) or the number of days before onset; the second number refers to days or weeks after onset. The CP for streptococcal disease is read as 3 days before to 3 days after onset. The CP for diphtheria is read as from the time of onset to 4 weeks after onset.

TABLE 4-5. Transmission and Control of Viruses Transmitted from Man to Man

Disease	Spread	IP[a]	CP[b]	Prevention
Smallpox	airborne spread	7–16D	O–3W	secondary
Infectious hepatitis	indirect, vehicular	15–50D	varies	secondary
Coxsackie virus	vehicular, indirect	varies	varies	none
Echo virus	vehicular, indirect	varies	varies	none
Polio virus	vehicular, indirect	7–12D	3D–4W	secondary
Reovirus	airborne	unknown	unknown	none
Adenovirus	airborne	5D	duration	secondary
Rhinovirus	airborne	12–74H	1–5D	none
Influenza	airborne	1–3D	O–3D	secondary
Mumps	airborne, direct, indirect	2–3W	7–9D	
Chickenpox	airborne, indirect	2–3W	1–6D	secondary
Measles	airborne, direct, indirect	10–14D	4–5D	secondary
Rubella	airborne, direct, indirect	2–3W	7D–4D	secondary

[a] *IP = incubation period: D = days; W = weeks; H = hours*

[b] *CP = communicable period: D = days; W = weeks; O = onset of disease. The first number stands for onset (O) or the number of days before onset; the second number refers to days or weeks after onset.*

approaches 40 percent. Prominent fungal diseases include troublesome skin lesions such as ringworm and athlete's foot, as well as more serious illnesses such as histoplasmosis and candidiasis. A fungal infection of the lung, histoplasmosis is often asymptomatic but can prove fatal if it spreads to other body organs. This infection is very common in the eastern and central parts of the United States. Candidiasis (moniliasis, thrush) is most commonly seen in patients who are on antibiotics and in whom the organism, *Candida albicans,* replaces the normal flora. The vagina is a common site of candidiasis in adults, while the oral cavity is favored in infants. Spread to other organs is rare.

Malaria is the most important protozoan disease, and it is one of man's most persistent and potent enemies. It is characterized by the parasitism of red blood cells and by severe fever as the red cells burst, releasing additional organisms. Malaria is often fatal, especially among infants.

Hookworm (discussed in Chapter 2) and schistosomiasis are helminthic diseases. The latter, which cannot be either satisfactorily prevented or

treated, shares with malaria the dubious honor of being the world's leading disease. Schistosomiasis is transmitted from both human and animal
reservoirs by certain species of freshwater snails. A chronic disease extending over many years, it affects virtually all body organs and is severely
debilitating and often fatal. Trichinosis is a helminthic disease which, in
the United States, primarily affects pigs. It is transmitted to man when
he eats inadequately cooked pork. Pigs develop disease from eating scraps
of pork in the garbage on which they feed. Sterilization of garbage before feeding it to pigs and thorough cooking of pork before feeding it to
humans prevent transmission of infection.

Arthropods (insects) are transmitters of disease such as malaria, yellow
fever, typhus, and plague. They are also pests in their own right. Chiggers,
mites, ticks, poisonous spiders, scorpions, lice, bees, wasps, hornets, and
mosquitoes are some of the arthropods which make human life miserable.
We will discuss some of these pests later.

Three Important Infectious Diseases

Because of their great importance as causes of disability and
because they are good examples of some of the principles we have discussed thus far, hepatitis, tuberculosis, and streptococcal infections are
covered here in some detail.

HEPATITIS

Hepatitis is an acute, infectious, viral disease whose manifestations arise from its effects on the liver. It is in reality comprised
of two separate disease entities: infectious hepatitis (IH) and serum
hepatitis (SH). They are caused by separate viruses, and though clinically similar they are quite distinct epidemiologically. Both are difficult to prevent and both lack a specific therapeutic drug. Being viruses,
neither infectious nor serum hepatitis responds to antibiotic therapy. Table
4-6 outlines the principal features of the two diseases.

Jaundice is the outstanding clinical characteristic of both SH and IH.
There may be wide variation in symptoms from patient to patient, although
loss of appetite (anorexia), hepatomegaly (enlargement of the liver),
light stools, dark urine, and abnormal laboratory tests of liver function are
almost always present. While both tend to be brief illnesses, either can
drag on for a prolonged period. Mild relapses occur in both illnesses, but
not commonly. The most serious complication is hepatic necrosis, a mas-

sive destruction of liver cells which is fatal in over 60 percent of cases. In general, the fatality rates are low in both diseases, but serum hepatitis is the more serious condition.

As Table 4-6 shows, the main differences between the two diseases are epidemiological. The key difference is perhaps the mode of transmission. By and large, infectious hepatitis is spread by the fecal-oral route. Far less common is vehicular transmission via contaminated water, or food exposed to contaminated water, especially oysters and clams. Transmission by way of contaminated blood, needles, or syringes is possible but considered quite rare. In contrast, man contracts serum hepatitis primarily through contaminated blood and blood products or by using needles and syringes which have contained contaminated blood. Because of this mode of transmission, serum hepatitis is most common in patients who have received blood transfusions and in "main-lining" drug addicts who frequently inoculate themselves in a group using a shared needle and syringe. Serum hepatitis is therefore a disease of adults, while infectious hepatitis is primarily a disease of children. The incidence of SH following transfusion is often as high as 1 percent per unit (1 unit is equal to approximately 1 pint) of blood received. There is no effective way to inactivate SH virus in blood. It was recently discovered that the blood of 25 to 50 percent of SH patients carries an antigen which is not present in the blood of IH patients. This "Australia Antigen" has been used to screen blood containing SH virus. Such screening is required by law in a few states, and its intent is to avoid the use of blood contaminated with virus. But not all SH carriers also have the Australia Antigen. Its validity as a screen is therefore low because it is a specific but insensitive test, and there are many false negatives.

Attempts to control the spread of SH by restricting blood donations from persons with a history of SH is ineffective because only 10 percent of cases are clinically apparent. A ban on blood donations from any person who had ever received a transfusion would be unwise, since the length of time that the virus persists in the blood is largely unknown and because blood donors in the United States are all too few in the first place. Some authorities recommend that persons receiving blood wait six months before being allowed to donate it.

The magnitude of the SH problem can be better appreciated if we consider a few of its social ramifications. New York City uses 300,000 units of blood each year. More than two-thirds of this blood comes from paid donors who receive 5 to 10 dollars per unit. Unfortunately, the people most likely to sell their blood are often the very people most likely to carry SH virus, i.e., drug addicts. Alcoholics are also frequent paid donors. As the prevalence of addiction rises, so does the prevalence of contami-

TABLE 4-6. Infectious versus Serum Hepatitis

	Infectious	Serum
CLINICAL FINDINGS		
Principal findings	abrupt onset; fever; anorexia; abdominal discomfort; jaundice; dark urine; light stools; enlarged liver; enlarged spleen; abnormal laboratory tests of liver function	insidious onset; anorexia; nausea, vomiting; abdominal discomfort; jaundice; dark urine; light stools; enlarged liver; enlarged spleen; abnormal laboratory tests of liver function
Treatment	activity restriction; high caloric diet	activity restriction; high caloric diet
Complications	chronic course; hepatic necrosis; relapse	chronic course; hepatic necrosis; relapse
Case fatality rate	less than 2%	about 10%
EPIDEMIOLOGICAL FINDINGS		
Distribution	worldwide; tends to cyclic recurrence at 5–10 yr intervals; most common in children, young adults, institutional populations, low-income areas, military forces, rural areas; autumn and winter	worldwide; more common in adults than children; most common in drug addicts, persons receiving transfusions
Reservoir	man; possibly primates	man
Transmission	fecal-oral contact; contaminated water and food; contaminated blood; contaminated needles and syringes	inoculation of blood and contaminated needles and syringes; rarely through contact with contaminated blood
Screening test	Australia Antigen not present	Australia Antigen present in 25–50% of carriers and cases
Ratio of subclinical to clinical cases	1:10	1:10
Incubation period	15–60 days (2–5 weeks)	60–180 days (2–6 months)
Communicable period	latter half of incubation period through first few days of jaundice	weeks before onset of symptoms and in some cases for years later
Prevention	health education to sanitary disposal of feces; disposable or sterilized needles and syringes; passive immunity with gamma globulin	disposable or sterilized needles and syringes; prohibit blood donation from patients with history of SH; prohibit blood donation by known addicts
Control	obligatory report of cases; isolation during first 2 weeks of illness	obligatory case report

nated blood. Blood donated voluntarily is 12 times less likely to transmit SH as blood acquired commercially. In other words, the relative risk of SH is far greater to patients receiving blood from a paid donor. Volunteers are in short supply throughout the United States. Unfortunately, less than 5 million Americans donate blood each year, and serum hepatitis is part of the social cost of this apathetic behavior. It is estimated that if an additional 2 percent of New Yorkers donated blood once a year, SH from transfusions would disappear from the city.

A new dimension was recently added to the problem when courts in Illinois and Pennsylvania handed down decisions making hospitals and blood banks financially liable for SH resulting from transfusions they provide. If this decision becomes general, it can be expected to greatly increase the cost of blood and to do much to stimulate the public, the hospitals, and the blood banks to procure more donated blood. SH exemplifies the close relationship between medicine and the society of which it is a part. SH is presently beyond the control of medicine because there is no way either to screen out contaminated blood completely or to inactivate blood containing virus. Another and equally important reason is the absence of a cure for addiction. At the same time, there is a potential nonmedical solution available for posttransfusion SH: increased voluntary blood donations. Testimony to the effectiveness of this approach is available from Britain where almost all blood is obtained through voluntary donation and where the incidence of posttransfusion SH is negligible. SH among addicts is a more complex problem, but it is probable that its solution is at least as much social as medical.

Like SH, the control of infectious hepatitis is limited by the problem of subclinical cases. In addition, IH virus in water supplies is resistant to chlorine, at least in the concentrations used among civilian populations. However, known contacts can be protected through passive immunization with gamma globulin, which is not effective against SH. Isolation is sometimes advocated in IH during the first two weeks of illness, but this measure is effective only insofar as it limits contact with a known infectious source. The communicable period in IH begins halfway through the incubation period, and, aside from members of the patient's household, systematic search for contacts is impractical. Reporting of both IH and SH is now required by law in all states, but underreporting is the rule, especially of SH among addicts. Nevertheless, 46,000 cases of IH were reported in 1968, and this made it one of the most commonly reported infectious diseases. In that same year, 5,000 cases of SH were reported, twice as many as in 1967. It is estimated that the true number of SH cases is about 55,000 per year.

TUBERCULOSIS

Tuberculosis has dogged the tracks of man throughout recorded history. Evidence of TB has been found in Egyptian mummies, and the disease was familiar to the ancient Greeks and Romans. In spite of its antiquity, tuberculosis was very poorly understood until the first half of the nineteenth century, when the French physician, René Laennec, recognized that a wide range of syndromes were simply different manifestations of the same basic disease. The communicable nature of TB was demonstrated in 1865, and the bacillus itself was identified by Koch in 1882. Eight years later Koch developed tuberculin, an extract of the tubercle bacillus, which is still the most valid screening test available. An equally important diagnostic tool came along in 1895 with the discovery of x-rays by Roentgen. The therapeutic value of rest and induced **pneumothorax** was recognized at the end of the nineteenth century. In the 1950s, isoniazid gained therapeutic acceptance and began a new era in the long struggle to control this persistent adversary.

Tuberculosis begins as a primary lung infection which is usually asymptomatic and which usually heals spontaneously. Occasionally, this primary lesion progresses directly to pulmonary tuberculosis. Full-blown pulmonary tuberculosis destroys lung tissue through the formation of tubercles, lesions which tend to enlarge in size until they become literal cavities within the lung. These cavities are filled with a cheeselike material consisting of bacilli and necrotic lung tissue. Tuberculosis is capable of spreading to any body organ, but lymphatics, bones, joints, intestines, kidneys, larynx, meninges, and skin are most commonly involved. Miliary tuberculosis is highly fatal and refers to a condition wherein virtually every organ is seeded with small tubercles. In the vast majority of cases today, tuberculosis is confined to the lungs and distant sites are rarely involved. Recovery from TB is characterized by the development of a fibrous wall around the diseased area. Tubercle bacilli often survive within this wall of isolation and become active again years later in the presence of lowered host resistance. For this reason it is most uncommon to declare anyone "cured" of tuberculosis; the more cautious term, "inactive," is used instead.

Figure 4-5 depicts the downward trend of tuberculosis mortality in New York City since the early 1800s and notes the important discoveries about

---

PNEUMOTHORAX: artificially induced collapse of a lung

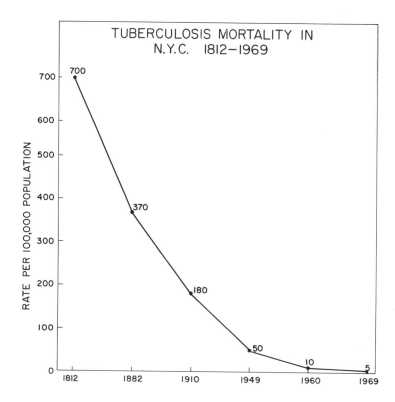

FIG. 4-5.   *TB rates dropped almost 50 percent between 1812 and 1882 even though methods to combat the disease were non-specific. Indeed it was not until 1865 that the disease was recognized as communicable and the tubercle bacillus itself was not discovered until 1882. The first truly effective anti-tuberculous drug was available after 1949 and most of the decline in death rates since that time is due to this drug, INH. (Based on statistics from The Tuberculosis and Respiratory Disease Association of New York City, and from Dubos, 1965. Man Adapting, Yale University Press.)*

the disease that have occurred in the past 170 years. When Koch discovered the tubercle bacillus in 1882, he estimated that about 15 percent of all deaths in Europe were caused by this disease. In both Europe and the United States the dramatic decline in mortality began in 1800, some 20 years before Laennec's contribution and 80 years before the discovery of the bacillus itself. Most students of this disease attribute the decline to general improvement in living conditions. Better working conditions, improved nutrition, and more adequate housing probably have contributed more to the eclipse of tuberculosis than anything directly related to public health or medical care. By 1948, when INH became available, tuberculosis

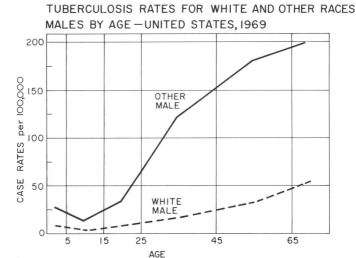

TUBERCULOSIS RATES FOR WHITE AND OTHER RACES
MALES BY AGE — UNITED STATES, 1969

FIG. 4-6.   *Even though fewer people suffer from tuberculosis than ever before, this encouraging fact should not obscure the unfortunate ethnic disparity in incidence rates between white males and "other" males. Also notice that age is an important factor. (After* Reported Tuberculosis Data 1969, *Public Health Service, U.S. Department of Health, Education and Welfare, 1971 ed.)*

mortality had fallen to 45:100,000. Twenty years of antituberculous drug therapy reduced this rate by 90 percent, to a low of 4:100,000 in 1968. Morbidity rates have fallen along with mortality. The incidence of tuberculosis declined from 54 cases per 100,000 in 1953 to 21 in 1968.

Mortality and case rates have fallen most rapidly among young people generally and among females in particular. However, as Figure 4-6 shows, case rates for non-white males over age 25 are still rather high. The death rate among blacks is almost twice as high as that among whites, and death rates in large urban centers are more than twice those in small towns and rural areas. Within large urban areas tuberculosis is primarily a disease of the poor, and in the United States death rates from TB are highest in those areas with large concentrations of poor people. In New York City, for example, the overall TB death rate was 5.2 per 100,000 in 1969, but 19.0 in Harlem and 11.4 in the Bedford section of Brooklyn, two areas which are predominantly black and poor. Other areas with high death rates include Washington, D.C., which is predominantly black; Puerto Rico, where living standards still lag behind those on the mainland; and Alaska, where the overall rate is pushed upward by an exceptionally high rate among Eskimos.

The tubercle bacillus exists as a number of strains. Those most important for man are the human and the bovine strains. As the name implies, the latter is primarily a disease of cattle. It is transmitted to man through cow's milk. Unlike the human strain, which tends to produce a primary lesion in the lungs, bovine tuberculosis often establishes its primary infection in the throat. This condition, known as scrofula, is still seen in developing countries. However, after 40 years of intensive tuberculin testing of cattle, bovine tuberculosis was eradicated in the United States about 20 years ago. This was achieved by slaughtering all positive reactors.

Man thus remains the only important domestic reservoir. The organism from a case of active pulmonary tuberculosis spreads from man to man by the airborne route. Primary infections are not communicable. The incubation period is four to six weeks. At the end of this period the primary lesion is established and the tuberculin test becomes positive. In most cases the former subsides and the individual remains free of active disease for life. The danger that the primary lesion will advance to pulmonary tuberculosis is greatest during the first year after its appearance. Those with active pulmonary TB often emit tubercle bacilli for years, although drug therapy can shorten the communicable period considerably.

Susceptibility to tuberculosis is general. Children under the age of 3 seem particularly susceptible, but in adults tuberculosis is abnormally common among diabetics, alcoholics, and those with chronic debilitating diseases. Patients on long-term **steroid** therapy are also especially susceptible, as are the malnourished and patients with measles. In the United States steroid therapy is commonly used for rheumatoid arthritis in older people, the very age group with the highest tuberculosis morbidity and mortality. These patients need very close medical supervision, and the danger of tuberculosis should not be underestimated.

The key to the diagnosis of tuberculosis is the tuberculin skin test. It is a superior diagnostic test which is both sensitive and specific. A positive test does not imply active disease, but rather infection with the tubercle bacillus in the recent or remote past. As the prevalence of tuberculosis has declined, the number of positive reactors has declined as well. Fortunately, the tuberculin test is inexpensive, and for this reason it is the best screening method in low-prevalence population groups. Screening

---

STEROID: the name applied to a family of chemical compounds produced by the adrenal gland; often used in medicine because they suppress the inflammatory process; unfortunately, they also suppress body resistance to infections and some other diseases; best known compound of this group is cortisone

yields are highest in the high-risk groups such as the poor, the institutionalized, alcoholics, migrant workers, and employees of medical institutions. People with positive tuberculin tests are followed up with a chest x-ray; if that is positive, the patient's sputum is cultured for tubercle bacilli. Those whose chest films are negative are treated prophylactically with INH for one year to prevent the development of active pulmonary tuberculosis, while those with positive sputum cultures are treated with INH, PAS, and streptomycin.

Tuberculin testing, with x-ray and laboratory follow-up when indicated, comprise the basis of tuberculosis control in the United States. It works because INH is very effective as a prophylactic measure. In countries with high tuberculosis prevalence, reliance is placed on an attenuated live vaccine known as BCG, which has been in use for about 50 years. The objective of BCG vaccination is to produce a mild primary infection which will increase host resistance to more virulent strains. BCG has been a source of controversy for years, but the prevailing view is that it is effective in preventing active tuberculosis. It is sometimes used in this country to protect people who are constantly exposed to tuberculosis, e.g., household contacts of patients, or inmates and employees of large institutions such as mental hospitals and prisons. The disadvantage of BCG lies in the fact that persons receiving it react to tuberculin, and the value of that very useful diagnostic test is therefore lost.

In contemporary America, active tuberculosis is usually **endogenous** in that it arises from an old primary lesion. Such lesions are most common in older people. In young men from 17 to 20, for example, only 3 percent react to tuberculin. Since most active cases arise from an endogenous source, it follows that the disease should be most prevalent in old people, among whom the rate of positive reactors is highest. Although tuberculosis was formerly a disease of children and young adults, its current prevalence in the elderly does not reflect a change in who is infected so much as it does the experience of a cohort in whose youth the original infections were acquired. The decline in primary infections among the young is probably most closely related to improved living conditions. In all likelihood, social and economic betterment remains the most potent weapon against this implacable adversary.

STREPTOCOCCAL INFECTIONS

Tuberculosis is a chronic infectious disease which sometimes lasts the better part of a patient's life. Streptococcal infections, in con-

---

ENDOGENOUS: arising from within the host

trast, are fleeting, but the ubiquitous Streptococcus may, if inadequately treated, leave its victim with either of two serious chronic diseases which can be every bit as devastating as tuberculosis.

Acute glomerulonephritis (or acute nephritis) is a noninfectious inflammation of the kidneys which, after a latent period of 10 days to 2 weeks, occasionally follows a streptococcal infection. The incidence of this disorder is difficult to quantify because many cases are subclinical; and, in addition, an identical syndrome sometimes occurs without a recognized antecedent streptococcal infection. Acute nephritis is characterized by **hematuria, edema** of the face and legs, and an elevated blood pressure. Most cases in children go on to complete recovery, but in about 10 percent the disease becomes chronic. Chronicity is more common in adults who contract acute nephritis. The case fatality rate for all age groups is approximately 10 percent. Chronic nephritis is the most common precursor of chronic renal disease, a condition in which the destruction of tissue is so great that the kidney ceases to function adequately and frequently ceases to function entirely. Chronic renal disease is an important cause of death. It leads to chronic hypertension, which is a significant contributory factor in myocardial infarction, cerebrovascular accidents, arteriosclerotic heart disease, and **congestive heart failure.** There are few better examples in medicine of a causal chain than that which begins with transient streptococcal infection, usually a sore throat, and progresses through glomerulonephritis to chronic renal disease, hypertension, and ultimate death from a stroke or a heart attack.

Rheumatic fever is a more common sequel to untreated streptococcal infection than nephritis. It follows the infection within one to three weeks in about 3 percent of cases. Rheumatic fever has become a less important cause of death in the past two decades, but it still kills over 10,000 Americans each year and cripples many others by permanently damaging the heart. It is by far the most common cause of heart disease in persons under the age of 40. The incidence of rheumatic fever is highest in children between the ages of 5 and 15. Poor people are most commonly affected, especially those living under crowded conditions. Like the streptococcal infections which precede it, rheumatic fever is a recurring condition. One attack is followed by another, each preceded by a streptococcal infection—usually pharyngitis, tonsillitis, or scarlet fever. Each successive attack

HEMATURIA: blood in the urine
EDEMA: swelling
CONGESTIVE HEART FAILURE: inability of the heart to pump out the blood returned
                          to it, with resulting congestion of the lungs and lower
                          extremities

increases the likelihood of permanent damage to the heart. In addition to its effect on the heart, rheumatic fever is characterized by an acute arthritis, the presence of raised, tender, skin nodules, and sometimes neurological symptoms.

Recovery from the attacks is the rule, but the duration of illness varies. Repeated attacks tend to scar and disfigure the valves of the heart permanently. In some cases the valves cease to function, a condition known as insufficiency, in which blood pumped from one heart chamber to another is partly regurgitated. In others, the valve is scarred and fixed in a manner which narrows it. This is known as stenosis, and it greatly increases the labor of the heart. The prevalence of rheumatic heart disease in the adult population approaches 1 percent.

The streptococci are a large family of bacteria which are classified into 15 groups. The vast majority of human infections, including those leading to nephritis and rheumatic fever, are of group A. Among the spectacular variety of infections produced by these organisms are pharyngitis, otitis, erysipelas, and puerperal fever. In childhood, streptococcal septicemia is a particular hazard following streptococcal otitis. In adults septicemia is most common in erysipelas and puerperal fever. Untreated, these septicemias are highly fatal, mortality being roughly 70 percent. Relatively uncommon today, erysipelas is an infection of the skin and most often involves the face and legs. Puerperal fever refers to a streptococcal infection of the uterus at the time of childbirth. Like erysipelas it is now uncommon, but it was at one time a leading cause of maternal mortality.

Streptococcal sore throat (pharyngitis, tonsillitis, or both) is far and away the most common infection produced by this organism. The condition is known as scarlet fever when it occurs in the presence of a skin rash. Streptococcal sore throat can be so slight as to go unnoticed, or severe enough to cause death. The human throat and nose comprise the chief reservoir of the streptococci, and asymptomatic carriers are common. Streptococci spread from man to man by direct contact, by indirect contact with contaminated objects, and by airborne droplets. Vehicular spread also occurs and usually produces explosive outbreaks. The usual source of infection is milk taken from a cow with streptococcal **mastitis**. Streptococcal infections are characterized by a brief incubation period—usually 1 to 3 days—and a communicable period which lasts as long as the particular infection—commonly 10 days.

Fortunately, the Streptococcus is very sensitive to penicillin. This drug has, so to speak, turned a lion into a pussycat. Virtually all streptococcal

---

MASTITIS: inflammation of the breast

infections will respond to penicillin, and early therapy is the best prevention against nephritis and rheumatic fever. People with a history of rheumatic fever are put on a prophylactic penicillin program. These programs vary in duration, but a common regimen for children is daily penicillin until the age of 18 and, for adults, five years after the last attack. The administration of penicillin prevents the streptococcal infection and protects the individual from recurrent attacks of rheumatic fever. For those allergic to penicillin, sulfa drugs provide an acceptable substitute. In spite of its susceptibility to penicillin, the Streptococcus remains an important disease agent. Streptococcal sore throat *alone* accounted for 435,000 cases in 1968 and was the second most commonly reported infectious disease.

The Partial Eclipse of Infectious Diseases

Table 4-7 compares the 10 leading causes of death in 1900 with those in 1965. In 1900, influenza-pneumonia, tuberculosis, and diphtheria were all leading causes of death; and gastroenteritis, chronic nephritis, and diseases of early infancy were intimately related to an infectious process. The last-mentioned diseases primarily included birth injuries, noninfective respiratory problems, ill-defined conditions, and infections occurring among newborns. Chronic nephritis, as we know, is a sequel of glomerulonephritis, but it also follows frank kidney infections and the chronic illness diabetes mellitus. By 1965, none of the first 10 causes of death was an infectious process except influenza-pneumonia and, in some cases, diseases of early infancy; mortality rates for these conditions had fallen 85 and 54 percent, respectively. With some notable exceptions, infectious diseases not only kill fewer people but seem to afflict fewer people as well. If one scans the list of reportable diseases, it is clear that only venereal disease, streptococcal sore throat, hepatitis, and salmonella infections are reported more frequently than they were a decade ago. Some, like measles and polio, have declined because of vaccines. Others, such as tuberculosis, typhoid, and rheumatic fever, have yielded to improved living conditions and drug therapy. The decline of still others—like **anthrax** and **brucellosis,** which tend to be diseases most

---

ANTHRAX: a disease of cattle which is capable of producing a fatal septicemia in man
BRUCELLOSIS: a disease of cattle and goats, usually transmitted to man through milk; it is a generalized infection which waxes and wanes over long periods of time

TABLE 4-7. Leading Causes of Death, 1900 and 1965,
with Some Comparative Death Rates

Rank	1900	1965
1	Influenza and pneumonia	Heart disease
2	Tuberculosis	Cancer
3	Gastroenteritis	Cerebrovascular lesions
4	Heart disease	Accidents
5	Cerebrovascular lesions	Influenza and pneumonia
6	Chronic nephritis	Certain diseases of early infancy
7	Accidents	General arteriosclerosis
8	Cancer	Diabetes mellitus
9	Certain diseases of early infancy	Other circulatory diseases
10	Diphtheria	Other bronchopulmonic diseases

Disease	Death Rate (per 100,000)		Change (in percent)
	1900	1965	
Heart disease	137.4	367.4	+268
Cancer	64.0	153.5	+240
Cerebrovascular lesions	106.9	103.7	...
Accidents	72.3	55.7	–22
Influenza and pneumonia	202.2	31.9	–85
Certain diseases of early infancy	62.6	28.6	–54

common in rural areas—is perhaps best attributed to the increasing urbanization of the population. Although their exact order cannot be specified (since it changes from year to year), the most commonly reported infectious diseases currently are gonorrhea, streptococcal sore throat, mumps, syphilis, and rubella. Behind these come hepatitis, tuberculosis, measles, Shigella infections, and salmonellosis. Viral infections of the upper respiratory and gastrointestinal tracts are by far the most common infections in terms of work and school absences; neither of these minor illnesses is reportable.

As we turn our attention to chronic diseases, it is worth noting (Table 4-7) the enormous increase in mortality from heart disease and cancer during the last 60 or 70 years, and the emergence of other chronic diseases, such as general arteriosclerosis and diabetes, as leading killers. Cerebrovascular lesions ranked fifth in 1900 and third in 1965, even though the death rate hardly changed at all during the 65-year period. This is explained by a lower overall mortality rate on the one hand, and the increasing importance of heart disease and cancer on the other. These last two diseases now account for more than half of all deaths in the United States.

The decline of infectious diseases in the United States, and in industrialized countries generally, should not obscure the fact that these diseases are still of great importance in developing countries, which encompass two-thirds of the world's people. In these areas, schistosomiasis, malaria, diarrheal diseases, and tuberculosis are leading killers, and their eventual control presents a tremendous challenge which involves not only drugs and vaccines but the more important problems of malnutrition, poverty, and rapid population growth.

Notes

1
>Ring around the rosie,
>Pocket full of posie,
>Ashes, ashes, we all fall down.

The "rosie" refers either to the site of the flea bite, which becomes swollen and surrounded by a reddened area of skin, or to the round, swollen lymph nodes which are also surrounded by a reddened area, a "ring." Posies are small bouquets of flowers that were allegedly carried to ward off the plague. "Ashes" is thought to be a corruption of "achoo," the sneeze which heralds the onset of a fatal pneumonia; or it may refer to the idea of "ashes to ashes, dust to dust."

References

Benenson, A. S., ed. Control of Communicable Diseases in Man. Washington, D.C., American Public Health Association, 1970.

Burton, L. E., and Smith, H. H. Public Health and Community Medicine. Baltimore, Williams and Wilkins, 1970.

Center for Disease Control, U. S. Public Health Service. Morbidity and Mortality Weekly Reports, Annual Supplement, Summary, 1970.

Deuschle, K. W. Tuberculosis. In Clark, D. W., and MacMahon, B., eds. Preventive Medicine. Boston, Little, Brown, 1967.

New York City Health Services Administration. Unpublished documents.

Jawetz, E., Melnick, J. L., and Adelberg, E. A. Review of Medical Microbiology, 8th ed. Los Altos, Calif., Lange, 1968.

Kilbourne, E. D. Approaches to the control of human infections. In Kilbourne, E. D., and Smillie, W. G., eds. Human Ecology and Public Health. New York, Macmillan, 1969.

Sartwell, P., ed. Maxcy-Rosenau Preventive Medicine and Public Health, 9th ed. New York, Appleton-Century-Crofts, 1965.

Weinstein, L. Chemotherapy of microbial diseases. *In* Goodman, L. S., and Gilman, A., eds. The Pharmacological Basis of Therapeutics, 3rd ed. New York, Macmillan, 1965.

Wintrobe, M., *et al.*, eds. Harrison's Principles of Internal Medicine, 6th ed. New York, McGraw-Hill, 1970.

CHAPTER
5

Chronic Diseases and Their Management

Eighty-five million Americans, more than 40 percent of the population, are afflicted with one or more chronic diseases. One million of these people are totally disabled, 5 million more are unable to work, and an additional 20 million must variously limit their activities because of a disability imposed by chronic illness. Table 4-7 pointed out the emergence of this type of illness as the nation's leading cause of death. In fact, as much as 75 percent of all deaths in the United States are attributable to chronic diseases; heart and **vascular** disease, in one form or another, account for 54 percent alone.

Chronic diseases include a large number of usually unrelated, heterogeneous conditions, which range in severity from mild and easily corrected visual defects to rapidly progressive and highly fatal cancers. Table 5-1 compares chronic and infectious diseases in a very general way. As the name implies, chronic diseases are long lasting and commonly permanent.

VASCULAR: pertaining to the blood vessels

TABLE 5-1. Infectious versus Chronic Disease
(A Very General Comparison)

	Chronic	Infectious
Duration	long, often for life	usually brief
Causative agent	usually unknown; usually considered nonliving	usually a known living organism
Treatment	usually symptomatic	directed against the causative agent
Course	usually progressive	usually self-limiting
Pathological changes	irreversible	commonly reversible
Goal of care	control, rehabilitation, and maintenance	cure
Prevention level	usually tertiary	primary, secondary, and tertiary
Occurrence	nonreportable	many are reportable
Incidence	high	high
Prevalence	high	relatively low
Mortality	high	relatively low
Morbidity	high	high
Age of patient	middle to old age	children and young adults
Duration of care required	long, usually many years or for life	relatively brief

Because the causative agent or agents are rarely known, chronic diseases must be treated symptomatically. Digitalis is a very important drug which is effective in the control of congestive heart failure, but heart failure is a symptom of arteriosclerotic heart disease, and digitalis has no effect whatever on this underlying condition. In other words, even when the symptoms can be controlled, the disease process itself remains unaffected. In consequence, the course of chronic disease tends to be progressive over years and often decades. Since the pathological changes which develop over these relatively long periods of time are usually irreversible, the goal of care is successful tertiary prevention, i.e., to maximize function, to minimize further deterioration, and to keep patient and disease in a state of equilibrium. With the knowledge presently available, one does not speak of cure but rather of control and management. Infectious diseases, in contrast, are usually self-limiting in that the patient either lives or dies, and the issue is decided within a relatively brief period of time. The development of antibiotics has made cure the therapeutic goal in most nonviral infections, and even viruses are often subject to prevention by immunization procedures.

Chronic diseases are not subject to medical control through either primary or secondary prevention. However, it is theoretically possible to prevent a few diseases for which risk factors are known. If the attributable risk of these factors is very high, much disease could be prevented by eliminating all contact between the risk factor and the population. This, of course, is primary prevention; its potential value in the control of chronic disease is best exemplified in relation to cigarettes. A total ban on cigarette sales throughout the United States, or a very high tax which would raise the price per pack to 5 or 10 dollars, would drastically reduce consumption and presumably have a preventive effect on lung cancer. However, a ban or a tax lies in the province of government, not medicine, and the prospects of such legislative action against cigarettes are very dim indeed. Legislatures are subject to pressure from a variety of groups endeavoring to protect economic interests. Drastic action against the tobacco industry would reduce incomes of growers, manufacturers, trucking companies, wholesale distributors, and retail outlets. Some people would lose their jobs, and local and state governments would lose a significant source of tax revenue. The question that the legislative bodies and the society they represent must answer is whether less lung cancer is worth the economic cost of less cigarette smoking.

Such difficult decisions are rarely encountered in the control of infectious diseases. For one thing, few, if any, infections must be controlled by the removal of products from the physical or social environment. Indeed, vaccines and antibiotics introduce new products into the economy. Most important, however, is that the control measure for many infectious diseases can be directed against the necessary cause itself. This simplifies things considerably. Protecting a man against smallpox by vaccination is quick, simple, and effective. Asking this same man to protect himself from heart disease by losing 25 pounds and jogging several miles a week is a complex request which demands a change in his entire style of living. In addition, it offers less certain protection than vaccination in that it deals not with a necessary cause but with a risk factor whose elimination may still leave the individual exposed to a number of risks, some or most of which have yet to be identified. Also, chronic diseases are progressive, and the removal of a risk factor may thus occur too late in the course of the disease to be of much help. Here again infectious diseases present less serious difficulties. Because they are commonly self-limiting and usually treatable, these diseases rarely produce bodily changes that are irreversible. As a result there are more opportunities for effective intervention.

There are several important principles implied in this discussion which

deserve mention. They are each applicable to chronic diseases and together account for most of the difficulty inherent in the control of these
ubiquitous illnesses. First, it is easier, less complicated, and more effective
to control a disease when there is a known causative agent. Manipulation of risk factors is complicated, difficult, and of uncertain value. Second, regardless of the kind of disease involved, control is easiest and most
effective when minimal or no human cooperation is demanded. Specifically, to change human habits and styles of living is enormously difficult;
and the more drastic the required change, the less probable is success.
Third, problems which are insoluble medically may nevertheless be
capable of nonmedical solutions. Unfortunately, the implementation of
such solutions usually involves legislation as well as alterations in human
behavior—two goals that are, as we have suggested, extremely hard to
achieve.

Because chronic diseases are difficult to prevent, slowly progressive,
more or less permanent, and usually incurable, people suffering with
these conditions require long-term and sometimes lifetime care. In the
absence of effective preventive or curative measures, the control of chronic
diseases depends on the availability, accessibility, and acceptability of
personal health services. The cost of care is thus exceedingly high, a fact
of great consequence and one which we will discuss later in this book.
Infectious diseases tend to be most devastating among children and young
adults. The eclipse of infections means that more people live on into
middle and old age, where chronic diseases are most likely to manifest
themselves. In spite of the billions of dollars spent annually on health
care, morbidity and mortality from these diseases remain generally high,
and there is little or no evidence of a downward trend in incidence or
prevalence (Fig. 5-1). The fact that annual expenditures on health have
increased each year serves to accentuate the cost problem. More and
more people are beginning to wonder what kind of return they are getting on this investment. Indeed, chronic disease lies at the heart of our
so-called "national health crisis," both medically and economically.

It would be an error to conclude from our discussion that those diseases which are not infectious are therefore chronic. In reality the two
categories are by no means exclusive. Tuberculosis, leprosy, malaria,
hookworm, and schistosomiasis are examples of infectious diseases which
are also chronic. In addition, as we learned from our consideration of
rheumatic fever, infectious diseases sometimes lead to chronic illness of
a noninfectious nature. We have also seen that debilitating chronic diseases often precede the onset of an infectious process. Thus, pneumococcal pneumonia is a common terminal event in a number of chronic re-

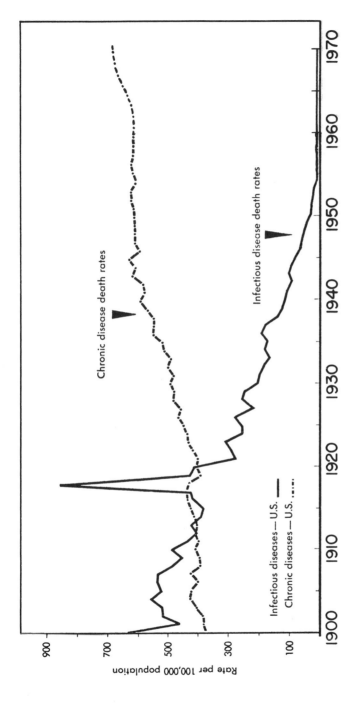

FIG. 5-1. *Mortality from infectious and chronic diseases in the twentieth century. The drop in the importance of infectious diseases as causes of death is matched by the equally spectacular rise of chronic diseases as the leading killers in industrialized countries. The sharp spike in the infectious disease death rate around 1918 reflects the worldwide epidemic of influenza which occurred in that year. Such worldwide epidemics are usually referred to as pandemics. (After Turner, 1971. Personality and Community Health, 14th ed. Courtesy of The C. V. Mosby Co.)*

spiratory diseases. Similarly, the damaged heart valves accompanying rheumatic fever are fertile ground for certain bacteria which are normal inhabitants of the throat. Bacterial infection of previously damaged heart valves produces an extremely serious cardiac infection known as **endocarditis.** Ironically, the most common bacterial invader is a streptococcus, *Streptococcus viridans.* In endocarditis, the chain of causation thus extends back to an initial streptococcal infection which was followed by chronic rheumatic heart disease which rendered the patient susceptible to yet another streptococcal infection.

Actually, the web or chain of causation in most diseases can be traced back to the social system and the way people adapt to it or are manipulated by it. Ultimately, each society generates its own pattern of disease through a large number of determinants, including poverty, customs, behavioral fashions such as smoking, and the range of technology that influences an individual's environment and to a large extent determines the disease agents to which he is exposed.

In our society heart disease ranks first as a cause of disability, arthritis second, and mental illness third; fourth are nonparalytic impairments of the back, spine, legs, or hip. Others, in descending order, include hypertension, visual impairments, asthma, genitourinary disorders, gastrointestinal diseases, and paralytic conditions. These round out the top ten. Note that the components of this list are not specific diseases but rather impairments derived from a number of disease entities. Visual defects are caused by a variety of independent diseases. Gastrointestinal diseases include stomach ulcers, colitis, cancers, and many other conditions whose relationship to each other is based solely on a common tendency to cause disability and a common locus in the gastrointestinal tract.

In the remainder of this chapter we will examine some of the important groups of chronic diseases. Each group represents an enormous subject better covered in entire books than in sections of a single chapter. For this reason our discussion will be aimed at essentials rather than details.

Cardiovascular Diseases

As we noted previously, diseases of the heart and blood vessels kill and disable more Americans than any other group of illnesses. The most important entities in this group comprise a trio of closely re-

---

ENDOCARDITIS: inflammation of the inner wall and valves of the heart, usually due to an infectious process

lated, highly devastating diseases: arteriosclerotic heart disease (ASHD), hypertension, and cerebrovascular accidents. Referable to all three is the arteriosclerotic process itself, which begins with the deposition of fatty material in the inner lining of medium and large **arteries.** The build-up of this material narrows the diameter of the artery and acts as a focus for the formation of a blood clot. This troublesome clot, or thrombus, may close off the vessel completely and thereby prevent blood from reaching any tissues beyond, a condition known as thrombosis. Often the thrombus, or a part of it, breaks free and travels in the bloodstream until it reaches a smaller artery where it blocks blood flow because it is too large to pass through the vessel any further. Such migratory thrombi are called emboli, and because thrombosis and embolism are sometimes hard to distinguish, they are often lumped together under the term "thromboembolism." Thromboembolism is not invariable in arteriosclerosis. Frequently the vessel is closed by the accumulation of fatty material, and this occludes the artery just as effectively as a thrombus.

Hypertension is both a disease and a disease process contributing to other maladies. It refers to an increase in the pressure exerted on the walls of arteries, particularly the very small ones known as arterioles. Transient elevations in pressure result from an increase in the rate at which the heart pumps blood. Thus, blood pressure temporarily increases when we are afraid, angry, or exercising. More serious increases in pressure occur when the resistance to blood flow within the vessels is permanently elevated. Commonly, the basis of this increased peripheral resistance is a narrowing of arterial diameter. It is therefore felt by some experts that hypertension results from an underlying arteriosclerosis. However, others feel that prolonged vascular narrowing more often results from overactivity by chemical mediators such as **epinephrine,** and that this precedes the development of arteriosclerosis. Which is cause and which is effect? We do not know. What is known is that the relationship between arteriosclerosis and hypertension is an intimate one which tends to be synergistic. Hypertension stresses the heart, which is obliged to pump blood against an increased pressure; long-standing hypertension leads to heart failure. It also stresses the vessels themselves, and these sometimes burst, producing a hemorrhage that is often severe and even fatal.

ARTERY: the thick-walled vessels carrying blood from the heart to other parts of the body; veins, in contrast, are thin-walled vessels which return blood from the periphery to the heart

EPINEPHRINE: a chemical secreted by the adrenal gland; also known as adrenalin, it constricts the arterioles, dilates the bronchial tree, and increases the heart rate

Hypertension is a very common disorder that affects roughly 15 percent of the adult population. In about 15 percent of cases an underlying, often correctible cause of elevated blood pressure can be identified. In the remaining 85 percent the disease is referred to as essential hypertension because the **etiology** is unknown. About 1 percent of the time, essential hypertension is rapidly progressive and, if untreated, leads to death within a relatively brief period—sometimes just several months. This comparatively rare form is known as malignant hypertension. The vast majority of patients, however, are little troubled by their disease for decades. Indeed, it is estimated that 40 percent of those with hypertension are unaware of their condition. Complications appear late in the disease and include heart failure, visual disorders, coronary artery disease, kidney failure, and cerebrovascular accidents. These are the same sequelae present in malignant hypertension, but in the malignant form they appear very early in the disease. A number of drugs are now available to reduce elevated blood pressure. While their effectiveness in essential hypertension is controversial, they have greatly improved the outlook in the malignant variety, the 5-year survival of which is now 50 percent. Over-all death rates from hypertension have fallen somewhat in the past 20 years. The average life span of untreated patients is more than 20 years from the time of the initial diagnosis. Since many, if not most, cases are diagnosed in middle age, hypertension is often compatible with normal life expectancy. Cases tend to cluster within families and among groups with a high dietary salt intake. It is slightly more common in women, but their **prognosis** is better than that for men. Hypertension is especially prevalent among blacks and perhaps among persons in low-income groups generally.

Of all diseases acting on the heart itself, arteriosclerosis is the most lethal. ASHD produces four very important cardiac syndromes, any or all of which may occur in a given patient. The most dramatic and most feared of these is the myocardial infarction, or "heart attack." Infarction develops from the sudden interruption of the blood supply to a portion of the heart muscle as a result of thromboembolism or arteriosclerotic occlusion. Deprived of its blood supply, the affected muscle becomes **necrotic.** Occlusion of a major coronary artery produces death, because there is not enough viable heart muscle left to carry on. Sudden severe chest and arm pain usually accompany infarction, but about 20 percent are silent and produce minimal or no symptoms. Thirty percent of patients having a

---

ETIOLOGY: a term commonly used in clinical medicine; synonomous with cause
PROGNOSIS: the probable outcome of a disease process
NECROSIS: death

first myocardial infarction die, and the fatality rate increases with each additional attack. The first couple of days following the attack are the most hazardous. Chances for survival go up dramatically thereafter. Those who recover with no residual symptoms have an 85-percent chance of surviving 5 years. In general, about half of the afflicted patients are able to return to work after infarction.

Angina pectoris is a temporary episode of chest pain. It is caused by intermittent narrowing of the coronary arteries or, what is essentially the same thing, the inability of already narrowed arteries to meet increased cardiac demand for oxygen as a result of exertion or excitement. Anginal attacks usually respond to nitroglycerin, a drug that dilates the coronary arteries. Closely related to angina is coronary insufficiency. This condition lies somewhere between angina and frank infarction. It is characterized by constant inability of sclerotic arteries to provide oxygen to the heart. Pain is often persistent, but is less severe than that of angina. Both angina and coronary insufficiency are often followed by infarction and disorders of heart rhythm. Congestive heart failure is common in hypertensive disease as well as in arteriosclerosis. Although this condition is compatible with many years of life, it frequently represents the terminal event in patients with infection, angina, or coronary insufficiency. Mild heart failure afflicts about 1 percent of the total population, including 6 percent of those over 65 and 10 percent of those over 70.

ASHD is as etiologically puzzling as arteriosclerosis itself. Prevention is difficult because there is no valid screening test, and efforts must be directed at known risk factors. As previously noted, these include obesity, hypertension, elevated serum cholesterol, cigarette smoking, and lack of exercise (Fig. 5-2). Other risks of importance are diabetes, **gout,** a family history of coronary artery disease, and familial hypercholesterolemia or hyperlipemia. There is some evidence to suggest that elimination of risk factors reduces the incidence of ASHD, but from our earlier discussion we know that it is extremely difficult to deal effectively with most risk factors. The prevalence of ASHD increases with age and is far more common in men than women; there is little racial difference. The incidence of this disease is estimated at 1 percent of the total population per year. The underlying arteriosclerotic process itself is even more common, being present in about 75 percent of young adults. The development of heart disease in later years is thus not surprising.

Cerebrovascular accidents (CVAs), or "strokes," are vascular lesions

---

gout: a metabolic disease characterized by inflammation of the joints and by the deposition of uric-acid crystals around them

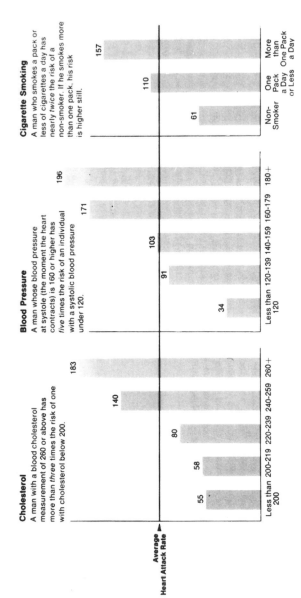

Cholesterol

A man with a blood cholesterol measurement of 260 or above has more than *three* times the risk of one with cholesterol below 200.

Less than 200 | 200-219 | 220-239 | 240-259 | 260+
55 | 58 | 80 | 140 | 183

Blood Pressure

A man whose blood pressure at systole (the moment the heart contracts) is 160 or higher has *five* times the risk of an individual with a systolic blood pressure under 120.

Less than 120 | 120-139 | 140-159 | 160-179 | 180+
34 | 91 | 103 | 171 | 196

Cigarette Smoking

A man who smokes a pack or less of cigarettes a day has nearly *twice* the risk of a non-smoker. If he smokes more than one pack, his risk is higher still.

Non-Smoker | One Pack a Day or Less | More than One Pack a Day
61 | 110 | 157

Average Heart Attack Rate

FIG. 5-2. *These charts depict the "heart attack" rate associated with levels of cholesterol, blood pressure, and cigarette smoking. The heavy black horizontal line represents the average heart attack rate among men aged 30-39 in Framingham, Mass. Higher serum cholesterol levels, blood pressure and heavy cigarette smoking are associated with above average risk of heart attack. (From Heart Facts, 1972. Courtesy of The American Heart Association.)*

of the brain which are distinguished from heart disease in listing causes of death. CVAs are the third highest cause of mortality in the United States and account for 12 percent of all deaths. Largely an affliction of the elderly, CVAs are rare before the age of 45. Risk factors are similar to those for ASHD and include hypertension, diabetes, high serum cholesterol, obesity, cigarette smoking, and family history of stroke. Unlike ASHD, however, CVAs are more common in females and blacks. About 80 percent survive a first CVA, but return to normal function is less certain. Weakness, paralysis, speech disorders, and disturbed mentation are frequent sequels to strokes, although much can be done to avoid these consequences by early efforts to rehabilitate the patient. Indeed, 85 percent of surviving stroke victims can regain the ability to care for themselves.

CVAs develop in either of two basic ways. The first is reduction of the cerebral blood supply, usually because of thromboembolism. Severe arteriosclerosis can also be responsible for this when it affects the large vessels leading from the heart to the brain. In years past, syphilis was a common cause but this is now rare. Cerebral thrombosis is secondary to hypertension or cerebral arteriosclerosis. Emboli are especially prevalent in those with rheumatic heart disease and are therefore the most important causes of strokes in younger people. Thrombosis and embolism together account for some 85 percent of all strokes. Hemorrhage, the second mechanism of CVAs, arises from hypertension and occasionally from defects in the walls of cerebral blood vessels. Hemorrhagic strokes are more often fatal than those due to thromboembolism.

As we learned from our consideration of rheumatic heart disease, cardiovascular diseases are not exclusively limited to the middle-aged and elderly. In addition, heart disease is often present at birth—in the form of **congenital** cardiac defects. These vary in kind and severity and are most common in mongoloids and children born to mothers who had rubella early in pregnancy. The current availability of rubella vaccine can be expected to reduce the incidence of this type of heart disease. Congenital heart defects were also reported in children born to mothers who had used thalidomide before it was taken off the market.

Circulatory disorders which affect vessels quite removed from either the heart or brain are known as peripheral vascular diseases. The most important of these is thrombophlebitis, an inflammation of the veins in the leg. This condition, whose etiology is unclear, is a common complication of pregnancy and a significant risk to women using oral contraceptives. Blood clots tend to form in the inflamed area, and though thrombophlebitis

---

CONGENITAL: existing at birth; this term is *not* a synonym for heredity

usually runs a self-limiting course, its principal danger lies in the possibility that an embolus might travel to the lungs, an event which is often fatal. Arteriosclerosis in peripheral arteries (arteriosclerosis obliterans) has the same effects on circulation in the leg as it has on circulation in the heart and brain. Severe cases lead to **gangrene** and often require amputation of the lower leg. An even more common, though less serious, peripheral vascular disorder is varicose veins. It occurs most frequently in women who have had several children and in people who stand for long periods. This condition, in which the veins are bulging, tortuous, and uncomfortable, is usually controlled by the use of elastic stockings or by surgical removal of the offending vein.

Cancer

Cancer, or carcinoma, is the second leading cause of mortality in the United States and accounts for about 16 percent of all deaths. It is primarily a disease of middle and old age, the average age at the time of diagnosis being slightly more than 60. Nevertheless, cancer is an important cause of death in childhood, ranking second only to accidents. In this period of life leukemia is the most common form of cancer, followed by **malignant** brain tumors and cancer of the kidneys. In addition, cancers affecting the lung, breast, bone, and colon are not uncommon in young adults. Because of the high incidence of cancers involving the female genital system, this disease is slightly more common in females, but mortality rates are somewhat higher in men. Apart from genital cancers, women enjoy lower incidence rates for all **neoplasms** except thyroid and colon (Fig. 5-3). The annual incidence of all cancers is about 300 per 100,000 population, which represents about 600,000 new cases yearly. The overall death rate approximates 13 per 100,000, which is less than half the mortality from cardiovascular diseases. Five-year survival is roughly 40 percent over-all, but this rate obscures a 35-percent survival rate for men compared with 45 percent for women. The first year following diagnosis is a crucial indicator of ultimate survival in that patients who live through this first year have a 5-year survival rate of 66 percent.

Cancer is characterized by neoplasia, the uncontrollable proliferation

---

GANGRENE: death of a body part
MALIGNANT: when used in reference to cancer, this term refers to tumors which
        spread to body organs other than the one in which the tumor first appears
NEOPLASTIC: referring to new growth, i.e., cancer

CANCER INCIDENCE BY SITE AND SEX

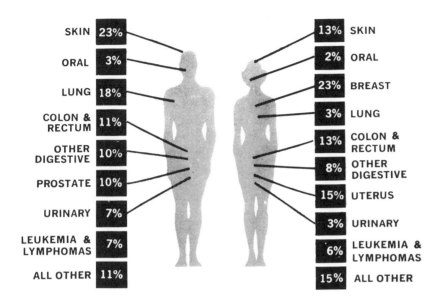

SKIN 23%
ORAL 3%
LUNG 18%
COLON & RECTUM 11%
OTHER DIGESTIVE 10%
PROSTATE 10%
URINARY 7%
LEUKEMIA & LYMPHOMAS 7%
ALL OTHER 11%

13% SKIN
2% ORAL
23% BREAST
3% LUNG
13% COLON & RECTUM
8% OTHER DIGESTIVE
15% UTERUS
3% URINARY
6% LEUKEMIA & LYMPHOMAS
15% ALL OTHER

FIG. 5-3.   *Note that the percentages for each sex refer to the proportion of all cancers occurring in that sex at that site, e.g., 13 percent of all female cancers involve the skin vs. 23 percent for men. This does not necessarily mean that skin cancer is more common in males than females. For instance, cancer occurs in certain sites that are peculiar to only one sex. For example, breast cancer necessarily lowers percentages of other cancer sites in females. (From* Cancer Statistics, 1971. *Courtesy of American Cancer Society, Inc.)*

of any of a number of different types of cells whose unrestricted growth produces a tumor which compresses, invades, and ultimately destroys normal tissues surrounding it. Most cancers develop from cells lining the outer or inner surface of a body organ. They tend to grow in a highly localized area for a time, but all too often cancer cells find their way into the bloodstream or lymphatics and spread to new sites distant from the original local growth. The spread of tumor cells to other body sites is known as metastasis. Strictly speaking, the term "cancer" refers to tumors which are capable of metastatic change. Tumors which do not metastasize are considered "benign," and these are relatively easy to treat because of their localization. The emphasis on early detection of cancer is important because early cancers are more likely to be localized, in which case they are essentially similar to benign tumors.

One of the curiosities of cancer is the wide range in its incidence from country to country. Stomach cancer is extremely common in Japan, but it is less common in the United States than it was 30 or 40 years ago. Cancers of the breast, uterus, prostate, and gastrointestinal tract are far more prevalent in this country than in Japan. Interestingly, these patterns often change with migration, i.e., people moving to a new country tend to develop a cancer pattern similar to that in the host nation. This observation suggests that the etiology of cancer is closely related to factors at work in the environment.

In spite of years of intensive research, little is known of the cause or causes of cancer. There is a growing conviction that leukemia may be caused by a virus, and viruses have long been implicated in some animal cancers. It is also known that certain substances are **carcinogenic**. Coal tar, pitch, and a number of oils have been implicated in skin cancers. Cigarette smoke and the tars it contains are associated with lung cancer, as are asbestos, chromates, and nickel. X-rays and radioactive materials are known to be potent factors in the development of cancer of the skin.

By and large, the best hope of reducing deaths from cancer lies in early detection (Fig. 5-4). However, the effectiveness of early detection depends on a public educated to its value. More than half of all cancers arise in the skin, breast, rectum, cervix, and oral cavity. All of these sites are easily examined, and all cancers discovered in such examinations are most treatable early in their course. Cancer prevention, like that of cardiovascular disease, depends on the avoidance of known risk factors. Breast cancer is least common in women who breast-feed their young and, not surprisingly, is most common in single women without children. Cervical cancer seems to be especially prevalent among women who commence sexual activity at an early age. Certain occupational groups are particularly subject to certain cancers. Bladder cancer is more common in chemical workers exposed to aniline dyes, and neoplastic bone disease is associated with workers who apply luminous paint to watch dials. Uranium miners are prone to lung cancer. Some cancers are associated with habits or social customs. The practice of circumcision apparently protects men against cancer of the penis. Alcohol is associated with esophageal cancer, as is cigarette smoking. Smoking is also related to cancer of the larynx and bladder. In India, where cigars are often smoked with the lit end in the mouth, oral cancer is a particular problem.

With the exception of skin cancer, the most common neoplastic disease in the United States is that of the colon and rectum. This cancer occurs with especial frequency in the elderly, and the prognosis is rather good

---

CARCINOGENIC: cancer-producing

CANCER STRIKES ONE IN FOUR

Of every 24 people
six will have cancer

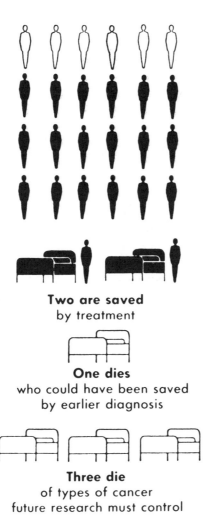

Two are saved
by treatment

One dies
who could have been saved
by earlier diagnosis

Three die
of types of cancer
future research must control

FIG. 5-4. *(From* Cancer Statistics, *1971. Courtesy of American Cancer Society, Inc.)*

if diagnosis is made while the tumor is localized. Sixty percent of these lesions are detectable by digital examination of the rectum, and another

20 percent are within range of the sigmoidoscope. The detection of bowel cancer is therefore relatively simple, and the 5-year survival in localized cases is 80 percent. With metastasis, survival drops to 40 percent. The incidence in both sexes is approximately equal. Familial polyposis is a condition occurring in several members of the same family and consisting of many small tumors (polyps) throughout the large intestine. These polyps are considered precancerous and their surgical removal is recommended. Fortunately, familial polyposis is a very rare condition.

Stomach cancer, unlike that of the bowel, is usually asymptomatic until late in its course. Five-year survival is only 12 percent. Persons who belong to blood group A are somewhat more susceptible, as are those with pernicious anemia. Male incidence and mortality rates are twice those for females. There is also reason to believe that cancer of the stomach is more common among the poor. The incidence of this disease has been decreasing in the United States, although it is very common in Japan, Iceland, and a number of other countries.

Breast cancer, though virtually limited to the female sex, is nevertheless the third most common cancer. Metastasis often occurs before the tumor is noticed by the patient. The prognosis for localized lesions is good, and in such cases the patient enjoys an 80-percent 5-year survival rate. Breast cancer is more common in whites than blacks and tends to be an affliction of older women who no longer menstruate. It is a form of cancer against which little progress has been made.

In contrast, considerable progress has been made against uterine cancer, the other major female neoplasm. The uterus is a pear-shaped organ composed of a rounded body and a slimmer neck, or cervix. The cervix extends into the posterior end of the vagina. Cancer can develop in either the cervix or uterine body, but the cervical form occurs at an earlier age and carries a less favorable prognosis. Cervical cancer is most common in lower socioeconomic groups, which perhaps explains its high incidence in blacks. Uterine cancer of both types is far more common in **multiparous** women. The Pap smear is credited with greatly improving the outlook in cervical cancer. This test consists of the microscopic examination of cervical mucus in a search for cancerous and precancerous cells. The death rate from uterine cancers has dropped by almost 40 percent in the past 30 years. In addition to the Pap smear, good obstetrical and gynecological care is important to early detection. Some experts feel that circumcision of the male sexual partner is a valuable preventive measure.

MULTIPAROUS: pertaining to a woman who has had more than one pregnancy; primiparous refers to women having a first child

The rise in the incidence of lung cancer began at about the time that the incidence of stomach cancer began to fall. Today lung cancer is the most common neoplasm in males, and its incidence in females is rising. It is associated with cigarette smoking, air pollution, and, as mentioned earlier, exposure to materials such as asbestos. The more one smokes, the higher the risk. Incidence is higher in cities than in rural areas, presumably because of the urban air pollution problem. The usual victim is a middle-aged male who lives in a large city and has a history of years of smoking. Chest x-ray is the only widely available screening procedure, and it is both imprecise and nonspecific. The 5-year survival in this disease is only 5 percent for males and 10 percent for females.

Among children, leukemia is the leading form of neoplastic disease. It is characterized by an abnormal proliferation of the white cells of the blood. The acute form, which is most common in childhood, has a 5-year survival of 1 percent. The chronic form most frequently afflicts older persons and often runs a course of several years' duration. The 5-year survival in the chronic form is between 15 and 20 percent. Patients suffering from leukemia usually succumb to heart failure, brain hemorrhage, or infection. In spite of its importance in children, leukemia is a comparatively rare disease, accounting for only 3 percent of all cancers. In children under 15, however, one cancer in three is leukemia. Exposure to radiation is a most important risk factor. Leukemia has long been identified as a significant occupational hazard of radiologists and others working in close proximity to sources of radioactivity. As might be expected, leukemia has been a major threat to survivors of the atomic holocausts at Hiroshima and Nagasaki. Leukemia is also particularly common in children born to mothers who are x-rayed during pregnancy. This disease is slightly more common in males than females; racial differences are negligible.

Prostatic cancer accounts for 10 percent of cancer deaths in males and is a disease of elderly men. About 75 percent of these tumors can be palpated on careful rectal examination, but more than half have metastasized by the time the diagnosis is made. Other cancers tend to be less common or less important as causes of death than those we have discussed. Table 5-2 summarizes some pertinent cancer facts.

Diabetes Mellitus

Diabetes mellitus is a disease the roots of which are deep in the historical past. The term itself comes from the Greek, meaning "sweet water." It is a chronic disease characterized by insufficiency of a body chemical secreted by the pancreas and known as insulin. Insulin is

TABLE 5-2. Some Facts on Cancer—Five Leading Causes of Cancer Death[a]

Rank	Men	Women
1	Lung	Breast
2	Bowel	Bowel
3	Prostate	Uterus
4	Stomach	Ovary
5	Pancreas	Stomach

Cancers which may tend to occur in families: breast, stomach, colon, prostate, cervix, lung.

Cancers with less than 35-percent survival over 5 years: breast (if not localized), leukemia, lung, stomach, bone, kidney, liver, ovary, and pancreas.

Cancers with more than 50-percent survival over 5 years: localized breast, lymphomas, oral cavity, prostate, localized bowel, skin, cervix, uterus, larynx, bladder.

[a]*Source: Blum and Keranen, eds. Control of Chronic Diseases in Man. Washington, D. C., American Public Health Association, 1966.*

vital to the metabolism of dietary carbohydrates. Normally, carbohydrates are broken down in the intestinal tract into simpler, sugar-like compounds, the most important of which is glucose. Glucose is absorbed into the bloodstream and transported to the liver, where it is stored in a modified form known as glycogen. Insulin is essential to normal glucose utilization; its principal action seems to be its ability to facilitate the entry of glucose into the cells of the liver. In diabetes the insulin supply is inadequate, and glucose levels in the bloodstream rise abnormally, a condition called hyperglycemia. Eventually, the levels of glucose get so high that it appears in the urine. This is known as glycosuria. Testing the urine for glucose is a common screening test for diabetes; but, because blood-sugar levels must be very high before glycosuria appears, some diabetics have sugar-free urine. Urine testing thus yields many false negatives and is a less sensitive screening procedure than determining the glucose levels in a blood sample.

When liver cells are denied glucose, they begin to manufacture it from fat. As by-products of this process, toxic fatty acids accumulate in the bloodstream; this leads to a very serious condition known as diabetic acidosis, which is usually fatal without vigorous treatment. Diabetics also develop arteriosclerosis earlier in life than others. The reasons for this are not clear, but it may be related to an abnormal amount of cholesterol and other fatty substances in the blood. Degenerative changes involving smaller arteries and **capillaries** also occur in diabetics, but this process is thought to be unrelated to arteriosclerosis. These vascular changes ultimately affect the kidneys, eyes, skin, and nerves. Finally, diabetics are especially prone to the development of certain infectious diseases, such as tuberculosis, staphylococcal skin infections, and kidney infections. These infectious processes are also more difficult to treat in diabetic patients.

The etiology of diabetes is not clear. It is equally unclear whether the requirement for insulin reflects insufficient production or increased demand. Many students of the disease feel that diabetes is genetically inherited as a simple autosomal recessive characteristic; but this view is controversial, although it has been known for years that the incidence of diabetes in children of diabetic parents is higher than that found in the general population. Diabetes is often subclinical and tends to be "unmasked" by a number of conditions. These include hyperthyroidism and obesity, as well as pregnancy and prolonged therapy with cortisone, cortisone-like drugs, and **thiazide diuretics.**

The cornerstone of diabetic therapy is, of course, insulin. In milder cases, blood-sugar levels can be reduced to normal by special diets or oral hypoglycemic drugs. These compounds have been used extensively for more than a decade, and their great advantage is that they can be taken by mouth. Recently, a controversy has erupted about their utility in diabetes. Insulin must be given by injection, and for this reason there is a real need for a safe and effective oral preparation. Unfortunately, there is little evidence that either insulin or a substitute for it does much to avert the many complications which plague diabetics. The basic effect and significant benefit of therapy is that it keeps the patient out of the highly fatal acidotic state.

One fairly common complication of diabetic therapy is hypoglycemic shock, which results from an overdose of insulin or oral drugs. It is characterized by a precipitous drop in blood pressure, sweating, agitation, and **palpitation.** Hypoglycemic shock is an excellent example of a break in the delicate balance required in insulin therapy. Too much produces hypoglycemia, while too little can lead to acidosis. Further, blood-sugar levels

---

CAPILLARY: the very smallest of the blood vessels, they connect the arterial and venous circulatory systems, deliver oxygen and nurture to the body organs, and carry away waste products

THIAZIDE: the name applied to a group of commonly used diuretic drugs

DIURETIC: a drug which increases urinary output

PALPITATION: a transient irregular heartbeat

depend on physical activity and on the size, composition, and regularity of meals. Exercise implies the need for more insulin; longer-than-usual periods between meals lowers the insulin requirement. In no disease is careful education of the patient more critical than in diabetes.

Because of vascular complications, a decrease in the blood supply to the lower extremities is common in diabetes and often precedes frank gangrene of the toes. Frequently, amputation of the affected toe, foot, or lower leg is required to alleviate this condition. Vascular complications which affect the eye make diabetes the third leading cause of blindness in the United States. Diabetics are at greater risk in surgery. Pregnant diabetics are also at greater risk, as are their babies, many of whom resemble prematures even though they tend to be heavier than most newborns. Renal failure, cerebrovascular accidents, and coronary artery disease are also common complications which often prove fatal to the diabetic patient.

It is estimated that 2 percent of the total population has diabetes, and that only half of these people are aware of their condition. Diabetes ranks eighth as a cause of death. Prevalence of the disease increases with age and reaches a peak at about 70 years. When compared to those in the general population, disability rates are three times higher in diabetics. Diabetes cannot be prevented, and the prognosis is worse in younger diabetics, who tend to develop complications sooner than older patients. Fortunately, only 5 percent of diabetics are under the age of 25. Average life-expectancy in diabetics is about 15 years from the time of diagnosis. Consequently, the effect of the disease on the longevity of a particular individual depends primarily on how old he is when the disease appears.

Chronic Respiratory Disease

This term is a very general one which covers a number of noninfectious, noncancerous illnesses of the respiratory system. The most important of these are chronic bronchitis and emphysema. Chronic bronchitis usually precedes emphysema, although it is an unresolved question whether they are separate entities or simply different phases in the development of the same basic disease process. Chronic bronchitis is an inflammation of the bronchial tree, characterized by the secretion of thick mucus. Cough and the production of sputum are the usual symptoms, and they tend to persist for months at a time. Colds and other URIs make the condition worse. Chronic bronchitis is more common in Britain than in the United States, but the great importance of the disease in this country is underscored by a prevalence of 15 to 20 percent among persons above 40 years of age.

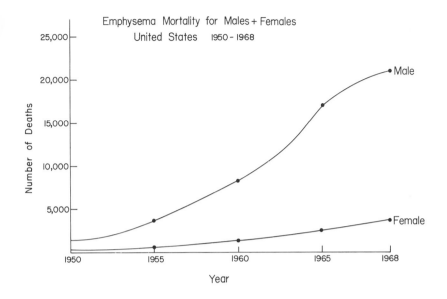

FIG. 5-5.   *Although this chart shows that emphysema primarily affects males, the attack rate among females increased more rapidly during the 1950-1968 period. (Statistics from National Tuberculosis and Respiratory Disease Association.)*

Emphysema involves a chronic and permanent loss of pulmonary elasticity. Small saclike structures (alveoli) in the lungs are severely damaged in emphysema, and their functional ability is greatly impaired. As a result, oxygen exchange is less efficient, and patients who suffer with emphysema are often persistently short of breath. Almost 70 percent of emphysema patients give a history of cough with sputum production, symptoms compatible with chronic bronchitis. Ninety percent are heavy smokers; males outnumber females 10 to 1. The causal role of air pollution in these chronic respiratory diseases is unclear, but it is well known that polluted air greatly aggravates the condition. The association of bronchitis and emphysema with urban areas and persons in lower socioeconomic groups probably reflects the greater exposure to air pollution in the poorer areas of cities.

Over-all mortality rates for bronchitis are low, but male rates are rising and female rates are decreasing. The low death rates from bronchitis are probably largely explained by the fact that so many of these patients die of emphysema. Death rates from emphysema increased 15 times in the 18-year period between 1950 and 1968 (Fig. 5-5). The 1968 rate of 12.1 per 100,000 may seem low, but it is sobering to consider that a second

15-fold increase in this rate would make emphysema the nation's third leading killer by 1980. The prevalence of emphysema increases with advancing age, and present estimates are that about 3 percent of the over-40 population is affected. Specific preventive measures are unavailable for those chronic respiratory diseases. Nevertheless, as we have seen with lung cancer and cardiovascular disease, abstinence from cigarettes eliminates at least one of the most significant risk factors. Once emphysema appears, cessation of cigarette smoking tends to slow down progression of the disease. The long-term prognosis in emphysema is poor, but careful treatment and avoidance of cigarettes can often prolong life and limit disability. Patients with emphysema most often succumb to heart failure, with pneumonia a common complicating factor.

Allergic Disorders

Earlier in this book we discussed immunity and the protective effects of antibodies. It was noted that exposure of an antigenic microorganism stimulates host production of antibodies specific for that particular antigen. Reexposure to the same antigen calls forth antibody and serves to remove the host from harm's way. This antibody-recall phenomenon is known as an anamnestic response. It occurs in individuals who have been sensitized by prior exposure to the antigen and are therefore hypersensitive to that antigen. Ironically, the obvious advantages of this protective mechanism are tempered by certain disadvantages, the most prominent of which are allergic reactions. Unfortunately, a number of materials besides microorganisms serve as antigens in some people. Examples include grasses, pollens, animal hair, dust, and a number of other commonly encountered substances. These antigens are often referred to as allergens. The term allergy refers to the antigen-antibody reaction that occurs when a hypersensitive host is exposed to antigenic substances. The terms allergy and hypersensitivity are often used interchangeably.

For our purposes we will distinguish two basic kinds of allergies—immediate and delayed. The immediate type refers to the swiftness with which the host's skin reacts to the injection or application of allergenic test material. These reactions usually occur within a half-hour. In the delayed type the reaction appears only after 24 to 72 hours. An additional point of distinction is that the antibodies produced in immediate reactions circulate in the bloodstream and can be passively transferred from the host to other individuals. The antibodies characteristic of delayed reactions are believed to exist at the cellular level, and they cannot be transferred from man to man through serum, although in some cases these antibodies can be transferred by means of cells or cell extracts. The runny noses, headaches, and sneezes of hay fever exemplify the immediate type of response. The tuberculin skin test, which is read after about 48 hours, is an example of a delayed reaction.

The most serious immediate reaction is anaphylaxis. It follows reexposure to certain kinds of allergenic materials, most prominent of which are penicillin and the venom introduced by the sting of a bee, wasp, or hornet. Anaphylaxis is characterized by spasms of the air passages, dilation of the vascular tree, **tachycardia**, and giant hives. The victim is short of breath and lapses into deep shock as his blood pressure falls. Anaphylaxis is often fatal but can be treated successfully with epinephrine, which dilates the bronchial tree and constricts the arterioles. This condition is most common in persons who suffer from other allergies. The number of anaphylactic deaths due to insect stings is unknown, but each year about 100 persons succumb to anaphylaxis following the injection of penicillin.

In terms of morbidity, hay fever and asthma are the most important allergic disorders of the immediate type. Hay fever, an inflammation of the nasal passages, is difficult to distinguish from the **rhinitis** accompanying the common cold. For this reason prevalence is largely unknown. A wide range of allergens can precipitate hay fever, but pollens are perhaps the most ubiquitous. It is for hay fever sufferers that radio and television broadcasts regularly announce a "pollen count." Hay fever is often relieved by any of a group of drugs known as antihistamines. Histamine is one of several body chemicals released as a result of the reaction of antibody and allergen.

Asthma is a condition characterized by bronchial spasm and oversecretion of mucus. Attacks follow the introduction of an allergen by way of the respiratory system. Asthma is commonly divided into **extrinsic** and **intrinsic** types. The former, a disease of childhood and early adult life, usually subsides by the age of 30. It is related to specific allergens and is most common in those with a family history of allergies. Attacks tend to be intermittent. Roughly half of all asthma cases are of this type. The intrinsic type has its onset after the age of 40, and its relationship to allergenic substances is uncertain. Attacks frequently follow upper respiratory infections, but mild symptoms are often present most of the time.

TACHYCARDIA: very rapid heartbeat
RHINITIS: inflammation of the nasal passages; most commonly used to describe a "stopped-up" or "runny" nose
EXTRINSIC: arising outside the host; similar to exogenous
INTRINSIC: arising within the host; similar to endogenous

This form of asthma is often difficult to distinguish from chronic bronchitis, and it is not an uncommon precursor to emphysema. Status asthmaticus is an intractable, sustained asthmatic attack which lasts several days and is a common cause of death in asthma patients. Heart failure and pneumonia are also important causes of death in asthmatics. About 5 million Americans suffer with hay fever or asthma, and about one-fifth of them must limit their activities as a result. About 200,000 are so severely disabled that they are unable to work. Almost all of the death and disability resulting from asthma occurs in persons suffering with the intrinsic type.

Less important immediate-type allergies include hives and eczema. Also known as urticaria, hives are large, raised, red, itching wheals which appear shortly after exposure to an allergen. Hives often occur only once in a lifetime, and it is estimated that 20 percent of the population has had at least one episode. Eczema is a disease of early childhood and often precedes hay fever and asthma. It affects about 2 percent of children and is a self-limiting skin condition which is characterized by reddening, thickening, and itching. When immunized against smallpox, eczema patients are very susceptible to a serious generalized vaccinia infection, and smallpox vaccination is therefore contraindicated in these children.

In addition to tuberculosis, a number of other infectious diseases—including histoplasmosis and typhoid—are capable of producing a delayed type of reaction when antigenic substances are injected into the skin. In a few diseases, notably tuberculosis and histoplasmosis, this reaction in persons previously infected with the disease agent forms the basis of a diagnostic test. Another type of delayed reaction is contact dermatitis. Undoubtedly the most familiar affliction of this group is poison ivy. A large number of industrial chemicals are capable of producing contact dermatitis, and the high prevalence of this condition in industry is an important cause of absenteeism. Another example of delayed hypersensitivity is the rejection of organs transplanted from one person to another. Heart transplants have received the most publicity, but kidney transplants are more common. In either case the donated organ represents an enormous mass of foreign protein against which the new host reacts. The rejection of donated organs is the main problem in transplant surgery.

Delayed hypersensitivity is also involved in the so-called "auto-immune" diseases. In these conditions the body forms antibodies against its own tissues for reasons which are presently obscure. It is suspected that an

---

VACCINIA: a virus which primarily affects cows; also known as cowpox; it is used to immunize humans against smallpox because immunity to cowpox produces immunity to smallpox as well

auto-immune process is at work in pernicious anemia, ulcerative colitis, glomerulonephritis, and a group of conditions known as **collagen** diseases. Most prominent among the collagen diseases is rheumatoid arthritis. This is a very common condition affecting about 6 percent of the population. It generally begins in the fourth decade of life and over the years contributes heavily to disability and invalidism. Arthritis affecting the spine is most common in men, but the more common disease of wrists, hands, knees, and so on, predominantly afflicts women. Rheumatoid arthritis is more than three times as common in persons with a family history of the disease. It is subject to long periods of **remission,** but recurrence is usual.

On the face of it, it would seem that many allergic disorders are subject to primary prevention. Obviously, the antigens involved in auto-immune disorders are not avoidable. Less obvious is the fact that avoidance of other antigens is often so difficult as to be impractical. One can escape ragweed pollens by migrating to Europe, but there is no assurance that European antigens will not cause just as much misery. The simple truth is that pollens, dusts, and other airborne allergens are almost impossible to avoid without literally sealing oneself off from the environment. Some foods can be successfully avoided, but it is extremely difficult to eliminate eggs and milk, the most common sources of food allergy. In one form or another these foodstuffs are present in virtually all processed foods. In addition, several vaccines are prepared with eggs or egg products. Drugs and the agents involved in contact dermatitis are easiest to avoid, the former by the use of substitute preparations and the latter by simple expedients such as the wearing of gloves.

Secondary prevention of allergic disorders entails the process of desensitization. It is sometimes of value in hay fever and extrinsic asthma, if the offending allergens can be identified. Desensitization involves the repeated injection of small amounts of material from the provoking antigen. For undetermined reasons, such injections stimulate the production of antibodies different from those associated with hay fever or asthma. These new antibodies combine with the allergen and thus "block" the harmful allergen-antibody reaction. This approach is effective only in some cases, and the prevention of allergic disorders in general is less than satisfactory. As for treatment, it is often difficult but can nevertheless be quite helpful. Antihistamines are effective against hives and hay fever but are of no value in asthma and eczema. Steroid drugs, because of their anti-inflammatory properties, are of value in a number of allergic disorders.

COLLAGEN: a protein that is a principal component of connective tissue
REMISSION: a period in the course of an illness, during which time the patient is totally free of disease manifestations

Dental Disorders

Dental disease is so common that its absence is abnormal. One reason for this high prevalence rate is the erratic way in which most people obtain care. Each year, about 45 percent of the population visit a dentist, even though 70 percent have untreated caries (Fig. 5-6). By the age of 35, 70 percent of the population need dentures to replace lost teeth. Among those over 55, at least half have no teeth at all. Dental disease is especially common among the poor, in whom prevalence exceeds 90 percent (Fig. 5-7). In some ways it is perhaps fortunate that public apathy remains at a high level. If all the people who need it decided to seek dental care, 5 to 10 times as many dentists would be required to meet the demand.

Dental caries is the most commonly encountered problem. It is a process through which tooth structure is broken down and a cavity is produced in the tooth enamel. It is believed that dental caries is caused by a type of streptococcus which is normally present in the oral cavity. The bacteria become part of a plaquelike calcified mass known as calculus, which forms on the surface of the teeth. The calculus is the precursor to dental decay. The bacteria thrive on carbohydrates, particularly sugar; and the elimination of foods with a high sugar content might do much to reduce the incidence of dental caries. Brushing the teeth after meals is also considered a valuable preventive measure.

As might be expected, the most effective way to prevent dental caries involves primary prevention, specifically the presence of fluorides in drinking water. Some communities enjoy naturally fluorinated water. Elsewhere, the addition of fluorides to water supplies is now common in the United States. Fluorides are also found in a variety of foods, including fish, meat, vegetables, and potatoes. The preventive benefits of fluoridation are maximized if intake begins at birth. Fluoridated water supplies reduce the prevalence of dental caries by almost 70 percent. Fluoridation provides a good example of the economics of prevention. The 70 million people who visit the dentist each year spend about $2.5 billion on dental care. Fluoridation costs roughly 10 cents per capita. Thus, the entire population of the United States could be served by a fluoridated water supply for less than the amount now spent on dental care by about one-third of the American people. Where water is not fluoridated, fluorides may be applied directly to the teeth. Topical fluorides reduce caries by 40 to 50 percent if started as soon as teeth appear.

Tooth loss is most commonly due to periodontal disease. The principal manifestations are gingivitis and periodontitis. Gingivitis is an inflamma-

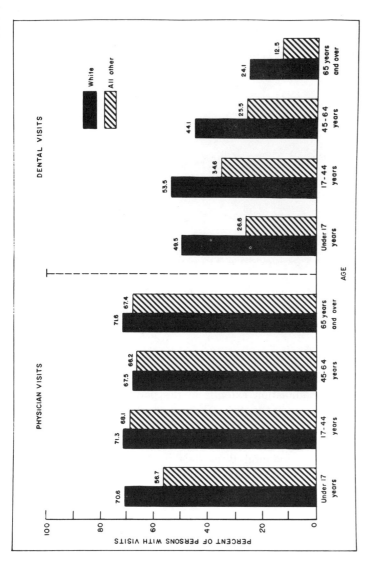

Fig. 5-6. *While approximately 69 percent of the total population received treatment from a physician in 1969, only 45 percent visited a dentist. Note that the difference in utilization of medical services by color is more striking for dental than for medical (From U.S. National Center for Health Statistics, Age Patterns in Medical Care, Illness, and Disability, U.S. 1968-1969, Public Health Service Publication, Series No. 10, No. 70, Washington, D.C., 1972.)*

153

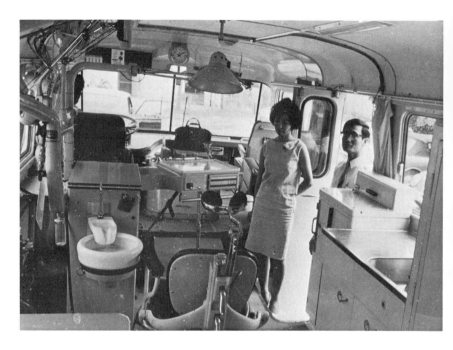

FIG. 5-7. *Mobile dental units are of value in rural areas without dental services. Ironically, they may have a role in urban areas where dentists and other health providers tend to be distributed at great distance from low income neighborhoods. (Courtesy of Dr. C. L. Marshall.)*

tion of the gums. This condition begins early in life and is due to bacteria, food debris, crowded teeth, incorrect teeth-brushing, and calculus formation. When the inflammation extends to the periodontal membrane, the condition is known as periodontitis. The periodontal membrane, the gums, and the underlying bone comprise the supporting tissues of the teeth. Once these supporting tissues are compromised, tooth loss follows as a matter of course. Periodontal disease is most common in low-income groups. It is believed that proper brushing of the teeth and regular visits to the dentist for professional teeth-cleaning are effective in preventing periodontal disease.

Visual Defects

The importance of visual disorders is apparent from the fact that half the United States population wear eyeglasses. In addition, over

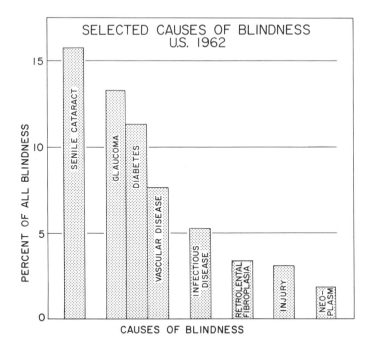

FIG. 5-8.   *Of the eight causes of blindness presented here, it is important to note that diabetes ranks third. Infectious diseases are a less important cause today than in years past. Most of these cases resulted from a gonorrheal infection of the eyes resulting from travel through the birth canal (vagina) of an infected mother. In developing countries, the viral eye infection, trachoma, is a common cause of blindness. Retrolental fibroplasia affects infants exposed to high levels of oxygen in incubators. Blindness developed in thousands of babies before the connection between retrolental fibroplasia and oxygen was discovered. Retrolental fibroplasia is thus an example of an iatrogenic disease. (From* Diabetes Source Book, *U.S. Department of Health, Education and Welfare, Public Health Service Publication No. 1168, 1967.)*

a million people must restrict their activities to a greater or lesser extent because of poor vision, and over 400 000 of these are legally blind. Legal blindness is a term used to denote **visual acuity** worse than 20/200 in the better eye. This means that the blind person must be within 20 feet of an object to see it clearly, while one with normal vision can clearly see the object from a distance of 200 feet. Blindness is a relative concept that includes people who literally see nothing at all, as well as those who per-

---

VISUAL ACUITY: sharpness or clarity of vision

ceive light but cannot differentiate objects. In one form or another, assistance to the blind costs the nation about $150 million a year.

Most of the 100 million American eyeglass-wearers need these devices to correct refractive errors. Light rays passing through the cornea and lens of the eye are focused on the rear-most part of the eye, known as the retina. Light rays entering the eye from the external environment must be bent, or refracted, to focus on a small area like the retina. Refractive errors thus refer to the bending of light rays in a manner that produces a blurred retinal image. The most common refractive errors result in myopia, or nearsightedness, and hyperopia, or farsightedness. The term presbyopia refers to the progressive loss of visual acuity with advancing age. Astigmatism is the abnormal warping of the lens of the eye, a condition in which part of the visual field is blurred. Most of these errors can be corrected through the use of eyeglasses, but very serious refractive errors are the fourth most common cause of legal blindness.

The leading cause of blindness in the United States is cataract (Fig. 5-8). Cataract refers to opacity of the lens of the eye, and it is usually present in both eyes. This condition is most common in the elderly and in diabetics. Cataracts also occur congenitally, in which case they are especially common in children born to mothers who had rubella during the first trimester of pregnancy. Almost all persons over the age of 60 have some degree of lens opacity, and almost all of these cases can be surgically corrected.

The cornea is the transparent anterior part of the eye. Infections, chemicals, and physical trauma sometimes lead to corneal opacities which cause blindness because they block light rays entering the eyes. These opacities can be corrected surgically by transplanting a cornea from a donor. Such transplants are usually successful because the cornea has no blood supply and is thus free of the antibodies which so often lead to rejection in other transplants.

Glaucoma is a disease characterized by an abnormal increase in the pressure of the fluid lying between the cornea and the lens of the eye. Most frequently glaucoma is a primary condition, but it is occasionally secondary to a tumor or an infectious process. Glaucoma is often a genetically inherited trait that manifests itself during the fourth decade of life. About 2 percent of people over 40 are affected, and, even though the condition is treatable, glaucoma presently accounts for about 15 percent of blindness. The disease can be detected by a simple test that is often included in multiphasic screening programs. Examination is most important for relatives of index cases.

Strabismus, also known as "cross-eyes," is a common condition of childhood and affects about 1 percent of school children. When the eyes cross, they do not focus on the same objects. This produces double vision. The

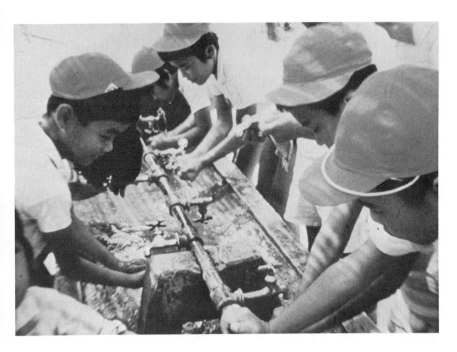

FIG. 5-9.   *These Okinawan children are required to wash their hands and faces at school. Commonly, however, they dry themselves on a towel shared by all. In this way, trachoma is transmitted from child to child. Unfortunately incomplete personal hygiene can be worse than none at all. (Courtesy of Dr. C. L. Marshall.)*

brain compensates by suppressing one of the images, and this, in effect, leaves one eye unused. Strabismus most commonly results from infections of the central nervous system or from injuries occurring at birth. Weakness of the muscles controlling eye movement is also a frequent cause.

On a worldwide basis, the most common cause of blindness is a viral disease known as trachoma. This is a condition which results in extensive scarring of the eyelid and cornea. It is transmitted from person to person by direct contact and perhaps indirect contact as well (Fig. 5-9). Although trachoma is easily cured by antibiotics, reinfection is usual. In the developing countries, where trachoma is most prevalent, it is highly unlikely that this disease can be controlled without the development of a vaccine or a massive improvement in sanitary and living conditions. In the United States, trachoma remains a problem only among American Indians living in the Southwest.

Hearing Defects

About 7 million Americans suffer some degree of hearing loss, and almost 4 million of these people are totally deaf. Deafness is defined as a hearing loss in excess of 30 **decibels**. In many cases hearing loss is apparently inherited; but there are many other causes, including diseases of intrauterine life (such as maternal rubella), perinatal conditions (such as **kernicterus**), and infectious diseases in early childhood (e.g., meningitis). Otitis media, a very common complication of a simple upper respiratory infection, often produces permanent hearing loss in young children. This is most likely to occur when otitis media becomes chronic, as it often does in children experiencing repeated upper respiratory infections. Adults with previously normal hearing often suffer hearing loss because of prolonged exposure to excessive noise (more than 100 decibels) or as a result of a disease known as otosclerosis.

Hearing loss can be divided into two basic types: nerve deafness and conduction deafness. Nerve deafness refers to a disorder of the nerve pathways leading from the ear to the brain. This is the more common type in children; it arises, as we have seen, from infection, birth injury, or perinatal toxic brain damage. Nerve deafness is incurable, but most children are helped by the use of hearing aids. It is important to distinguish deafness from mental retardation, a distinction often more difficult to make than might be expected. Hereditary hearing loss is thought to be fairly common; but its prevalence is hard to establish, because hearing deficits that might be considered hereditary may also be caused by some unknown nonhereditary factor. It is estimated that 50 percent of hearing losses in children are either hereditary or of unknown etiology.

The second basic type of hearing loss is conduction deafness. This condition occurs when the three bony structures in the middle ear fail to operate properly in transmitting sound from the external environment to the nerve endings of the middle ear. Otitis media and otosclerosis are common causes of conduction deafness. Otosclerosis is a disease of adults that is most common in white females. In about 1 percent of cases it causes hearing loss by immobilizing the bones of the middle ear.

Hearing ability normally decreases with increasing age. This conse-

---

DECIBEL: the unit of sound volume or loudness
KERNICTERUS: a condition of newborns which is characterized by severe jaundice and
   which often results in brain damage

quence of aging is most common in males, and both ears are usually affected. Sometimes this natural process is accelerated when certain drugs are used, particularly streptomycin, kanamycin, and the antimalarial drugs quinine and chloroquine.

Disorders of speech are closely related to hearing loss, especially in childhood. It is difficult to teach a person to speak if he cannot hear. About one-half of all speech problems in children are mild disorders like lisping or stuttering. The other half are due to a number of conditions, including congenital deafness, **cerebral palsy**, mental retardation, head injuries, and cleft palate. Speech disturbances in adults are commonly associated with diseases affecting the brain. These include cerebrovascular accidents, **multiple sclerosis**, brain tumors, **Parkinson's disease**, and an uncommon hereditary illness known as **Huntington's chorea**. People at all ages with speech disorders can usually benefit from professional speech therapy.

Chronic Disease and the Common Good

Although it is unquestionably true that medicine deals most effectively with acute illnesses and infections, it would be erroneous to conclude that current medical skill and knowledge are impotent or of little value against the challenges of chronic illness. Despite the many battles yet to be won, remarkable progress has been made in the extent to which death can be delayed, discomfort eased, and disability avoided. Indeed, it is the very possibility of these benefits that serves to focus attention on the long waits, high costs, fragmented services, and other problems so prominent in the continuing national concern with the "health care crisis."

The fact that chronic illness is managed rather than cured points up an issue of greatest importance to the society at large. Long-term management of a disease requires the constant and permanent assignment of re-

---

CEREBRAL PALSY: a number of conditions which have in common a deficit of neurological function; include defects of speech, hearing, and vision as well as convulsions and mental retardation

MULTIPLE SCLEROSIS: a chronic degenerative disease of the spinal cord; produces a variety of neurological symptoms and is most common in young adults

PARKINSON'S DISEASE: a chronic illness characterized by rigidity of the limbs and a fine tremor of the hands

HUNTINGTON'S CHOREA: a hereditary disease with onset in early adult life; produces dementia and bizarre, involuntary movements of the body

sources (money, drugs, equipment, and so on) both to the disease and the afflicted individual. Since even the richest country on earth does not have unlimited resources, some person or agency must decide who shall receive the benefit of what is available and, of equal importance, who shall not. The considerations involved in such decisions are complicated, difficult, and controversial. There are more critical questions than satisfactory answers. But for every health professional the questions—some of which we will raise here—are unavoidable, and the search for acceptable resolutions is an ongoing part of professional effort.

Each year approximately 50,000 persons in the United States find themselves in the unenviable position of requiring permanent, frequent, and expensive medical intervention to prevent death from kidney failure. In these people the ravages of chronic renal infection, chronic glomerulonephritis, or congenital kidney defects have rendered the kidneys useless. The functions of this vital organ must be provided by a kidney transplant or by a complex machine which makes possible a process known as dialysis. For a number of reasons renal transplants are often difficult to obtain, and dialysis is thus the sole alternative for most patients. Several times each week these patients must spend most of the day "on the machine." A permanent shunt in the arm directly connects an artery to a vein; and, when the patient is "hooked up," blood from the artery is routed through the dialysis machine where it is cleansed of the accumulated toxic waste products normally excreted by a healthy kidney. Following its trip through this machine, blood reenters the patient's body by emptying into the vein. When the process is completed, the arterial-venous shunt is reestablished, and the patient can look forward to a day or two of normal existence before he must again be dialyzed.

In addition to being permanent and frequent, dialysis is very expensive. It therefore presents a classic example of the difficulties encountered in deciding how resources should be allocated. It costs about $40,000 per year to be dialyzed three times a week in a hospital. If dialysis is carried out at home (where the spouse, relatives, or friends do the work), the cost is reduced to about $3,500 yearly. Home dialysis, however, requires an investment of $10,000 to purchase the machine, and the constant and frequent demand on family members to attend the machine precludes the possibility of their full-time employment.

Whether treatment occurs in the home or the hospital, the costs of dialysis are obviously sufficient to wipe out the savings of most middle-class families. Partly for this reason, only about 15 percent of the patients who would benefit from dialysis actually receive it. In some cases, in order to protect the financial integrity of the family, patients refuse to begin or fail to continue dialysis. In others, patients dislike living tied to a machine and choose not to undergo endless treatment sessions which can only maintain an unsatisfactory status quo.

Let us consider the hypothetical case of a man who opts to discontinue dialysis and dies as a result of his decision. Let us further imagine that this patient was a poor man who had received his dialysis treatment at public expense. Can we say that the patient committed suicide when he discontinued dialysis? If budget cuts had forced the Welfare Department to discontinue financial support for treatment, could we say that murder had been committed? With funds to care for indigent patients in short supply, is it proper to spend large sums on this patient and thus consume money which, for example, might be used to treat curable conditions in school children? Who should make such a decision and upon what criteria should it be based? Should doctors decide? lawyers? politicians? theologians? a representative committee?

The simplest, though perhaps most cynical, basis for such decisions would be money. Agonizing choices would be eliminated, at least for the providers of care, and a person could either afford to buy life or not. To a large extent this is what happens with regard to dialysis. In the absence of an insurance plan or a public obligation to bear the costs of therapy, the law of supply and demand would seem to be the order of the day. However, there is widespread dissatisfaction with this situation and a growing feeling that a better decision-making mechanism is needed. But if one decides the matter of survival on grounds other than financial, who bears the cost for poor patients? If it is decided that a given patient shall live and this decision is later changed, who turns off the machine? Does a physician face a murder charge if he stops therapy? And if the physician stops therapy at the request of the patient, is it murder or suicide?

Thus far we have asked whether the expenditure of resources to maintain life in the face of incurable disease is justified when there is a competing need to allocate resources for the prevention or cure of more tractable illnesses. We have also asked which incurable patients should be maintained if resources to maintain all cannot be found. Both questions involve issues of an ethical, a moral, and a philosophical nature. Beyond these questions, however, lies the still larger question of whether more resources should be allocated for direct patient care at all. Will more doctors and more hospitals reduce the incidence and prevalence of heart disease or cancer? To date, the answer seems to be a negative one. The life expectancy of men in the United States has remained essentially unchanged for over a decade; yet during this same period expenditures for medical care increased tremendously. Middle-aged Swedish men have a mortality rate half that of American men of similar age. This is in spite of the fact that Swedes visit physicians less regularly than Americans, and Americans are served by one physician for every 700 citizens, while Swedes must get by on one for every 1,200.

Although health seems almost independent of physicians, it is strongly correlated with poverty and factors significantly related to poverty, i.e., nutrition, sanitation, population density, and so on. Poor people tend to have poor health. We have provided medical care for the poor, sometimes in the belief that ill health causes poverty. Perhaps it would be worthwhile to attack poverty with the expectation that health would improve. The more than $60 billion spent annually on medical care is enough to provide about $300 per year for every man, woman, and child in the United States. Would the interests of health be better served by an annual government subsidy of $300 paid to each individual or, in the case of children, to their parents?

It was noted at the outset that many questions would be raised to which the answers are unclear, although the need to pursue them is urgent. The difficult issues implicit in this brief discussion arise from the present status of medical technology—both its limitations and its ability, given ample resources, to prolong life. Recognizing that these issues exist and must be dealt with is the first step toward solutions; further, an awareness and appreciation of one's technology is the essential difference between a professional and a technician.

References

Blum, H., and Keranen, G., eds. Control of Chronic Diseases in Man. Washington, D.C., American Public Health Association, 1966.

Burton, L. E., and Smith, H. H. Public Health and Community Medicine. Baltimore, Williams and Wilkins, 1970.

Sartwell, P., ed. Maxcy-Rosenau Preventive Medicine and Public Health, 9th ed. New York, Appleton-Century-Crofts, 1965.

The New York Times. February 28, 1971.

The New York Times. October 24, 1971.

Wintrobe, M., et al., eds. Harrison's Principles of Internal Medicine, 6th ed. New York, McGraw-Hill, 1970.

CHAPTER

6

Health Problems of Mothers, Children, and the Elderly

By and large, all persons in the general population are prey to specific diseases and environmental conditions hazardous to health. However, a number of illnesses are distinctly associated with certain sub-populations within the whole. The health problems of the largest and most important of these sub-populations comprise the subject of this chapter.

Maternal and Child Health

MATERNAL HEALTH

This term refers specifically to the health of pregnant women and of mothers during the **postpartum** period. Until the relatively recent past, the hazards of childbirth were awesome, and maternal mor-

---

POSTPARTUM: occurring after childbirth

TABLE 6-1. Maternal Mortality Rate (per 100,000) by Race
(United States, 1915–1968)

Rank	White	Black	Total
1915	601	1,056	608
1925	603	1,162	647
1935	531	946	582
1945	172	455	207
1955	33	130	47
1966	20	72	29
1968	17	64	24

aSource: United States Department of Commerce, Historical Statistics of the United States,
Colonial Times to 1957; and Statistical Abstracts of the United States, 1971.

tality was the leading cause of death among young adult women. The
spectacular decline in maternal mortality during the twentieth century
is without question a major factor in the present longevity advantage
women enjoy over men in industrialized countries. Unfortunately, maternal deaths are still very high in much of the nonindustrialized world.
Table 6-1 reveals the trend in maternal mortality in the United States
since 1915. It shows a decline of 95 percent in white mortality and an
impressive but less pronounced decline for blacks, whose rate is almost
four times higher. The higher mortality among blacks is closely related
to their economic status; thus, to a large extent, the real challenge of
maternal health is the task of securing adequate medical care for low-
income pregnant women.

Three conditions account for more than 90 percent of all maternal
deaths. In order of importance these are hemorrhage, infection, and
toxemia, a disease unique to pregnant women. Hemorrhage during the
postpartum period is the most serious threat to maternal survival. It
occurs as a result of difficult labor or injury ensuing from labor. In addition, postpartum hemorrhage is commonly related to uterine bleeding
associated with retained **placental** fragments. Maternal infection may be
caused by a number of different bacteria, but streptococci account for
about two-thirds of cases. **Puerperal sepsis,** as this type of infection is

PLACENTA: an organ developed by the fertilized ovum and adherent to the uterine
wall; serves the fetus as its organ of nutrition, respiration, and excretion;
sometimes known as "afterbirth"
PUERPERAL: pertaining to the 6-week period following childbirth
SEPSIS: infection

often called, is essentially a wound infection. Septicemia and peritonitis are the most serious complications, and they are occasionally fatal even in this era of antibiotics. Puerperal infections are most common in women who are exhausted after prolonged labor or those in whom hemorrhage or incomplete placental separation has occurred.

Toxemia is also known as eclampsia. It is a condition which develops in the latter third of pregnancy and is characterized by hypertension, edema, rapid weight gain, and **proteinuria**. In severe cases these symptoms and signs are followed by convulsions or coma or both. Mild or severe toxemia occurs in about 10 percent of all pregnancies. Like hemorrhage and infection, toxemia is most commonly encountered in low-income women from minority groups.

It is a quiet tragedy that almost three-quarters of maternal deaths are probably preventable. The key to prevention lies in adequate prenatal care, but studies have shown that the extent to which women seek and receive such care varies directly with family income and education. It is not unusual for 40 percent of maternity patients in large municipal hospitals to have entered with no previous prenatal care whatever. The particular value of prenatal care is in the opportunity it affords to identify potential problems early, when they can often be easily corrected. This care generally includes an initial visit to the physician, who takes a history, does a physical examination, and arranges for a series of laboratory tests—all of which enable him to evaluate the health status of the expectant mother accurately. Return visits to the physician at monthly, bi-weekly, and, finally, weekly intervals provide ample opportunity to detect any changes in the condition of the patient. Three groups of women are at particularly high risk during pregnancy: those with a history of previous abortions or stillbirths; those with a history of difficult pregnancies; and those with known medical complications such as heart disease or diabetes.

Induced abortion, which is illegal in most states, is an important factor in the problem of maternal mortality (See Appendix 7). Although it is estimated that more than one million abortions are performed illegally each year, the cloak of secrecy that drapes this very common practice obscures the incidence of maternal and infant deaths from this cause. The legalization of abortion in an important issue in the intensifying struggle toward full equality for women. Whether or not abortions should be legal is a controversial question morally and politically (Fig. 6-1). From a health standpoint, however, there seems little doubt that the medical care which tends to accompany legalized abortion substantially reduces what for many women is a health hazard of major proportions.

PROTEINURIA: protein in the urine

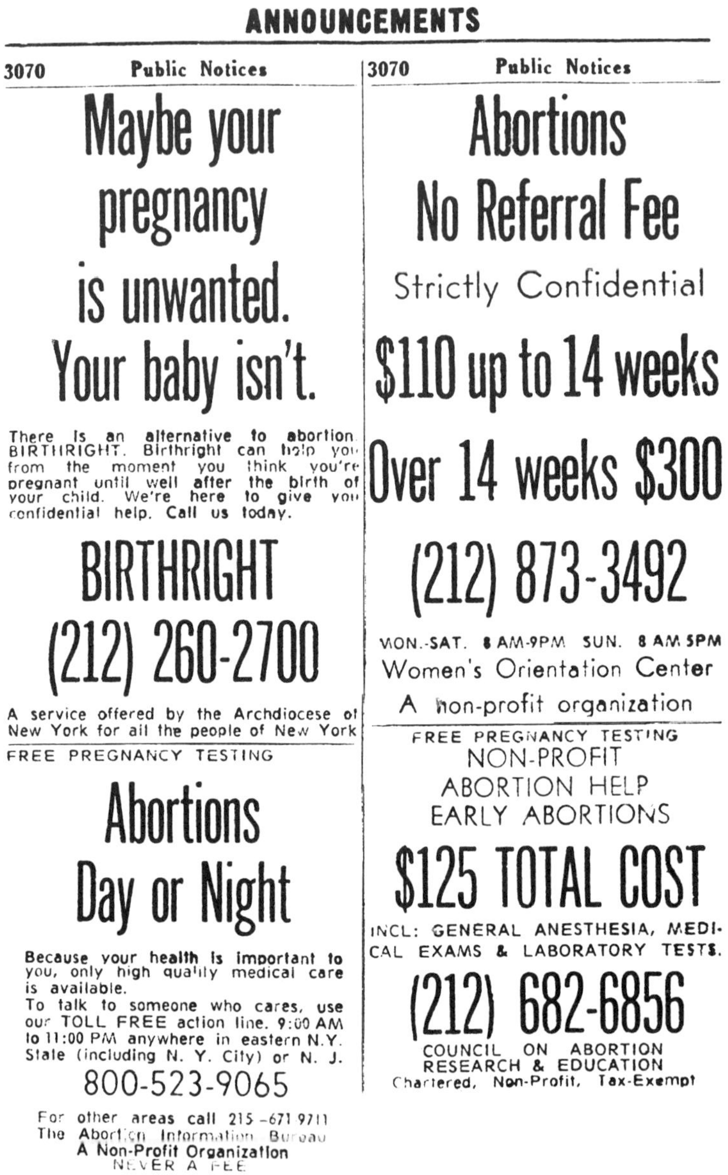

ANNOUNCEMENTS

3070 Public Notices

Maybe your pregnancy is unwanted. Your baby isn't.

There is an alternative to abortion. BIRTHRIGHT. Birthright can help you from the moment you think you're pregnant until well after the birth of your child. We're here to give you confidential help. Call us today.

BIRTHRIGHT

(212) 260-2700

A service offered by the Archdiocese of New York for all the people of New York

FREE PREGNANCY TESTING

Abortions Day or Night

Because your health is important to you, only high quality medical care is available.
To talk to someone who cares, use our TOLL FREE action line. 9:00 AM to 11:00 PM anywhere in eastern N.Y. State (including N. Y. City) or N. J.

800-523-9065

For other areas call 215-671 9711
The Abortion Information Bureau
A Non-Profit Organization
NEVER A FEE

3070 Public Notices

Abortions No Referral Fee

Strictly Confidential

$110 up to 14 weeks

Over 14 weeks $300

(212) 873-3492

MON.-SAT. 8 AM-9PM SUN. 8 AM 5PM
Women's Orientation Center
A non-profit organization

FREE PREGNANCY TESTING
NON-PROFIT
ABORTION HELP
EARLY ABORTIONS

$125 TOTAL COST

INCL: GENERAL ANESTHESIA, MEDICAL EXAMS & LABORATORY TESTS.

(212) 682-6856

COUNCIL ON ABORTION RESEARCH & EDUCATION
Chartered, Non-Profit, Tax-Exempt

FIG. 6-1. *Notices like these appear regularly in New York City newspapers. Apparently it pays to advertise. (Reprinted by permission of The New York Post. Copyright © 1972 by the New York Post Corporation.)*

After the passage (in July, 1970) of a very liberal abortion law in New York State, its deaths from abortion were reduced to one-third the number reported in the year prior to the law's enactment. Since the number of illegal abortions performed during that year is unknown, it is not possible to determine a mortality rate; but as of September 1971 the New York mortality was 4.8 deaths per 100,000 abortions, a figure that compares favorably with recent overall maternal mortality rates (Table 6-1). In the first 15 months of the new law, 200,000 women (60 percent from out of New York State) had abortions. To date, fewer than 20 states have liberalized abortion laws, and in a few states abortion is impossible to obtain under any circumstances.

Abortion is safest and easiest when performed during the first trimester of pregnancy. Later than this the procedure becomes increasingly difficult and risky. Abortion is usually performed using one of three methods. Dilatation and curettage (D&C) is the most commonly used technique early in pregnancy. It consists of dilating the cervical opening and passing into the uterus a curette which is then used to scrape away the newly conceived embryo. Vacuum aspiration, a more recently developed method, is basically similar to the D&C and is also used early in pregnancy. The cervix is dilated, and a thin tube attached to a vacuum pump is inserted into the uterus. The vacuum removes the embryonic material much like a curette. Abortions later in pregnancy, up to the twenty-fourth week, are performed by a method known as saline induction. A long needle is inserted through the patient's abdomen and into the uterus. **Amnionic fluid** is removed and a salt solution injected in its place. The salt solution kills the fetus, and this is followed by a period of active labor during which the fetus is expelled.

The state of the medical art is such that childbirth need not pose a significant threat to maternal health. The magnitude of this threat is in large measure determined by other factors, particularly the socioeconomic status of the woman in question. Similarly, the hazards of induced abortion depend less on dangers inherent in the procedure itself than on its legality, i.e., the ease with which the abortion can be obtained significantly affects when, where, by whom, and how safely it is carried out.

AMNIONIC FLUID: the clear liquid in which the fetus is immersed within the **amnion** (a membrane, within the uterus, which forms a sac surrounding the fetus)

CHILD HEALTH

The health of pregnant women is so closely entwined with that of their unborn children that attempts to separate the two are totally unrealistic and extremely misleading. Abortion is the classic example of this interdependence, but a number of maternal factors have a major effect on fetal well-being. Both fetal and infant mortality are influenced by maternal age; the very young girl and the very old mother run higher risks of fetal loss than women in their twenties or early thirties. Women who are pregnant for the first time, and those with many previous children, are also poorer risks. As we have already noted, socioeconomic status is of major importance as well. Women with uterine abnormalities are more likely than normal women to abort spontaneously or to deliver prematurely. Abnormalities of the pelvic bone structure can make for very difficult labor, which often poses a severe threat to fetal survival. Fortunately, the prevalence of pelvic disproportion has decreased with the decline of rickets (see Chapter 2).

In addition, various maternal illnesses are known to affect the unborn child adversely. Syphilis in the mother is often transmitted to the child, who is then born with the disease; spontaneous abortion and stillbirth are also more common in these mothers. German measles (rubella) in the first trimester of pregnancy results in fetal death or a malformed child in one-third of cases. Cataract, deafness, and heart defects are the most common malformations occurring in the offspring of mothers exposed to this otherwise mild infection. Maternal polio sometimes results in fetal death or defect but rarely leads to paralysis of the infant. Measles and infectious hepatitis late in pregnancy can produce premature labor. Cytomegalic inclusion disease and toxoplasmosis are a pair of maternal infections that may be passed on to the fetus, in whom they produce a wide range of effects which often lead to permanent retardation if the infant survives.

Maternal anemia may lead to fetal **anoxia,** since the reduced oxygen-transporting ability of the mother's blood compromises the only source of fetal oxygen. The prenatal mortality of babies born to diabetic mothers is nine times that of babies born to normal mothers. These infants are characterized by higher-than-average birth weight coupled with the developmental status of a premature. Perinatal mortality is also excessive

---

ANOXIA: lack of oxygen

when the mother suffers from severe heart disease.

During pregnancy smallpox vaccination is **contraindicated,** since it results in fetal death about one-quarter of the time. Steroid drugs such as cortisone can masculinize a female fetus and thus should be avoided during pregnancy. If the pregnant woman is exposed to x-ray, there is heightened risk that the child will get leukemia or cancer of the central nervous system during childhood.

Strictly speaking, fetal death refers to the death of the unborn child at any time from the moment of conception to birth. It is estimated that 10 to 12 percent of all pregnancies end in the death of the fetus. Fetal deaths due to abortion usually occur early in pregnancy and are under-reported save in the handful of states with liberal abortion laws. Those deaths close to the time of delivery are more accurately reported. A stillbirth is a fetal death occurring after the twentieth to twenty-eighth week of **gestation.** (The confusion surrounding the state-by-state definition of fetus was discussed in Chapter 3.)

The various threats to life during the intrauterine period are matched by the dangers of the neonatal period, that crucial time which covers the first 28 days of life. The importance of the neonatal period to the survival of the newborn child is underscored by the fact that 70 percent of all infant deaths occur in this period, most of them in the first week. The leading causes of neonatal and infant deaths are thus the same.

As we know from an earlier discussion, mortality after the twentieth to twenty-eighth week of gestation, plus that occurring during the neonatal period, is known as perinatal mortality. Mortality during the perinatal period equals that of the first 40 years of the life span. A handful of conditions account for about half of all fetal deaths. Table 6-2 lists these conditions and the major causes of neonatal death.

Abruptio placentae refers to the abnormal separation of the placentae from the inner wall of the uterus. A complication of late pregnancy, this condition is most common in women with chronic renal disease, and is also a frequent companion to toxemia. Since the placenta serves as a kind of fetal lung, abruptio placentae results in fetal anoxia. At this point, recall that the uterus is a pear-shaped organ with its opening where the pear's stem would be. It lies upside down in the pelvis, with its opening at the posterior end of the vagina. In the condition known as placenta praevia, the placenta lies astride the uterine **os,** where it is very likely

---

CONTRAINDICATION: that which rules out a particular treatment
GESTATION: the intrauterine development of the newly formed individual
OS: the orifice of the uterine cervix

TABLE 6-2. Leading Causes of Fetal, Neonatal, and Infant Deaths
1960s, New York City and Great Britain[a]

Fetal Deaths	Neonatal and Infant Deaths
Abruptio placenta or placenta praevia	Prematurity
Congenital malformation	Postnatal asphyxia and atelectasis
Rh incompatibility	Congenital malformation
Toxemia	Birth injuries

[a]*Sources: City of New York Health Services Administration. Infant Mortality, New York City—Miscellaneous Tables. December, 1967. Also, Lightwood, R., Brimblecome, F., and Barltrop, D. Paterson's Sick Children. Philadelphia, Lippincott, 1971.*

to bleed into the vagina. Placenta praevia is a far greater threat to the fetus than to the mother and is more common in multiparas than among primigravidas. Abruptio placentae and placenta praevia account for about 18 percent of all fetal deaths.

Prematurity is the leading cause of neonatal and infant mortality. A premature infant is one who weights less than 5½ pounds (2,500 grams) at birth. Nationally, about 8 percent of births are premature, and prematurity is far more common in black than in white babies. Survival among prematures is directly correlated with weight. Virtually all infants weighing less than 2 pounds at birth succumb, while 90 percent survive who weigh between 4½ and 5½ pounds. The most common cause of death in prematures is respiratory failure, and those who survive are more likely than infants of normal weight to be mentally retarded or to have cerebral palsy or **epilepsy.** In about 50 percent of cases of prematurity, no apparent cause is recognized. In the other half, multiple pregnancies, toxemia, hypertension, abruptio placentae, and placenta praevia have been causally implicated. It is estimated that between 10 and 15 percent of premature births are preventable with adequate prenatal care.

Congenital malformations are responsible for about 12 percent of stillbirths and 16 percent of neonatal deaths. These impairments are present at birth, but some, such as deafness or heart defects, are often not apparent until considerably later in the infant's life. Between 1 and 2 percent ·of all newborns have a visible congenital defect. Those fetuses with defects incompatible with extra-uterine survival die before birth and thus account for the stillbirth.component of this important cause of perinatal mortality.

EPILEPSY: a neurological disease characterized by convulsive seizures and loss of
    consciousness

Congenital malformations are more common in white babies than in black, although perinatal mortality is generally higher among the latter. Maternal age is also an important factor; defects such as **hydrocephaly**, **harelip**, mongolism, and some cardiac abnormalities are most common in infants born to older women. In general, the risk of delivering a malformed child is also higher in women of low income.

The Rh factor is a normal constituent in the blood of about 85 percent of the population. Its presence is genetically determined and it is transmitted as a dominant characteristic. It is not uncommon for a woman without the Rh factor (i.e., Rh negative) to carry a child who is Rh positive. The Rh factor present in the fetal blood acts as an antigen if fetal blood enters the circulatory system of an Rh negative mother. In this case, the mother forms antibody against fetal Rh; and this results in the destruction of fetal red blood cells, a condition known as erythroblastosis fetalis. Now, it so happens that fetal blood is most likely to enter the maternal circulation after the birth of the fetus and during the normal separation of the placenta from the uterine wall. A bit of reflection at this point will bring to light an important aspect of Rh incompatibility: the mingling of fetal and maternal blood, a necessary cause for the formation of maternal antibody against the Rh factor, occurs *after* the birth of the child. Moreover, that child's blood has sensitized his mother against Rh, and she is subject to an anamnestic response if she becomes pregnant with another Rh positive fetus. Thus, the first Rh positive child of an Rh negative mother escapes erythroblastosis unless the mother has been sensitized through transfusion with blood from an Rh positive donor or by a previous pregnancy that ended in spontaneous or induced abortion. The importance of erythroblastosis as a cause of perinatal death is expected to decline since a substance has been developed which, when administered to the mother during **parturition**, prevents the formation of maternal antibody.

Asphyxia and atelectasis are closely related. Asphysia is simply starvation for air. Atelectasis refers to the failure of the lungs to expand and exchange air. Consequently, atelectasis is a frequent precursor of asphyxia. Atelectasis is most commonly present at birth and can result from any of a number of etiologic factors. Asphyxia is produced by a variety of conditions and, as such, represents not so much a cause of death as a terminal event. Like asphyxia, birth injuries have multiple causes. By and

---

HYDROCEPHALY: abnormal distension of the skull due to retention of cerebrospinal fluid, the watery liquid that bathes the brain
HARELIP: failure, during fetal life, in the formation of that part of the face between the upper lip and the nose
PARTURITION: birth of the fetus

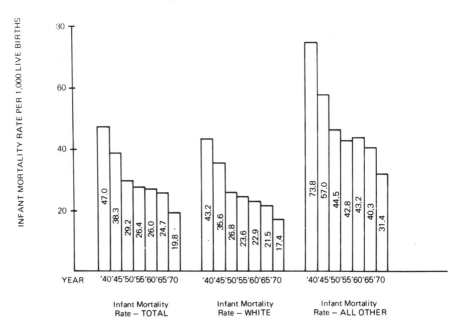

Infant Mortality Rates by Age and Color, Selected Years 1940-1970

Fig. 6-2. *(From* Reference Data on Socioeconomic Issues of Health, *1972 revised edition, American Medical Association.)*

large these injuries occur at the time of delivery, and the most serious cause intracranial hemorrhage. Infants who survive such injuries frequently have cerebral palsy or epilepsy.

In addition to the causes of mortality listed in Table 6-2, staphylococcal infections, especially of the umbilical stump, and diarrhea due to a number of bacteria are important causes of infant deaths during the neonatal period. Later in infancy, diarrheal diseases and pneumonia become the principal killers. Figure 6-2 presents the mortality rates for white and non-white infants in the United States during various years since 1940. Most notable is the decline of over 50 percent in the rates for both ethnic groups, and the fact that the ratio of white mortality to non-white has expanded slightly since 1940. Presently, the United States ranks somewhere between eleventh and fifteenth in the world in infant mortality, a standing far worse than most of the industrialized nations. Since about 1950, infant mortality in the United States has remained around 25 per 1,000 live births, a figure which is one-third higher than Denmark's and almost

TABLE 6-3. Five Leading Causes of Death by
Age Groups in United States, 1967

Rank	Cause of Death	Rate per 100,000 Population
	1–4 Years (over-all death rate 86.3)	
1.	Accidents	32.4
2.	Congenital malformation	9.7
3.	Influenza and pneumonia	9.2
4.	Cancer	8.2
5.	Meningitis	2.0
	5–14 Years (over-all death rate 41.4)	
1.	Accidents	19.3
2.	Cancer	6.6
3.	Congenital malformations	2.4
4.	Influenza and pneumonia	1.7
5.	Heart disease	0.8
	15–24 Years (over-all death rate 116.9)	
1.	Accidents	67.1
2.	Homicide	9.1
3.	Cancer	8.3
4.	Suicide	7.0
5.	Heart disease	2.6

Source: Facts of Life and Death, National Center for Health Statistics, Publication No. 600, 1970.

twice that of Sweden. Because it is unaffected by the age distribution of the population (as is the crude death rate), infant mortality is widely regarded as the best single index of the overall health of a nation's population. As the wealthiest nation in the world and the country with the most advanced technology, our infant mortality record leaves much room for improvement.

Table 6-3 identifies the five leading causes of death throughout the childhood years. Notice that we have switched our frame of reference from 25 infant deaths per 1,000 live births to—in the case of ages 1 through 4—86.3 deaths per 100,000. This figure is equal to 0.863 deaths per 1,000, a mortality rate more than 25 times less than that in infancy. Once the age of 1 year is reached, the remainder of childhood is a period of very low mortality. It is also a period when accidents are the leading cause of death, and the only time of life when homicide and suicide are major factors in mortality. Since most of these important causes of childhood mortality are discussed elsewhere in this book, we will concentrate here on a type of accident unique to youngsters under the age of 5: the unintentional ingestion of poisoning substances.

Each year, 300 to 400 children in this age group die as a result of accidental poisoning, although nonfatal poisoning episodes are far more common, numbering 73,000 in 1967. The peak age for poisonings is in the toddler stage—between 12 and 36 months. More than half of these poisonings involve medications, especially aspirin tablets. Household cleansers and polishes account for 17 percent, with pesticides, cosmetics, petroleum products, and even plants making substantial contributions. The kitchen is the most common site of occurrence, and usually the ingested substance is out of its customary storage place and often in a container other than the original. Almost all of these accidental poisonings are preventable (See Appendix 8).

Early childhood is often identified with the immunizations which are customarily given during the first year of life. Table 4-2 lists the vaccines in common use. Of these, six are especially important in childhood and should be given by the end of the first year of life. DPT is a combined vaccine which simultaneously immunizes the child against diphtheria, whooping cough (pertussis), and tetanus. DPT immunization should begin at about 2 months of age, with two additional doses at monthly intervals. However, it should be deferred if the child has **intercurrent** infection, and used with caution on children with a past history of convulsions. DPT should be postponed also in the presence of an epidemic for which a vaccine is available. Measles vaccine is given at age 9 months and provides protection lasting at least 5 years. Smallpox vaccine traditionally has been given at age 7 months and repeated when the child enters school. However, in 1971 the Public Health Service announced that vaccination against smallpox is no longer recommended, since the risk of contracting the disease in the United States is so low that there is no further justification for the slight risk involved in vaccination. Nonetheless, more than one-half of the 50 states require smallpox vaccination by law, and, until the legislation is changed, such vaccination can be expected to continue. It is, of course, still recommended for Americans travelling to parts of the world where smallpox remains endemic.

The successful quest for an effective vaccine against polio is one of medicine's great success stories. Prior to the advent of polio vaccine in 1955, paralytic polio affected roughly 15,000 children and young adults each year. By 1967 this number had fallen to only 41 cases. Polio vaccine is of two types, live and killed; the former, taken by mouth, is much

---

INTERCURRENT: occurring at the same time as another event

superior. The development of antibody response to the vaccine may be blocked by the presence of other enteric viruses, such as Echo, Coxsackie, and adenovirus. Since infections with these agents are most common in summer, polio vaccine is administered during cool months. None of the live vaccines should be given to persons allergic to eggs, since the vaccines themselves are prepared with the use of egg products. To avoid risk to the fetus, pregnant women should not be vaccinated. Conditions such as widespread cancers lower body resistance, as do steroid drugs and exposure to therapeutic radiation; live vaccination should thus be avoided in people who fall into these categories.

The Elderly

Persons over age 65 comprise nearly 10 percent of the population. In 1900, when life expectancy was only 47 years, less than 5 percent of the population reached what we euphemistically call the "golden years." The growth of this segment of the population is as spectacular in absolute terms as it is in percent. From 3 million persons at the turn of the century, this group increased to 20 million by 1970; it is projected that it will number 23 million people by 1980 (Fig. 6-3). The "senior citizen" represents a social paradox in that society, having labored long and hard to achieve an extended span of life, seems unwilling to provide much satisfaction for those at the top end of the span and unable to meet many of their needs. It is a supreme irony that this very society which so values long life also tends to regard the aged as liabilities.

But if the aged are a liability to society, it must also be recognized that advanced age is too often a liability to the individual. In terms of health, when compared with younger age groups, the elderly have a higher prevalence of illness, visit the physician more, spend more time in the hospital, endure more days of restricted activity due to illness, have less money with which to purchase care and have costlier illness (Fig. 6-4). The principal goal of **geriatrics** is to keep the patient functioning through proper management of chronic illnesses, which are rarely curable and which seem to be the inevitable companion of advancing age.

There are no diseases that are peculiar to the geriatric age group. Rather, the aged are subject to virtually every condition known, and in most cases they run a greater risk of being affected than the general

---

GERIATRICS: the specialty of medicine concerned with the diseases of advanced age; compare to gerontology, which is the study of the aging process.

TABLE 6-4. Five Leading Causes of Death for the Aged
in United States, 1967

Rank	Cause of Death	Rate per 100,000 Population
	65–74 Years (over-all death rate 3,750)	
1.	Heart disease	1,669.5
2.	Cancer	768.8
3.	Strokes	412.6
4.	Diabetes	94.2
5.	Accidents	91.2
	75–84 Years (over-all death rate 7,900)	
1.	Heart disease	3,670.6
2.	Strokes	1,216.7
3.	Cancer	1,102.1
4.	Pneumonia and influenza	207.0
5.	General arteriosclerosis	249.6
	85 Years and Over (over-all death rate 19,420)	
1.	Heart disease	9,240.5
2.	Strokes	3,592.5
3.	Cancer	1,482.9
4.	General arteriosclerosis	1,298.5
5.	Pneumonia and influenza	971.1

Source: National Center for Health Statistics: Vital statistics report, final mortality statistics, 1967, vol. 17, no. 12, March 25, 1969.

Statistical Abstract of The United States, U. S. Department of Commerce, 1971.

population (Table 6-4). Diseases of the gastrointestinal tract represent a case in point. Carcinoma of the colon is the most common cancer in the elderly and accounts for one-third of all cancer deaths in the over-65 age group. Among non-neoplastic gastrointestinal conditions, diverticulitis is especially common among the elderly. Saclike bulges (diverticula) tend to appear in the wall of the colon. When fecal matter becomes impacted in these pocket-like protrusions, colonic **spasm** and localized infection produce abdominal pain, fever, and sometimes **abscess** formation. These symptoms and signs are characteristic of diverticulitis, and severe cases require surgical correction. Diaphragmatic hernia is another gastrointestinal problem which is especially prominent in the elderly. The diaphragm is a thin, flat, dome-shaped muscle which separates the chest from the abdomen. The esophagus, which transmits food from the throat to the stomach, passes through a hole in the diaphragm. In some

SPASM: the involuntary contraction of a muscle; essentially a cramp
ABSCESS: a cavity resulting from tissue destruction which is filled with pus

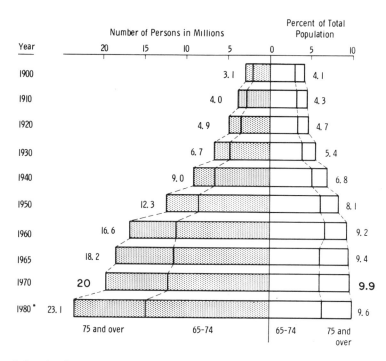

FIG. 6-3.   *Aged persons by age group: number and percent of total population (U.S.A., 1900-1980). (Adapted from* Medical Chart Book, *University of Michigan, School of Public Health, Third Edition, Revised 1968.)*

people this hole becomes abnormally large, and the stomach tends to protrude through it into the chest. This gives rise to a number of symptoms, including belching, chest pain, and "heartburn."

Peptic ulcer is by no means restricted to the elderly, but it is a more important cause of death in this than in any other age group. Ulcers are small craters which occur in the wall of the **duodenum** and, less frequently, the stomach. They can obstruct the duodenum and are subject to perforation and hemorrhage, all of which are life-threatening medical emergencies. Why ulcers occur is not clear; and while most can be treated by diet and drugs, about 10 percent require surgical intervention. Cholelithiasis, or gallstones, is another condition which frequently leads to the operating table. An etiologic mystery, gallstones can produce severe abdominal pain, nausea, and intolerance for fried or fatty foods. Most cases are asymptomatic, and the condition is one of the few diseases which is more common in women than men.

DUODENUM: the section of the intestines that is located just below the stomach

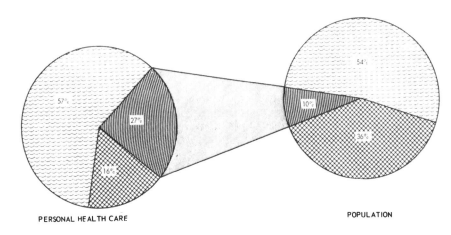

PERSONAL HEALTH CARE   POPULATION

FIG. 6-4.   *Medical care outlays for the aged (U.S.A., 1970). While the aged comprise
only one-tenth of the population, more than one-quarter of the 1970 personal health care dollar was spent for this group. The aged require relatively large outlays because they have more and costlier illnesses than the
younger population. (From* Basic Facts on the Health Industry, *Committee
on Ways and Means, U.S. Government Printing Office, Washington, 1971.)*

Surgery is a special hazard in the aged, largely because of respiratory
distress. The elastic resiliency of the lungs diminishes with advancing
age, and the once-flexible rib cage becomes relatively fixed and immobile,
a situation favorable to the development of pneumonia and atelactasis.

Less serious gastrointestinal conditions include irritable colon and
simple constipation. The former is the single most common cause of
chronic gastrointestinal symptoms; these cover a wide range, including
constipation, diarrhea, pain, gas, belching, and so on. Chronic constipation is one of the complaints traditionally associated with old age. This
symptom is exploited to such a degree in television commercials for
laxatives that many a nonconstipated oldster must regard himself as
abnormal. The primary significance of constipation is that it is a source
of continuous concern to the patient and of unending frustration to the
health workers involved in his care.

Of course, the medical problems of old people are not limited to a single organ system. Genitourinary disorders—such as kidney stones and diverticula of the bladder—plague both sexes, while **hypertrophy** and carcinoma of the prostate gland are problems peculiar to older men. Women, as we know, are subject to uterine neoplasms and, at times, prolapse of the uterus. Arteriosclerosis creates vascular insufficiency which reduces blood flow to the various tissues and organs. In older persons, years of hypertension and advancing arteriosclerosis lead to the myocardial infarcts and cerebrovascular accidents which often result in death or in permanent disability such as **hemiplegia**. Among elderly diabetics, peripheral vascular disease is quite common and often requires amputation of a toe, a foot, or an entire lower leg.

The importance of accidents as a cause of mortality among the aged is seldom stressed, but fully a quarter of all accidental deaths and three-quarters of all accidental deaths due to falls occur in persons over the age of 65. The elderly are also involved as pedestrians in a disproportionate number of auto accidents.

In addition to the disability, if not death, attributable to accidents and vascular disease, three additional problems are also significant as causes of disability among the aged: rheumatoid and other kinds of arthritis, hearing loss, and visual difficulties. Hearing loss affects almost 20 percent of people over age 65, and half of all visual defects occur in this age group.

Although physical impairments must figure prominently in any consideration of the elderly, it is probably true that on a day-to-day basis the most important difficulty encountered in getting old is mental deterioration. Part of this has a physical basis. With advancing age, the number of viable brain cells may diminish along with a general decrease in the total mass of brain tissue. Arteriosclerosis may compromise the blood supply to the brain. Whatever its cause, senility is characterized by increasing forgetfulness and an overall slowing of mental processes. These problems are compounded by feelings of loneliness, uselessness, and rejection by relatives. These feelings tend to be magnified if there is a seemingly endless supply of time with which to do nothing. In many cases the elderly face serious financial difficulties, and the anxieties and problems attendant upon this complicate what is often an already distressful situation. Because of senility, apathy, physical impairment, and financial constraints, the aged are frequently malnourished. Meals are skipped entirely in some cases; in others, food requiring more than a minimum of chewing are avoided because of missing teeth or poorly fitting dentures.

HYPERTROPHY: non-neoplastic, nonedematous increase in the size of an organ
HEMIPLEGIA: paralysis affecting one side of the body

At times it is impossible for the elderly person to buy groceries because of difficulties in getting to the store. As the individual becomes older, it is not uncommon for him to reach a point where he can no longer care for himself. In the absence of an adequate number of long-term care facilities, many of the elderly ultimately end up in mental hospitals. Indeed, almost 25 percent of admissions to these institutions are elderly people. An expanded discussion of problems related particularly to the elderly can be found in Chapter 7.

References

Bakst, H. Prevention in geriatric practice. *In* Clark, D., and MacMahon, B., eds. Preventive Medicine. Boston, Little, Brown, 1967.

Benson, R. Handbook of Obstetrics and Gynecology, 4th ed. Los Altos, Calif., Lange Publications, 1971.

Blum, H., and Keranen, G. Control of Chronic Diseases in Man. New York, American Public Health Association, 1966.

Buck, C. Prenatal and perinatal causes of early death and defect. *In* Clark, D., and MacMahon, B., eds. Preventive Medicine. Boston, Little, Brown, 1967.

City of New York Health Services Administration. Infant Mortality, New York City—Miscellaneous Tables. December, 1967.

Lightwood, R., Brimblecombe, F., and Barltrop, D. Paterson's Sick Children. Philadelphia, Lippincott, 1971.

MacMahon, B. Mental illness. *In* Clark, D., and MacMahon, B., eds. Preventive Medicine. Boston, Little, Brown, 1967.

Public Health Service Publication. Teaching Poison Prevention. Washington, D.C., Public Health Service, 1966.

Sartwell, P., ed. Maxcy-Rosenau Preventive Medicine and Public Health, 9th ed. New York, Appleton-Century-Crofts, 1965.

Shapiro, S., Schlesinger, E., and Nesbitt, R. Infant, Perinatal, Maternal, and Child Mortality in the United States. Cambridge, Mass., Harvard University Press, 1968.

Silver, H., Kempe, C., and Bruyn, H. Handbook of Pediatrics, 9th ed. Los Altos, Calif., Lange Publications, 1971.

Time Magazine. September 27, 1971.

U. S. Department of Health, Education, and Welfare. Soc. Sec. Bull., April, 1970.

Verhulst, H., and Crotty, J. Childhood poisoning accidents. J.A.M.A. 203:12, 1968.

Willson, J., Beecham, C., Forman, I., and Carrington, E. Obstetrics and Gynecology. St. Louis, The C. V. Mosby Co., 1958.

CHAPTER
7
Mental Illness

Virtually all forms of life are subject to some form of disease. More-over, many animal species share man's susceptibility to specific diseases. Thus, for example, dogs develop diabetes; parrots, elephants, cats, and dogs all may suffer from arthritis and die of cancer, heart disease, or stroke. Although complex behavior has been observed in many species from ants to apes, it is only man, *Homo sapiens,* who is known to "eat when he isn't hungry, fight when he isn't angry, and copulate the year round."

Man is also the only animal who looks around him and concludes that "everyone is strange but me and thee, and sometimes I am not so sure about thee." Whatever "strange" means in this context, it is in most minds but a short step to "crazy" or "insane" or "freaked out." Of all diseases, only mental illness seems to be peculiar to man. The individual described below, for example, is suffering from an illness to which we are all to some degree susceptible because of our humanity.

[Mr. X.] . . . was a skilled mechanic, 32 years old, intelligent and educated, who had made good headway in life. . . . The decisive event that brought him to the hospital was an attempt to rape his sister. He was in a straightjacket, in a bed with railings; nevertheless he was thrashing about violently; his face was covered with saliva and nasal mucous which he tried to swallow; he was smearing feces; he held his breath and puffed himself up; he rolled his eyes which seemed to protrude from their sockets. At the same time he was thinking volubly and loudly; he shouted occasionally, then suddenly he would assume an unctuous tone as though he were giving a sermon. The content of the "sermon" was, briefly, the following: There is an ideal heavenly love, not only between the two sexes but between all human beings, including the love of men for men; there is no sinful love, for all are brothers and sisters; one must renounce, be abstinent, and make sacrifices, so that humanity may reach its goal; . . . the ancient Indians had also renounced, had abstained from taking meat, had made sacrifices, and therefore men had perfected themselves by the migration of the soul from the lowest animal to ever-higher beings . . . He (the patient) would redeem the world, since he had solved the problem of eternal life; and he alone was capable of propagating mankind. This sermon was interrupted by trivial phrases uttered in full earnestness. The patient offered himself sexually to the male psychiatrist . . . for instance, with the following words: "You may push from the front and from the behind as you like." At times he complained that his thoughts were taken from him, that it had been suggested to him that he relieve himself in bed, that he was being scorched by a fire, that he was in Hell, in the underworld; it seemed to him that he was eating human flesh from dead bodies; he feared that he was changing into an animal, a worm. The patient heard voices, names long forgotten from his childhood and so on.

This description of our skilled mechanic and the details of his activities is most likely to produce a strong reaction in the reader. Rape, incest, the act of smearing feces, religiosity—all tend to invoke emotional responses. The idea that someone is hearing voices, or thinks he is turning into a worm, or losing his thought provokes puzzlement if nothing else. However, the fact is that this account is in a medical textbook. For the reader, the intellectual process of absorbing the material and learning from it is quite isolated from the feelings he might have were he in the room with Mr. X., who is suffering from a disease as old as man and yet still of unknown etiology.

Equally old is man's struggle to keep his sadistic drives in check when dealing with Mr. X. and those who share his suffering. Man has had and still has great difficulty treating the mentally ill as fellow men with the same rights and privileges as his "normal" comrades. Too often, the "insane" are regarded as victims ripe for dehumanizing and sadistic torture, which is **rationalized** as curative or palliative medical treatment

---

RATIONALIZE: to justify or explain one's actions as reasonable and estimable in situations where one is unwilling or unable to deal with his true motives (see Figs. 7-1, 7-2). This tendency is well expressed in the statement, "I tied him to a chair and repeatedly dunked him in cold water until he nearly drowned, because it helps him grow calmer and will eventually bring him to his senses." Sometimes the rationalization is expressed in terms of an understanding of the cause of behavior, thus: "I tied him to a chair and repeatedly dunked him in cold water until he nearly drowned, because it was necessary that he confess his possession by the devil." Or it may be expressed in "practical" terms: "All the chronically insane were ordered to be used for medical 'experiments' and then to be sent to the gas chambers because they are a financial burden on the state." It is never put in frank terms: "I beat him because I like it."

It is worth considering how Mr. X. might have fared a few centuries ago. He has surrendered to sexual lust for his sister. He reacts violently to those in authority; he speaks loosely of the Lord and makes comparisons between Christianity and pagan religions; he proclaims animals to be the hosts of men's souls; he proclaims himself the redeemer (i.e., the

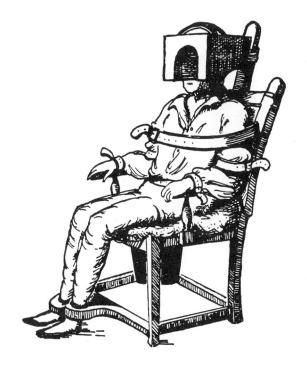

FIG. 7-1. *The "Rush Chair" was used to "quiet" the insane. Note that Benjamin Rush (1745-1813) is considered by many to be "The Father of American Psychiatry." Among his other "contributions" were bleeding patients to stages of exhaustion, and the gyrating chair for increasing the blood supply to the head. (Courtesy of Bettman Archives.)*

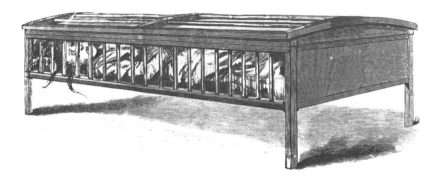

FIG. 7-2. *Insane patient in "The Crib" at New York Institution in 1882. (Courtesy of Bettman Archives.)*

Saviour). He is possessed of the devil. There are even physical signs. The evil spirit causes his body to puff up. Fearful that it may lose some strength

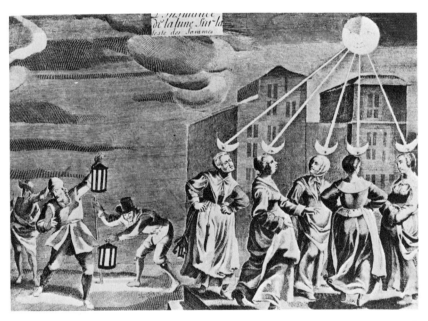

FIG. 7-3. *Moonstruck (lunatic) women dancing in 17th century town square. The word "lunatic" is derived from the Latin word for moon (lūna). People of the Middle Ages believed that lunacy fluctuated with the phases of the moon. (Courtesy of Bettman Archives.)*

through the running of his nose, this spirit commands that he eat the secretion, dead flesh, and so on. He must be made (through torture) to confess his possession by the devil; one may pray that his burning might be avoided, but wisdom leads one to doubt it. As to how this possession came about, serious and careful investigation must be undertaken at once, adhering to *Malleus Maleficarum*, the authoritative treatise which teaches that daemonic possession is the work of witches and that "all witchcraft comes from carnal lust which in women is insatiable" (see Fig. 7-3).[1] The sister must also be summoned and rigorously examined! So might a "witch hunter" have reasoned and proceeded at any time between the year 1487 and June 18, 1782, the date of the last recorded execution of a witch.

Mr. X. would have fared considerably better in the hands of Hippocrates (460–377 B.C.), the father of medicine, who wrote that "life is short, science is long, opportunity is elusive, experiment is dangerous, judgment is difficult. It is not enough for the physician to do what is necessary, but the patient and the attendants must do their part as well, and circumstances must be favorable." This approach was rational, if somewhat primitive by modern standards. Hippocrates accepted his lack of knowledge, divorced himself from superstition, and formulated a motto which might well benefit many a modern health worker: "If you can do no good, at least do no harm." Accordingly, he prescribed a **purgative** for madness, and **bled the patient** moderately in an attempt to soothe and reassure him. The Greeks bequeathed to the world a strong rational tradition in medicine. Nevertheless, the Greek who suffered from a mental or physical illness was free to seek treatment from the priests at a temple of Aesculapius, the god of healing. Unfortunately, since the temple was a sacred place, those judged in danger of death or near childbirth were excluded for fear that the god might be offended. Priestly healing was based on a process called incubation, which included purification (ritual washing), discussion with the priest (catharsis), and sleeping in holy areas of the temple. A cure was effected by a dream which included some sign of divine intervention and was then decoded by the priest and recorded in honor of the god. The altar was a small, round, shallow pit in which holy snakes were kept. It is said that the most difficult cases were placed in the pit to be licked or bitten by these sacred symbols of the god. Hence, the first "snake pit" was located among beautiful open

---

PURGATIVE: an agent, e.g., castor oil, which produces violent, watery evacuation of the bowels
BLEED A PATIENT: to let blood; the procedure of cutting a vein and thus allowing blood to leave the body; practiced by physicians and barbers

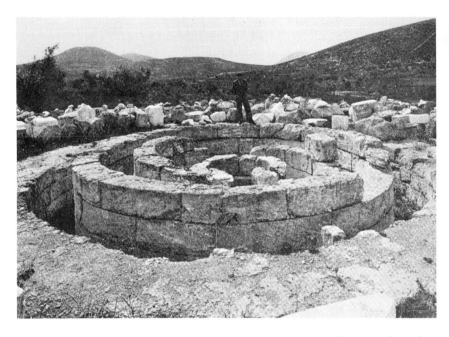

FIG. 7-4.   *Original Snake pit. This ancient Sanctuary of Aesculapius, is located in Greece at Epidaurus. The center circle was the altar wherein the "sacred" snakes were kept. (Courtesy of The New York Public Library.)*

buildings surrounded by pine woods and hills on the Peloponnesian peninsula (see Figs. 7-4 and 7-5). Access was limited, but one could leave any time.

How might Mr. X. have fared in other hands? If he had fallen ill in Valencia, Spain, around 1410, he might very well have found himself in a hospital which relied more on "free exercise, games, occupation, entertainment, diet, and hygiene" than chains. For some reason, this innovation did not become known to the rest of Europe for some time. Had our skilled mechanic fallen ill in Paris in the 1760s, he would have been treated at the Hotel Dieu, the general receiving hospital. There, bloodletting, **emetics, cuppings,** and purgatives would have been administered to a point where the patient was totally exhausted. If he feared this sort of treatment—as well anyone might—and if he grew more agitated and

EMETIC: a drug which produces vomiting
CUPPING: the application of a glass (heated to exhaust the air) to the skin so that suction brings blood to the surface

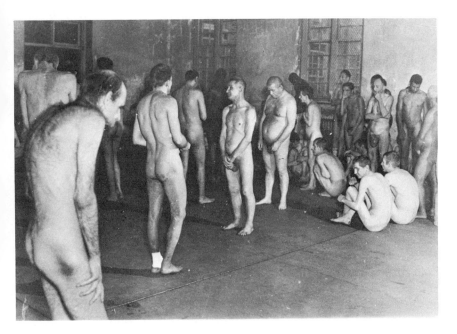

FIG. 7-5.   *Modern Snake pit. Depicted is a chronic male disturbed ward in an eastern state hospital. Although this stark neglect is still in evidence today, it is decreasingly typical of state hospital wards. (Courtesy of The National Association for Mental Health.)*

resisted more violently, he would have been kept chained, perhaps naked, and been given another course of the same treatment, often with the addition of some caustic chemical to burn his skin. For many, this amounted to a "kill or cure" treatment. Hippocrates, no doubt, was stirring in his grave.

If a patient neither died nor improved at the Hotel Dieu, he was transferred to the Bicêtre, an asylum for men suffering from chronic physical and mental illness. Here he was automatically considered hopeless and incurable; and, while he probably escaped further drastic therapy, he might well have spent the rest of his days in the most desperate of circumstances.

Lest one imagine that the rich and powerful were treated very differently, a brief examination of the therapeutic ordeal suffered by England's King George III (1738–1820) is instructive. Poor George was purged, bled, painfully restrained, and in constant terror of his physicians. He was particularly embittered because his complaints of pain were scarcely heard or were given little, if any, credence. There is good evidence that he probably suffered from porphyria, an inherited metabolic disease which causes severe abdominal pain and, sometimes, a toxic **psychosis.**

Although it did George III no good, things were to brighten all over the world as the result of the work of a very interesting man named Jean-Baptiste Pussin.[2] A tanner by trade, Pussin himself was treated at the Hotel Dieu. Twenty-five years of age and suffering from **scrofula,** he was judged incurable and was transferred to the Bicêtre on June 5, 1771. The hospital records make no further reference to his illness but note that on April 27, 1780, he was placed in charge of the children; and on October 3, 1785, he was made superintendent of the Saint Prix Division of the hospital. In this position, he was the administrator in charge of the daily life, care, feeding, restraint, and so on of the male insane patients, who, like himself, were considered incurable.

Pussin and his wife lived in the hospital with his 200 or so patients and 13 attendants, the latter personally trained by him and often recruited from among recovered patients. Pussin forbade his attendants to strike patients and fired those who did. He did his best to keep the inadequate facilities clean and orderly. He is described as a man of wisdom, calmness, compassion, firmness, bravery, and sensitivity. He demanded that patients control their behavior; those who became violent he restrained either with a straightjacket or, in the last resort, chains (see Fig. 7-6).

In addition to treating patients firmly and humanely, Pussin did something quite new—he listened to them. He thus learned about their lives and illness and attempted to discuss their problems with them. In short, he sought to treat them by providing decent conditions, minimal restraints, much understanding, constant reassurance, and what might best be called the force of his personality and position. Pussin's approach to treatment was psychological rather than physical. This innovation came to be known as "moral treatment." By 1790, when a governmental committee began to investigate the conditions in chronic disease hospitals, the Bicêtre was found to be the best hospital by far, and Pussin had obtained a cure rate of 20 percent. This was indeed something of an accomplishment for a tanner ignorant of psychiatry!

In 1793, the Bicêtre received its first physician-in-chief, and mental illness its first hero. He was Phillipe Pinel, and it was he who received the credit for "striking off the chains" of the insane and instituting moral treatment. In his book, *Treatise on Insanity,* Pinel describes (somewhat

---

PSYCHOSIS: a severe mental disorder in which the disorganization of the personality
is extensive, and perception and adaption to external reality is disrupted
SCROFULA: an infection of the lymph glands which is produced by tuberculosis

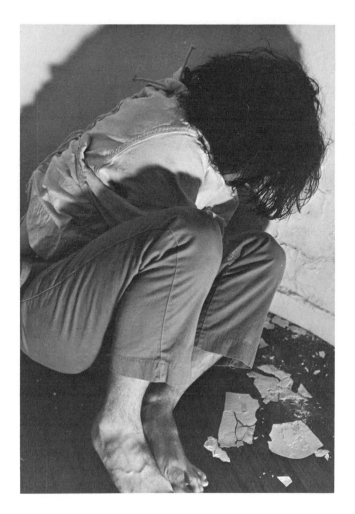

FIG. 7-6. *A great innovation in psychiatry which replaced chains. However, it is still far from a pleasant garment to wear. (Courtesy of Dr. C. L. Marshall.)*

apologetically) how he arrived at the Bicêtre and proceeded to learn psychiatry from a source other than the books of the time: "How could I neglect what the observation of mental patients over a great number of years and the custom of reflecting on his observations could teach a man, M. Pussin, endowed with good sense, devoted to his work, and entrusted with the superintendence of the mental patients of the hospital?" Nonetheless, it was the physician who wrote the book, and it was the

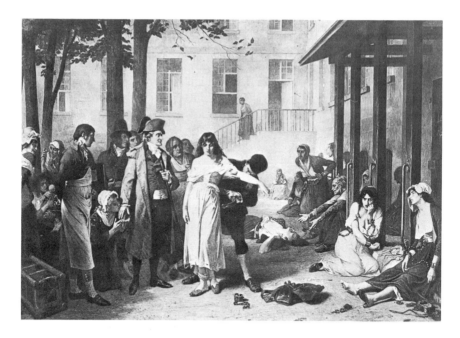

FIG. 7-7. *The aristocratic and famous Pinel "striking off the chains" of the insane at the Salpetriere in Paris. One wonders whether the aproned man (to his left) might be the historically overlooked, simple tanner named Pussin. (Painting by Robert T. Fleury, courtesy of Bettman Archives.)*

physician who became famous for what he learned from the skilled layman (see Fig. 7-7).

"Mightier than all the armies is an idea whose time has come," quoted the late Senator Everett M. Dirksen in support of twentieth-century civil rights legislation. In the late eighteenth and early nineteenth centuries, this dictum would have been equally applicable to the idea that humane conditions must prevail for the mentally ill. In Italy, Grand Duke Pietro Leopold of Tuscany, in the course of instituting enlightened reforms in his absolute monarchy, built a new mental hospital and, in 1774, promulgated the first liberal "law of the insane." In 1789, he appointed a physician, Vincinzo Chiarugi, to carry out reforms very similar to those of Pussin and Pinel. Chiarugi actually published before Pinel but remained virtually unknown. In 1796, William Tuke opened the York Retreat in England with much the same approach to treatment as that evolving in France.

Soon the reforms were spreading throughout Europe and, somewhat later, to America. From about 1817 to 1850, the moral treatment pioneered by Pussin and Pinel prevailed in the asylums and state hospitals which were being built in this country. Most of these were in rural areas, and the patients were allowed out of the buildings for recreation and for what today would be called occupational therapy. They worked in the fields, dairy barns, and blacksmith shops with attendants who were skilled in the various tasks and had been trained to respect and help the patients. In some of the hospitals there were at least rudimentary patient organizations which had responsibility for some activities and which represented the beginnings of hospital group therapy. Mr. X. could have done much worse than this!

The doctors in charge of these hospitals advocated that they contain no more than 250 patients so that each could be known to the staff. Further, they kept records of admissions and discharges; these records indicated that between 60 and 70 percent of those who had been ill less than one year were discharged as recovered (i.e., cured), and 5 percent as improved. Thus, it had been discovered that mental illness was not incurable. Unfortunately, this important information remained even more obscure than Pussin himself, because the idea of moral treatment proved to be shortlived. After the brief period of progress, conditions worsened again in Europe and, later, in America.

Among the many factors responsible for this in the United States was, ironically, the growth of scientific and medical knowledge. America's hospitals began to increase rapidly in size (i.e., number of patients), and they were soon run by physicians whose greater knowledge of the anatomy of the nervous system and use of the microscope made them feel vastly superior, scientifically, to their predecessors. These physicians believed that mental illness was the incurable result of some irreversible anatomical changes within the brain. They began to pamphleteer against what they called "the cult of curability." Despite their proclaimed scientific orientation, these misguided physicians based their widely accepted views upon belief, not objective observation. Some of this group, aware of the high rate of discharge from hospitals employing moral treatment, began a 50-year retrospective study of patients discharged as cured from the Worcester (Mass.) State Hospital in the years 1833 to 1846. The study was conducted from 1882 to 1893 and revealed that, in the half-century studied, *48 percent of those discharged as cured never had a relapse,* and only 20 percent ever again became a burden on the Commonwealth of Massachusetts. Since these results failed to prove that mental illness was incurable, they were not published until 1956!

Developments in the Care of the Mentally Ill— 1890 to Present

While the Massachusetts study was gathering dust, important developments occurred in the field of mental health. Sigmund Freud (1856–1939) began his medical career doing research in the anatomy and physiology of the nervous system. However, financial pressures forced him to abandon his microscope, and he turned to the practice of clinical **neurology**. While he made several important contributions to this field, he also used his practice to make careful and skillful observations about his **neurotic** patients. Beginning in 1893, he formulated and published a number of theories about the human mind and, in the process, originated **psychoanalysis**. Many of these theories are well known: the **unconscious**, the interpretation of dreams, the existence of sexuality in childhood, and so on. For our purposes, the importance of Freud and the many who have come after him, both disciples and dissidents, is that they have given us a dynamic psychiatry. There have been many professional disagreements and modifications of Freud's original work. However, there has been virtually unanimous acceptance of one basic idea: that the personality itself and symptoms *per se* are the result of various forces within the personality, or psychic structure, a part of which is not immediately available to our conscious awareness. Thus, symptoms and illness have meaning within the broader context of the patient's life. The contemporary therapist has a much more sophisticated understanding of the causes and meaning of the patient's behavior than was accessible to those providing treatment in the eighteenth and nine-

---

NEUROLOGY: the branch of medicine devoted to the organization, function, and diseases of nervous tissues—peripheral nerves, spinal cord, and brain

NEUROTIC: relating to or affected by neurosis; neurosis or psychoneurosis: any of a number of mental disorders characterized by anxiety and various symptoms. In contrast to psychosis, there is not a gross disorganization of the personality nor a gross disruption in adaptation to external reality.

PSYCHOANALYSIS: 1. a procedure for investigating mental processes and treating mental disorders, especially neuroses, by means of free-association, dream interpretation, and interpretation of resistance (the instinctual opposition to the process), and transference (the projection of feelings, thoughts, and wishes onto the analyst). Classically, a couch is used, and the patient is seen four or five times per week for a period of years. 2. a theory of psychology or mental functioning which applies to all humans, sick or well

UNCONSCIOUS: part of the psyche, or personality, which is not immediately available to conscious awareness

teenth centuries. Moreover, the therapist is now aware of the reasons why his "force of personality" has an effect on the patient and on the therapeutic relationship. The concept of an equilibrium of contending forces within the individual also paved the way to an understanding of group dynamics and family dynamics as well as to the development of their respective therapies.

In addition to the birth of dynamic psychiatry, there was a tremendous growth in knowledge about the disease entities and their classification. Kraepelin (1855–1926) had separated **manic-depressive psychosis** from the disease which Bleuler (1857–1939) was to name schizophrenia [3] and describe definitively in 1911. The description of Mr. X., a victim of schizophrenia, was first presented by Herman Nunberg (1884–1970), a brilliant young student of Freud's in 1920—a date still too early for Mr. X. to have benefited from some of the treatment now available. Freud's work dealt primarily with neurosis; those who came after him described psychosis in dynamic terms and worked with psychotic patients. In this country, Harry Stack Sullivan (1892–1949) made important contributions in this and other areas.

A further area in which significant developments have occurred is that of organic therapy. The belief that all mental illness is produced by some structural or chemical alteration in the brain, or, in other words, is organic rather than psychological in origin, has existed for a long time. Although there certainly are some conditions (such as that suffered by King George III) which are in fact due to an organic cause, this orientation seems all too often accompanied by a conviction of incurability or by injudicious, if not irresponsible, actions. It is to be hoped that the increasingly more sophisticated techniques of chemical research into brain and body will provide further helpful insights into the nature and treatment of mental illness. Unfortunately, virtually every advance in our knowledge of human physiology or biochemistry has produced some bizarre theory of mental illness or form of "therapy" which often has been implemented without any careful attempt to compare results with other forms of treatment and yet with an absolute conviction that it is of benefit to the patient. Thus, people suffering from psychosis have been subjected to castration, have had their teeth pulled, their adrenal glands excised, and their colons and sections of their small intestine removed by physicians

---

MANIC-DEPRESSIVE PSYCHOSIS: a mental disorder characterized by a severe disturbance in mood (either depression or elation), which so dominates the patient that life, personality, and contact with reality are disrupted

who were confident, on the basis of little or no scientific data, that such procedures would produce a cure. In the 1940s, an operation known as a lobotomy was introduced and popularized. This operative procedure involves cutting the connections between all or part of the frontal lobes of the brain and the rest of this organ. In theory, the lobotomy renders the patient placid, calm, and less aggressive. However, it also produces a tendency toward uncontrolled impulsiveness which makes it difficult to predict the patient's behavior. Not only was this operation performed without careful comparative studies, but no efforts were made for long-term follow-up of the patients. Before it was discovered that its efficacy was questionable, this procedure had been suggested for a great many different illnesses and even performed on children—sometimes more than once if results were not good the first time. Some forms of lobotomy had been considered simple enough to be performed in the doctor's office, and various people now predict that improvement in surgical techniques will renew the popularity of this procedure.

Fortunately, other organic therapies have proved less harmful to the patient, even if their value was open to question; some have been therapeutically helpful regardless of whether their mechanism or the origins of the illness were clearly understood. Shortly after the discovery of insulin, psychiatrists began to use it to increase the appetite of patients reluctant to eat. In the thirties, insulin shock treatment (or the production of an insulin coma) was introduced. Though the theoretical grounds for this were vague, it appeared to be of some benefit to young schizophrenics who had only recently become ill. However, no really well-controlled studies comparing it to other forms of treatment were done. It remained controversial and has now all but been abandoned, mainly because of its cost.

Joseph von Meduna introduced Metrazol shock treatment in 1933. Based on his microscopic observation of different cell changes in the brains of patients suffering from both epilepsy and schizophrenia, he theorized that the two diseases were incompatible. (No one else has ever been able to see the same changes, and many people have both diseases.) The drug Metrazol, when injected in the correct dosage, first causes a period of excitement and dread in the patient, which is often severe enough for him to offer his wife and fortune to the administering physician to buy escape. This phase is followed by a convulsion. For quite some time many attributed the clinical improvement in the patient to the first reaction, or "shock," rather than to the convulsion. The shock idea persisted even after it was discovered that the production of a convulsion by a small electrical current was easier, safer, and cheaper. Electroconvulsive treatment, or electric shock treatment, is still in use today and is a particularly valuable tool in severe depression, where it can be life-saving. Its use in schizophrenia is controversial, but it can certainly be used safely in a number of conditions if all else has failed. Now that the shock idea has been abandoned, the treatment is administered to patients after they have been anesthetized. However, it is still not understood what it is about the convulsion which helps the patient.

In 1952, Thorazine, the best known of a group of drugs called phenothiazines, was introduced for the treatment of mental illness. This and other drugs, all of which have similar actions and side effects, are often referred to as the major tranquilizers ("anti-psychotic" drugs is perhaps a better term). They are not addicting, and they can be of dramatic benefit to the acutely ill and, sometimes, to the chronically ill. They are occasionally thought of and used only as chemical restraints, but their value goes far beyond this. Although they are certainly not a panacea, the phenothiazines have enabled many patients to leave the hospital.

In about 1956, two classes of drugs were found to be not only helpful in depressions but almost specifically counteractive to them in many patients. These drugs are referred to as anti-depressants. The most recent addition to the psychopharmacology of mental illness is lithium carbonate, which is now the treatment of choice of the manic phase of manic-depressive psychosis; the use of this drug in the depressive phase has had varied results and remains controversial. Unlike the other drugs mentioned above, the use of lithium must be extremely carefully supervised, since it can be highly dangerous—even fatal—if the amount of the drug contained in the bloodstream increases only slightly over that necessary to produce the therapeutic effect.

The minor tranquilizers such as Librium, Valium, and Miltown are meant for symptomatic relief of anxiety and tension in neurosis and less serious emotional problems. They are prescribed by the hundreds of thousands, if not millions; this is not surprising when we realize that many doctors estimate that 50 percent of the complaints for which they are consulted are functional. Although prescribed for relatively mild problems, Miltown can become severely addicting if taken in large amounts.

The state mental hospitals (discussed later in this chapter) were virtually unaffected by the progress in dynamic psychiatry. However, its impact was strongly felt in general hospitals with psychiatric wards, in private psychiatric hospitals, and particularly in those hospitals associated with universities. The dynamics of the whole hospital began to come under observation. It was realized that the many intra- and inter-group reactions between patients, attendants, nurses, doctors, and administrators can produce movement toward illness as well as toward health. The knowledge, insights, and theories of sociology were added and applied with what had been learned from dynamic psychiatry; there is now a general attempt to coordinate all activities within a hospital (i.e., recreational activities, occupational therapy, staff meetings, individual and group therapy, and so on) so that they can most effectively serve the goal of producing health. Moreover, there is a growing move to enlist the patients as at least part-time therapists. Such developments are often referred to as the process of creating a total therapeutic milieu.

Another new development which has gained rather widespread acceptance is the concept of partial hospitalization. Thus, patients who are able to work but need the hospital outside of working hours may be in a "night hospital," and those able to be at home at night are placed in "day hospitals" (the first of which was founded in Moscow in 1936). Such partial hospitalization may be used independently or as a method whereby the patient in a traditional hospital can be gradually returned to the community. A few halfway houses now exist which serve as supportive residences and similarly help in this transition.

In recent years there has been much more emphasis on the need to recruit and train more paraprofessionals, or mental health workers, and to expand their areas of responsibility in the care and treatment of the mentally ill both in and out of the hospital. Perhaps, in addition, we have become more sophisticated in our understanding of the limitations of hospitals and no longer expect them to provide total cures. Indeed, it has been recognized that a large percentage of those who suffer from severe mental illness do not need to be hospitalized at all, particularly when there are adequate outpatient facilities.

Linked to many of the new developments and thinking in the field has been the emergence of what is called community psychiatry. In many ways, the cornerstone of this innovation is the Community Mental Health Centers Act of 1963. This federal legislation makes funds available for states to set up comprehensive mental health centers. Designed to serve a population of about 150,000, these centers are intended to provide preventive services, treatment (inpatient and outpatient), and rehabilitation programs for persons of all ages, classes, and ethnic groups. In addition, the act includes provisions for nursing homes for the senile elderly. The hospitals associated with these centers must be kept small and must include partial hospitalization. Central to the concept of community psychiatry are two important principles: (1) facilities must be carefully planned to meet the needs of the target population; and (2) those suffering from mental illness must be kept as close as possible to their home community and, whenever feasible, should reside within that community in their own home. Although it was hoped that such measures would eventually do away with the larger, isolated custodial state hospital, this has not yet come to pass. In addition, no extensive evaluation has yet been made of such questions as the effects of keeping a severely disturbed parent in the home with children. A problem which can be anticipated for any such new program in psychiatry is that institutional readmissions of unimproved, chronically ill patients gradually build up, and the need to provide custodial care for such sheer numbers of persons inhibits or makes impossible the treatment of those whose chances for cure are good.

It has been mentioned that the state mental hospitals have been relatively immune to the progressive contributions of dynamic psychiatry. From 1893 until well into the 1950s, these hospitals continued to increase in size. They have remained grim, cheerless places, overcrowded, under-staffed, providing only minimal custodial care, often little interested in helping anyone, and unable to attract a high caliber of physician. The incident, in 1942, of 25 senile patients in one New York State hospital being washed from a single basin of water and with the use of a single towel was typical of the dismal conditions which led to a series of "snake pit" exposés in the public media.

Recently, large numbers of psychiatrists who trained in these hospitals complained that the certification examinations of the American Board of Psychiatry and Neurology were discriminatory. The response of that specialty board was that most of those who complained were sufficiently lacking in English language skills to explain their failure on this basis alone. Such persons, it was argued, would have difficulty with most examinations. In addition, the only previous American certification earned by these psychiatrists was a passing grade on the examination which enables graduates of foreign medical schools to obtain a license to practice medicine in the United States. It was further pointed out that graduates of American nursing schools did as well, if not better, on these examinations than did the doctors taking them. The American Board of Psychiatry and Neurology finally decided simply to exclude graduates of foreign medical schools from taking the examination for specialty certification. Whatever conclusions may be drawn from this, it certainly confirms the state hospitals as the low institutions on the psychiatric totem pole.

Nevertheless, the state institutions serve a most important function in the treatment of the mentally ill by preventing other institutions and treatment facilities from becoming inundated by unmanageable numbers of incurable patients. Perhaps there will always be a need for places which provide custodial care for those patients who under no circumstances will get well. The state institutions also provide a place for those patients who find refuge and solace in chronic hospitalization, who regard any treatment as a demand from the outside that they improve, and who need to make a basic discovery that no one and no treatment can make them well against their own wishes.

It is implicit in this discussion that good care for the few is often bought at the expense of poor care for the multitudes. To the extent that state hospitals relieve the pressure on private institutions and university centers to admit patients indiscriminately, we have a dual system of care for the mentally ill. It is to be hoped that the efforts and programs of community psychiatry and such services as those provided by the community mental health centers will lessen the impact of this duality and reduce the number of institutionalized patients.

Some of the difficulties and complexities in the treatment of the mentally ill can be illustrated by the following case history:

Mr. J. was 60 years old when he came to the hospital. He had been admitted after threatening to jump from a 12-story window in order to get relief from the excruciating abdominal pain which had plagued him for 12 years. Mr. J. had sought the help of countless physicians because of the pain, and over time a clear pattern had emerged.

First, he went to a leading university medical center where a large number of diagnostic tests were performed, including an exploratory **laparotomy**. No abnormalities were found. At the urging of his wife, he then went to a private surgeon who removed part of an abdominal organ, but the pain persisted. In this way, he eventually underwent seven abdominal operations, only one of which was necessary—he was bleeding from an ulcer produced partly by his excessive use of aspirin for the abdominal pain and partly by steroid drugs which had been prescribed for another, unrelated complaint.

As the result of a relative's well-intentioned efforts to relieve his suffering, Mr. J. became addicted to narcotics and was subsequently referred for **psychotherapy**. Eighteen months of weekly sessions, augmented by tranquilizers and antidepressants, helped him to get off narcotics but had no effect on his persistent abdominal pain.

He was eventually readmitted to the university hospital, and this time a **chordotomy** was actively considered. To evaluate what effects could be expected from this surgical procedure, he was given

---

LAPAROTOMY: the surgical procedure of opening the abdomen

PYSCHOTHERAPY: the art of treating mental disorders; the establishment, by a trained person, of a professional relationship to explore part or all of the personality and its symptoms. The term is broader than psychoanalysis and connotes more limited objectives, greater attention to the conscious level of functioning, and shorter duration of treatment.

CHORDOTOMY: a surgical procedure which attempts to relieve pain by severing certain nerve tracts at the point where they leave the spinal cord.

spinal anesthesia. Although this physically blocked the ability to feel pain, Mr. J. nevertheless still complained of severe pain. It was thus clear that the operation would not help, and it was not performed. Later, however, he found a surgeon who did it. As a result, Mr. J. felt no pain when jabbed with a needle anywhere between his nipples and his toes, nor could he tell the difference between extreme heat and cold against his skin. The abdominal pain, however, persisted.

As a last resort, he underwent his ninth operation, a lobotomy (which, it will be remembered, was once thought to be a cure for mental illness). Although this procedure tends to make the patient "indifferent" to pain, it brought no relief to Mr. J. Indeed, he developed a psychosis which lasted for five weeks and which was felt to be a reaction to the operation.

During the next year the pain persisted undiminished and, if anything, became worse. At this point, Mr. J. declared his intention to commit suicide and was brought to the hospital, where it was noted by all who saw him that he was obviously in severe pain. In addition, he had the appearance of someone who had been physically ill for a long time. Emaciated, depressed, and desperate, he begged for some relief from his suffering.

He was given electroshock therapy because it was felt that the pain might well be caused by an underlying severe depression. The results were dramatic. The pain disappeared! His psychiatrist and the hospital staff were delighted that Mr. J. was relieved, and he was moderately happy for the first 48 hours. Then a strange thing happened. He began to complain of the same pain. This time, however, his psychiatrist, the nurses, and the members of his family were all puzzled by their unanimous observation that he was only pretending to have pain. The next day he said he wanted to go to a state hospital because the pain was so bad, although he could give no reasons for why a state hospital would help. He was told that this would be arranged if he wished but was asked to wait 10 days to see "how things went." He accepted this, but within an hour irate relatives called the psychiatrist because Mr. J. had told them he was being sent to the state hospital the next day. The psychiatrist was further puzzled, and scheduled a second session with the patient for later in the day. Mr. J., however, unable to wait that long and driven by his own inner motives, decapitated himself.

Mr. J. was a constant source of frustration to his family, his numerous physicians, and to himself. All attempts to cure, heal, or simply help his pain ended in failure. When his final psychiatric treatment did "help," he could not tolerate the situation. Thus, cure itself contributed to Mr. J.'s ultimate self-destruction. It is unfortunate that an often significant component of mental illness is a resistance to improvement or cure; and, in the end, an individual can defeat any techniques, actions, and efforts mobilized on his behalf. This is an important point to remember when we attempt to judge any therapeutic modality.

There seems to be a pendulum which swings between progress and neglect in psychiatry, and each innovation has its roots in what preceded it, e.g., the role of the dream in the "incubation" of the ancient Greeks preceded Freud's work on the interpretation of dreams, and the idea that the mentally ill are fair game for any experimentation came before the idea of trying to cure them by castration. It would seem that the philosopher Santayana's warning that we must remember the past lest we be doomed to relive it is particularly applicable to psychiatry.

The Extent of Mental Illness

Mental illness is the leading health problem in the United States today. In 1963, President Kennedy stated that "mental illness and mental retardation are among our most critical health problems. They occur more frequently, affect more people, require more prolonged treatment, cause more suffering by the families of the afflicted, waste more of our human resources, and constitute more financial drain upon both the public treasury and the personal finances of the individual families than any other single condition."

At any one time there are more people in hospitals because of mental illness than for all other illnesses combined. On any given day, this amounts to about 770,000 persons in state, private, and veteran's hospitals. About 1.5 million people receive treatment in these institutions in any one year, and 50 percent of those admitted for treatment each year have had one or more prior admissions. It is estimated that 10 percent of the total population is in need of psychiatric treatment—roughly 20 million people. Staggering as this figure is, it hardly gives a complete picture of the problem. Some prevalence studies indicate that between one-third and two-thirds of the population have some psychiatric disorder. Whether or not many people are sick enough for there to be a public responsibility for their treatment is an unanswered question. Recently, one large study found that only 19 percent of the population could be considered to be well, and 23 percent were considered to have impaired functioning (i.e., they were in trouble in the study's terms); the remaining 58 percent, having symptoms to a lesser or greater degree, provided a continuum between the "well" 19 percent and the "sick" 23 percent. Note that we are speaking in terms of *percentages*. Unless there is an unlikely change in those percentages during the coming years, population growth will account for an ever greater *number* of people seriously in need of treatment and/or hospitalization.

The cost of mental illness provides further staggering numbers. The direct costs include almost $2 billion a year spent for care in community, state, private, and federal hospitals. Over $93 million is spent on community mental health programs, including outpatient clinics. Two-hundred million dollars goes for private psychiatric treatment, and approximately $100 million has been spent annually on research in past years.

Industry also picks up a large tab for mental illness. It is estimated that hospitalized persons represent a loss of $2 billion a year in purchasing power. In addition, 50 percent of all absences from work are credited to emotional disturbances or mental illness, with an annual cost to industry of $5 billion. Emotional problems are extremely important contributory factors, if not the prime cause, in 75 percent of all accidents, which cost industry $3 billion a year in injury to workers and damage to equipment. (In view of these last two sets of figures, it is surprising that psychiatric consultation is not sought more often by industry.) It should be noted that the above statistics include only a portion of those whose principal problem is alcoholism (see Chapter 8) and that, further, we have not considered any of the statistics concerning mental retardation.

There are now 238 state hospitals and 46 county medical hospitals (a total of 500,000 beds) in the United States. Despite their serious limitations, these institutions are still the only psychiatric facilities available for a large part of the population. About 75 percent of their buildings were constructed before World War I, and 20 percent of these have been declared fire hazards. Some of the larger hospitals have over 14,000 patients. The average physician-to-patient ratio is less than 1:100, and, in some instances, there is only one psychiatrist per 360 patients. Over 45 percent of the patients in these institutions have been continuously hospitalized for over 10 years. The average daily expenditure for maintenance is $17.59 per patient. Although this is a decided contrast to the rough figure of $95.00 per patient per day in short-term general hospitals, the funds needed to maintain the state hospitals represent a significant financial burden to the states and a tempting target for budget-cutting in times of decreased tax revenues.

The 237 private psychiatric hospitals have approximately 16,000 beds and account for 70,000 admissions per year. These institutions range from hospitals providing short-term treatment at a cost of about $50 per day to facilities offering intensive long-term therapeutic care at an annual cost of about $28,000. Many of the short-term private psychiatric hospitals are geared mainly to giving electroshock treatment, and most insurance coverage is written to favor this type of treatment. Aside from their exorbitant costs, the impact of these facilities is limited by geographic restrictions, since nearly half of them are located in New York or California.

Another 10,000 beds are available in psychiatric wards of 495 general hospitals. The average stay is only three weeks, and there are thus almost as many admissions to these institutions each year as to the state hospitals. The alliance of the psychiatric treatment facility and the general hospital is undoubtedly beneficial, provided the former functions as a general psychiatric ward rather than simply a ward for electroshock treatment. Insurance policies are also written to favor this type of facility, and the length of stay is almost certainly influenced by the standard 21-day contract.

It has been mentioned that $200 million is spent annually on private psychiatric treatment. This sum includes the costs of maintenance electroshock treatments, brief supportive visits, drugs, psychotherapy (about two visits per week), psychoanalysis (four to five times per week), group therapy, family therapy (in which couples or entire families, including children, are seen), and various combinations of all these treatment possibilities. The fees paid for any one of them can vary widely. In general, however, the costs are such that these services are restricted to the upper-middle and upper socioeconomic groups. Although there has been some movement toward health insurance coverage for psychotherapy, it is still very difficult to obtain insurance which covers outpatient psychiatric treatment, even under the extended benefit or major medical type of policies. However, group policies obtained by industry and unions are improving in their coverage of both inpatient and outpatient care. IBM deserves special mention for its pace-setting plan which provides 80 percent coverage for outpatient treatment.

Another important source of outpatient treatment are the approximately 2,000 private and public clinics, which treat about 900,000 persons (adults and children) annually. Unfortunately, many (and not just the best) have long waiting lists. These clinics vary from high-quality facilities which are part of universities and hospitals to profit-oriented agencies, some of which have poorly trained personnel. Operating funds are supplied by states, communities, and private sources and are usually in short supply. Typically, the medical and nonmedical staffs of such clinics average only three years of professional training. In addition, these facilities are geographically limited to certain areas of the country because most states have not provided funds for community mental health programs. Of the $93.5 million spent for such programs, 50 percent is absorbed by New York, California, and Illinois.

Although this discussion has been about psychiatric treatment and psychiatrists, the reader has probably noted that the word *psychotherapy* has appeared, as it did in our case history of Mr. J. Not all psychotherapists are psychiatrists, and not all psychiatrists are psychotherapists. Indeed, there are only about 15,000 psychiatrists in the United States, 12,000 of whom are members of the American Psychiatric Association. There are an additional 1,000 psychiatrists who are members of the American Psychoanalytic Association. (Some of these psychiatrists hold membership in both organizations.) The Clinical Division of the American Psychological Association has about 3,000 members, and, in 1963, 1,300 of them had passed the board examination of the American Board of Examiners in Professional Psychology. However, surveys indicate that there are probably closer to 8,000 psychologists involved in clinical services. There are also about 3,000 psychiatric social workers, many of whom are psychotherapists; and, of the 600,000 employed nurses, about 18,500 are working in psychiatric settings. Few of these nurses, however, are trained as psychotherapists. In addition, there are some people who fit into none of these categories, but are self-designated psychotherapists. In New York State, for example, anyone can hang out a shingle identifying himself as such.

In all of the above disciplines, there are, of course, good psychotherapists as well as ones whose competence is questionable. Insurance coverage has tended to discriminate against psychologists and social workers, mainly on economic grounds. There has been some improvement in the criteria for certification of these and other groups, and, in the interests of quality care, this is a positive and welcome development. The geographic restriction which we have encountered before also applies to these professional groups, since they are generally located in or near urban centers. Again, New York and California tend to have the lion's share, and rural areas are deprived. In addition to advantages such as greater opportunity for continued professional education and stimulation, and a larger demand for psychiatric services, the cities offer a degree of anonymity which is often beneficial to patient and therapist.

Selected Mental Disorders

Each of us is unique; yet we are more alike than we are different. Each of us is born to parents who, consciously and unconsciously, have various expectations of us; and, in turn, we each relate to our own children in terms of what we are and what we expect. Some babies at birth are forceful squirmers, twisting and turning in their mother's arms; others are quiet, soft little lumps. Some nurse vigorously, some languidly. Some mothers are distressed by quieter babies, some by more active ones. Some mothers experience a vigorous, active nurser as "attacking" or "devouring"; others feel that a slow or listless nurser is rejecting or refusing them. Even these few examples make apparent the many possible variations in parent and child, and one can see how diverse and complex are the possibilities of interaction in just the first few months of life. Indeed, at each stage in an individual's life—childhood, adolescence, adulthood, old age—he is exposed to different variables. The development of his personality—who he is, what he feels, how he behaves—is determined by forces within him, by forces within his personal and societal environment, and by what happens when all the forces mutually interact. It is in the search to understand these dynamics that we find clues to why people and societies are strong or weak, sick or healthy, disturbed or integrated, and so on.[3]

In the discussion which follows, only a few illustrative examples of mental disorders will be considered. These include certain organic brain syndromes commonly associated with other illnesses, syndromes related to the deterioration which occurs in aging, and the disease entity schizophrenia.[4] (See Fig. 7-8.)

The term *organic brain syndromes* is used to describe one class of mental disorders. They are so named because they are caused by or associated with impairment of brain-tissue function. The brain is the body organ most sensitive to changes in the chemical environment which supports it. For example, a decrease in its blood supply—and therefore a decrease in oxygen and nutrients—will grossly impair the function of the brain long before any other organ is seriously affected.

Acute delirium is a classic organic brain syndrome. By definition, this means that there has been an *acute* impairment in the functioning of the brain tissue. This condition is so commonly associated with trauma, serious illnesses, anesthesia, and the effects of drugs that probably 10 to 15 percent of all patients on acute medical and surgical wards have some degree of delirium. Indeed, most people so recognize its connection with other illnesses that they rarely call a psychiatrist because of the symptoms, but rather an internist, general practitioner, or pediatrician. The first symptoms of acute delirium usually are restlessness, irritability, and confusion. The patient may appear quite bland or withdrawn or be panicky and difficult to control. The confusion ordinarily first shows itself in slowed and/or vague responses to questions, but soon progresses to gross *disorientation*. By this we mean that the patient does not know where he is; he is confused as to the year, month, day, or hour; and he misidentifies people around him. *Memory is defective or impaired* in that the patient is unable to recall what was said to him only moments before, nor can he remember what he has done or whom he has seen recently. There are usually *gross impairments in intellectual functions* such as the ability to comprehend concepts, do arithmetic, answer questions related to gen-

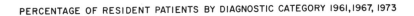

PERCENTAGE OF RESIDENT PATIENTS BY DIAGNOSTIC CATEGORY 1961,1967, 1973

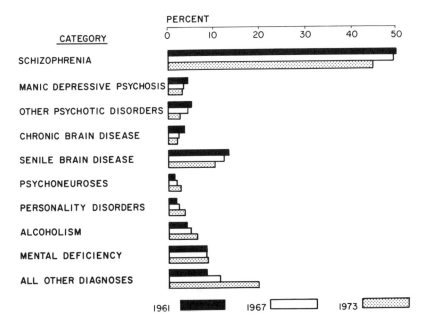

FIG. 7-8.   *Percentage of resident patients by diagnostic category—1961, 1967, 1973. The government figures are only for the* resident *patient population not the* incidence *of cases in each disease category.* (*From* Statistical Notes 1-25, *National Institute of Mental Health, Public Health Service, Department of Health, Education and Welfare, December 1971.*)

eral learning, and so on. There is a *general misinterpretation of sensory experience* or input, such that voices of strangers are firmly held to be those of relatives, and shadows on the wall are interpreted as people or animals. Night hours are thus very likely to intensify delirium. Frequently, there may be frank **hallucinations** (usually visual) involving insects, animals, people, or objects, and frank **delusions,** such as a conviction that the other patients are all "communist agents" pursuing him.

A most important point to remember is that this is usually a very frightening, often terrifying experience for the individual undergoing it. Secondly, it is noteworthy that the content of the delirium is rather spe-

HALLUCINATION: an apparent perception of an external object (sound, sight, smell, and so on) when no such object is present
DELUSION: a false belief; one that is obviously contrary to demonstrable fact

cific to the individual and related to his personal history. Both these points are illustrated in the following case summary:

Mr. H., a man in his fifties, was admitted to the hospital with an intense abdominal pain that was diagnosed as a dissecting aneurysm of the aorta. Before it was possible to arrange surgery on a planned basis, his aorta ruptured. This resulted in his requiring 80 pints of blood and a seven-hour emergency operation.

Seventy-two hours later, a medical student entered the patient's room and found him talking to himself. He was restless and pulling at the bedclothes and hospital gown. He thought the student (in a white coat) was his butcher and expressed amazement at seeing him in "this rotten hotel." Mr. H. insisted that his wife was calling to him from downstairs and that he had to get to her. When asked why, he explained that green turtles were walking up and down the wall and had been doing so for some time. Now they were starting across the ceiling and beginning to fall onto the bed. At that, he became terrified and lept out of bed, trying to free himself of all restraint, including his surgical dressing. The frightened medical student tried to block the way and get the patient back to bed, only to find himself pinned beneath a now nude man, with the stands and bottles (attached to the various tubes keeping the man alive) crashing around them both. Screams for help finally brought a head nurse—who was dismayed at the mess to be cleaned up—and an intern—who foresaw a long, tedious task of replacing needles and catheters. Both indignantly inquired of the student why he had not kept the patient in bed.

A few weeks later, the patient supplied the following information: When he first became ill with abdominal pain, he attributed it to food poisoning from bad meat from his butcher. Furthermore, during a time of crisis in his life, he had spent a night in a cheap hotel and had awakened to find the wall crawling with bedbugs. Mr. H. also revealed an important childhood memory: At age five, he and a much older brother were swimming in a pond. The brother found a green turtle, came out of the water with it, and badly frightened the patient, who thought that the turtle would bite him; the brother then threw the turtle at the patient's feet. The brother had been a butcher.

Beyond the obvious need to correct the underlying cause of his condition, the delirious patient should be kept sedated in a lighted room and restrained if necessary. Reassurance as to the cause of his difficulty is also most helpful, especially if it can come from a trusted person whom the patient is able to recognize:

ANEURYSM: a defect in the wall of an artery, such that the artery may balloon out and, frequently, burst. Congenital aneurysms affecting vessels in the brain are often the causes of stroke in young people.

A young woman who had recently terminated a rather successful psychotherapy became ill and was hospitalized. As her delirium began, she insisted that a friend call her (the patient's) psychiatrist. When he telephoned two hours later, she was obviously delirious and agitated but recognized his voice. He explained that the cause of what she was experiencing was her high fever, that it was called delirium, and that it would go away. He then called the nursing station to make sure that the hospital staff was informed of her condition. The nurse and intern found her sleeping quietly.

One of the problems which often confronts those treating a person who has both a physical illness and manifestations of a mental disorder is that the one can precipitate the other. In the case of delirium, this is a relatively identifiable sequence. However, when the organic brain syndrome resembles a less clear-cut psychiatric illness, it is much more difficult to establish the precipitating organic cause; among other things, this can have significant implications for treatment.

A 50-year-old man became depressed, i.e., he felt and looked sad and rather hopeless, had difficulty sleeping, experienced a decrease in appetite, and lost weight. These developments occurred one year after the irradiation of an inoperable carcinoma of his lung. He confided to his internist that he was certain his cancer had been caused by his wife and that he had left her. The internist examined him carefully, found nothing indicating a lesion in the brain, but referred him to a neurologist to be sure. The neurologist also could find nothing, and the patient was then referred to a psychiatrist for a consultation. The latter was somewhat puzzled by the symptoms of depression as this man described them—they didn't seem quite right somehow. Though odd and unusual, the idea that his wife had caused the cancer grew out of a long and troubled marriage that was filled with more hatred than love. The psychiatrist attempted to elicit some of the patient's feelings about having been ill and about the success of the x-ray therapy. The patient responded by recounting his recent difficulty with remembering the names of places and finding the right word. He felt that these things went far beyond normal "slips" and feared he was going crazy.
   This information, which the patient had withheld from the other doctors, prompted the psychiatrist to make some quick, crude mental tests for signs of a brain lesion and to confirm them with psychological tests. He told the patient what the correct diagnosis was and expressed his interest in helping him to deal with whatever feelings or fears might come up about his illness. Within 72 hours, x-ray therapy for the spread of the lung cancer to the brain was begun. The patient's symptoms disappeared, he remarried, and he lived productively and relatively happily for the next four and

one-half years. There were no signs or symptoms of cancer in his brain, and he died of other complications of his disease.

We have thus far considered two organic brain syndromes: acute delirium and a nonpsychotic acute brain syndrome due to metastatic cancer of the brain. Another group of mental disorders are those associated with aging. The words *senile, senescent,* and *senility* are derived from Latin roots meaning "to grow old" and "old one." They all convey (in English, at least) the idea of degeneration, feebleness, or infirmity. In no sense are they complimentary, particularly in our society.

As we grow old, our brains also tend to "age" and to function less well. For example, older people characteristically become forgetful or absentminded about recent events, although they often remember the less recent past quite clearly; or one may notice that an older person needs to repeat the time or day of an appointment a number of times. In addition to some difficulty in memory, there is usually a "set-in-their-ways" tinge to the personality and an increase in concern about bodily functions. Much behavior may become ritualized. Often, for example, each personal item is carefully placed and must not be moved, because the task of finding it or remembering where it has been put has become much harder.

There may also be a decrease in intellectual functioning, and previous personality patterns or traits may become exaggerated. Thus, someone who has always tried to control those around him may become even more insistent and demanding. Change, which is not really easy for any of us, can present a serious threat to the aged. Conservatism, or even a wish to turn back the clock to the "good old days," is often an expression of the individual's concern that he will not be able to cope with change. Moving to a new dwelling or town is an upsetting experience for many people. For the aged it is often traumatic. They may be overwhelmed by the loss of familiar surroundings and the simultaneous need to adapt to new living quarters, new people, new stores, and so on. The elderly also often tend to live in a state of chronic frustration because, myths aside, sex dies hard; and being old and alone makes the attainment of gratification difficult. At any age, the loss of a loved one or close friend creates such stress in so many people that it is one of the major precipitating factors in all emotional illness. As is true in so many other of their experiences, the aged face such losses at a time when their inner resources are often at a minimum.

Despite the decrease in their mental and physical functioning, many aging people remain productive and valued by family and society. For these persons, the concept of the "golden years" is perhaps applicable; for many others, however, there is increasing loneliness and a pervading sense

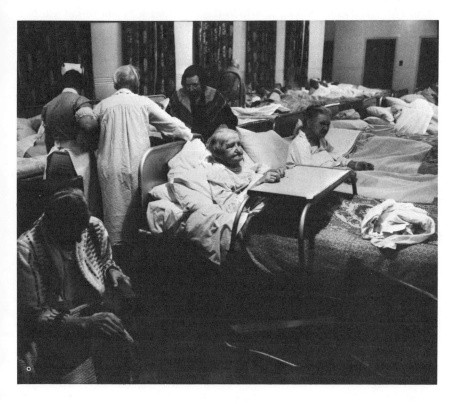

FIG. 7-9. *This overcrowded senile women's ward is certainly not an environment encouraging hope or recovery. (Courtesy of John Brooke.)*

of uselessness (Fig. 7-9). Retirement, which in our society commonly comes well before the expected age of death, often intensifies these feelings and thus can be a stressful, even feared event. When society was still predominantly rural, and such simple tasks as gathering kindling were important to a family, "granny" could still find a way to be useful. And if she paced about the house at night and left the door open, neither she nor the rest of the family were in great danger. The situation is quite different today in, for example, an apartment in New York City; such an accommodation rarely allows for much "pacing around" without disturbing other family members and, possibly, neighbors as well.

One or two other points should be added to this rough conceptualization of the aged. The legendary reverence afforded to the old in some cultures is virtually nonexistent in our society. On the contrary, we commonly have and communicate (verbally or otherwise) the feeling expressed in Albee's play, *The American Dream,* in which the daughter and son-in-law caution granny to watch herself lest they call the "van man" to take her away. It is not often that we are motivated to look at our elderly and share Dylan Thomas' "rage, rage against the dying of the light." Indeed, children often find themselves somewhat bewildered when they are mourning the loss of a grandparent's warm companionship, and their parents seem only to be relieved of a burden.

In psychiatric terms, "senility" refers to organic brain syndromes associated with aging and, specifically, to the clinical entity called senile dementia. Basically, this condition is an exaggeration of the aging process. The brains of old people normally develop abnormalities known as senile plaques. However, the brains of persons with senile dementia contain many more plaques and, in addition, are shrunken and have a decreased number of cells. The basic process of the degeneration is not understood; nor is it known why some people should show the onset of senile dementia at 65, some at 90, and many others not at all.

The onset is subtle and gradual, so that the brain and personality have a chance to adapt within their restricted limits. Again, there is progressive memory loss, first for recent and then past events. There is also progressive disorientation and confusion, with increasing impairment in intellectual functioning and the ability to make reasonable decisions. In the early stages, the person may manifest a previously uncharacteristic tendency to act impulsively. In more specific terms, the unfortunate individual suffering from this illness begins to regress, his I.Q. drops, and his ability to function diminishes until he is literally in diapers—unable to recognize his surroundings, unable to carry on even the most elementary conversation, unable to remember if he has eaten an hour before or to tell someone if he is hungry. Sometimes years are spent in some sort of repetitive childhood activity like rocking a rag doll. The mental deterioration is accompanied by progressive aging and feebleness of the body; there is unsteadiness of gait, wasting of muscle, and shrinkage of soft tissue. Death sometimes comes within a year, but often the disease lasts for as long as 10 years.

Because of its insidious onset, senile dementia may not be noticed by relatives for a long time, unless they have been away from the patient for a while. Occasionally, some intervening crisis produces an outburst of strange behavior in the individual and thus forces attention to the problem:

A well-dressed man, appearing to be in his early sixties, was brought to the emergency room of a hospital. He had been found wandering the streets, obviously lost. There was nothing in his pockets, and he refused to speak, except to mumble a few words. The police noted a small bump on his head and theorized that he had been mugged. He was resistant, negative, and fearful with both the police and the psychiatrist in the emergency room.

Unable to be identified, he was admitted to the psychiatric ward. Although efforts to communicate with him continued, the patient refused or was unable to carry on any conversation or state his name, address, age, occupation, or telephone number. However, he was able to feed himself and use the toilet. He spent the day walking up and down the halls with his hands held behind his back. Every so often, he would walk up behind a nurse or a resident physician and either mumble or say very clearly, "Um hm, very good!" Something about this behavior gave the staff an eerie feeling. When he tried to leave the ward and was restrained from doing so, he resisted and screamed, "Take your hands off me! How dare you!"

When his anxious family found him, it was learned that he was actually 72 years old and a retired surgeon. His memory difficulty had been known to the family for about two years. They were aware that over the past six months he had been talking less and becoming a little more confused. He had kept busy puttering in his rose garden, which hadn't looked as good as usual but was still the best on the block. On the day of his disappearance, he had set out for the hardware store only two blocks away. He had probably gotten lost when he tried to return home.

The other major clinical form of degeneration of the brain is called psychosis with cerebral arteriosclerosis. It is also referred to as arteriosclerotic cerebral degeneration. This degeneration is linked to decreased blood flow to the brain because of the arteriosclerotic process in the vessels supplying that organ. Clinically, these patients show a much more abrupt onset of symptoms than do those with senile dementia. There may be an acute delirium related to a small stroke; or there is often a sudden and sometimes dramatic change in behavior or personality. This is accompanied by memory disturbance, disorientation, poor judgment, and a **labile** and shallow **affect.** After the acute episode, a temporary plateau is usually reached; then another episode ensues, followed by another plateau at a lower level of functioning, and so on downhill.

The individual suffering from this form of brain degeneration is considerably more aware that something is wrong with him. He is threatened

LABILE: describing the emotional condition wherein a person may seem quite happy one minute and angry or sad the next, with little or no apparent reason for the change

AFFECT: the feeling-tone which is attached to or accompanying an idea or mental representation; more loosely, the term means feeling, emotion, or mood

and upset by his memory defect and often resentful and frightened about his infirmity and approaching death. In his attempts to cope with these feelings and with the increasing complexity of the world around him, he may begin to hallucinate; or he may become suspicious that others are out to destroy him, take his money, put his false teeth where he cannot find them, and so on. Sometimes, frank paranoid delusions appear, e.g., that the phone is tapped or that a 75-year-old spouse is fornicating daily with dozens of men. Again, the course of the illness is marked by progressive degeneration, but often not to the same point of disability as is seen in senile dementia. It is significant that occasionally an elderly person develops full-blown "arteriosclerotic type senility," and with proper treatment recovers completely! Indeed, in a supportive environment and with appropriate help, many people with the arteriosclerotic type of illness do very well for many years.

A 75-year-old self-made investment banker, who made daily decisions involving millions of dollars, required a minor hernia operation and was admitted to the hospital for the first time in his life. Accustomed to the best scotch at bedtime, he packed a bottle; but he failed to so inform his physician. Routine sleeping medication was ordered for him, and the net result of the drink combined with the medication was a "Mickey Finn." This unaccustomed "kick" from his scotch, the strange environment, the pain of the operation, and his fears that it would somehow damage his potency, all helped to trigger a behavior disturbance. He became suspicious, angry, bellicose, confused, and sexually exhibitionistic with the nurses and aides. Reproached by an intern for this last behavior, he hit the "young wise-ass" on his chin. The patient's family and physician were alarmed, even horrified by the sudden change and acute manifestation of senility. When seen in psychiatric consultation, the patient did not know the month or the day or the name of the hospital. He had trouble remembering simple objects for 15 minutes, and his grasp of general information was far below what one would expect from an executive at his level. Although reluctant to discuss it, he clearly indicated his conviction that his entire hospitalization was the result of a plot on the part of some of his business associates.

Because of the sensitive nature of the patient's professional responsibilities, there was considerable concern about how to handle him. However, with the aid and support of the psychiatrist and a physician-friend (also 75) who promised to make daily visits to the patient at home, the family agreed to his rapid discharge from the hospital. Once home, the patient made a remarkably speedy return to normal and went back to work. Two years later, he slipped on the ice while getting out of his limousine and fractured his wrist. He was again hospitalized and within a few hours appeared almost the same as he had on the previous hospitalization. This time, however, his physicians were alert to the problem, and he was quickly discharged home. The entire episode lasted only 24 hours, and he was back at work in less than a week.

It must be emphasized that elderly people develop psychiatric illnesses other than senility, and these should also be appropriately treated. The result can be years of restored health.

A brief return to statistics will help highlight the importance of both senile dementia and the psychosis with arteriosclerosis. It is estimated that by the year 2000 these illnesses will account for between 20 and 30 percent of all first admissions to public mental hospitals. Autopsy studies done on the brains of patients with these diagnoses reveal that 35 percent have changes primarily associated with senile dementia, 45 percent have arteriosclerotic changes, and 20 percent have evidence of both. Arteriosclerotic illness is more common in men and begins about five years earlier than senile dementia, which occurs more frequently in women. Of these patients, those not sent to mental hospitals are often in nursing homes, which are hard to find for this type of patient, expensive (up to $2,000 per month), and all too frequently substandard in care even when compared with that available in state hospitals. Although much has yet to be learned about the causes and treatment of these diseases, some correlations have been found. Both forms of senility are more common among those in lower socioeconomic groups, those with lower educational background, those living alone, and those living in urban centers with high concentrations of multiple-family dwellings.

SCHIZOPHRENIA

Schizophrenia is by far the most prevalent of the illnesses not attributed to physical conditions. In the United States, the odds are 1 in 100 that any given individual will be hospitalized with this illness at least once in his lifetime. Between 100,000 and 300,000 new cases are diagnosed each year, and there are at least 400,000 persons hospitalized with this illness on any given day. Thus, schizophrenia accounts for about two-thirds of the mental-hospital beds and over one-fourth of all hospital beds in the United States. Worldwide, probably over 4 million new cases are diagnosed each year, and the total world population of schizophrenics is approximately 9 million.

Schizophrenia is a fascinating and puzzling disease. Roughly 16,000 books and professional articles have been written on the subject. Nevertheless, there is still not enough factual knowledge available to confirm any of the various hypotheses or speculations about the etiology of the disease. Most of these boil down to being on one side or the other of what is called the "nature vs. nurture" controversy. In other words, is the illness the result of nature (i.e., a person's heredity, biochemistry, physiology, or anatomy) or nurture (i.e., the effects on the individual of his sociocultural environment, learning, and family interaction)?[5] No matter which side one tends to take, there remains a concern that those suffering from schizophrenia will produce schizophrenic or otherwise severely disturbed children. The incidence of the disease has remained stable over the last 100 years at least. In the past, marriage and reproductive rates have been distinctly lower for those with schizophrenia than for the general population. However, recent studies indicate that schizophrenics are now marrying more often and that their rate of reproductivity is approaching that of the general population. It is thus possible that there may be a higher incidence of the disease in one or two generations.

Considerable variation exists among patients with schizophrenia. The "classic" schizophrenic is one whose first psychotic episode occurs in his teens or early twenties. The onset may be quite abrupt, i.e., the individual's personality and functioning may become disorganized over a period of just a few days or weeks. On the other hand, there may be a slow and rather insidious development of the psychosis over a period of years. The more insidious the onset and the longer the psychosis has existed prior to treatment, the worse is the prognosis. Classically, the disease process continues with a steady deterioration in functioning until the patient has regressed to an infantile-like state. It was for this reason that Kraepelin gave the illness the name *dementia praecox*, or early mental deterioration. It is interesting to note, however, that 14 percent of Kraepelin's original series of patients did not deteriorate.

There are other seeming paradoxes about this illness. It is associated with long or recurrent hospitalizations, but there are many schizophrenics who never see a psychiatrist, let alone the inside of a mental hospital. Moreover, there are patients who have a single psychotic episode and never have a recurrence. There are also those who do have recurrent episodes of psychosis but who do not deteriorate and in fact function effectively or even at a high level between episodes. And, finally, there are those who very closely approximate the classic description of schizophrenia and slowly but inexorably deteriorate, become chronically ill, and ultimately require permanent hospitalization.

The primary symptoms common to all cases of schizophrenia are often referred to as "Bleuler's four A's": association, autism, affect, and ambivalence. The first refers to a disturbance in thought association. Most simply, this means a loosening in the logical associations which lead from one thought to another. As a result, spoken or written sentences may be vague, oddly constructed, or characterized by incomplete thoughts or ideas. "New" words (neologisms) are sometimes made up and are either amalgams of existing words or simply a combination of nonsense syllables. These patients also have general difficulty in understanding or dealing with abstract concepts. In the 60 years since Bleuler first called attention to this disease entity, the language and thought of schizophrenia has been studied rather intensively. Problems in these areas reflect what is now referred to as *thought disorder*. In its most extreme form, the verbal or written communication becomes highly individualized, bizarre, and chaotic. This is sometimes called "word salad," and it is, needless to say, very difficult to understand.

Cameron quotes some helpful examples. An acutely ill patient completed the statement "My hair is fair because . . ." with "because of something else, it's on my head, it comes from my mother." Compare this with his response after recovery: "because I inherited from my parents." Patients are often aware of some difficulty and try to describe it, as does this young school teacher quoted by Cameron: "I just exactly can't talk as clearly. I'd give a pretty dime to talk like I like or place my words in talking with people noticing."

Here are two longer examples from Bleuler (in neither case is the patient trying to "put anyone on"):

Dear Mother, Today I am feeling better than yesterday. I really don't feel much like writing. But I love to write to you. After all, I can tackle it twice. . . . I am writing on paper. The pen which I am using is from a factory called "Perry & Co." This factory is in England. I assume this. Behind the name of Perry & Co. the city of London is inscribed, but not the city. The city of London is England. I know this from my schooldays. Then I always liked geography. My last teacher in that subject was . . .

And the second example:

The Golden Age of Horticulture

At the time of the new moon, Venus stands in Egypt's August-sky and illuminates with her rays the commercial ports of Suez, Cairo, and Alexandria. In this historically famous city of the Califs, there is a museum of Assyrian monuments from Macedonia. There flourish plantain trees, bananas, corn-cobs, oats, clover and barley, also figs, lemons, oranges, and olives. Olive-oil is an Arabian liquor-sauce which the Afghans, Moors and Moslems use in ostrich-farming. The Indian plantain-tree is the whiskey of the Parsees and Arabs. The Parsee or Caucasian possesses as much influence over his elephant as does the Moor over his dromedary. The camel is the sport of Jews and Arabs. Barley, rice, and sugar-cane called artichoke, grow remarkably well in India. The Brahmins live as castes in Beluchistan. The Circassians occupy Manchuria in China. China is the Eldorado of the Pawnees.

The second primary symptom is autism. This term is applied when one's inner life assumes pathological predominance over the external world, with the result that daydreams, hallucinations, and delusions are more "real" than the real world, or they cannot be distinguished from it. Another way of stating this is that it is impossible for a schizophrenic to consider any viewpoint but his own or to take into account evidence which runs counter to a delusion. Thus, the patient who maintains that he is Jesus or Napoleon remains blind to logical arguments or evidence which contradict his belief. When external reality does have an impact on the patient, it may well be within the context of his inner life. For example, a college student who had become schizophrenic hallucinated his mother's voice calling him a "bad boy." This was so disturbing to him that he was unable to study. However, he formed a strong attachment to a psychiatrist, reported that the hallucination had gone away, and was soon able to resume his studies. Some years later, he and his former psychiatrist accidentally met on the street. When the patient was asked what had most helped him get well, he rather shamefacedly revealed that he had begun to hallucinate the psychiatrist's voice calling him a "good boy."

The third A is disturbance in *affect*, i.e., feeling, mood, or emotion. The affectual disturbance may take the form of being an inappropriate response to the subject under discussion. The patient may appear wooden-faced or indifferent while talking about the most emotionally laden experiences, or he may be able to feel, express, or show only the most limited range of emotion. In other cases, there may be abrupt changes in affect— e.g., within the span of minutes, the patient may swing from gaiety to rage and back to gaiety again. This is called lability of affect, and it was mentioned previously as a symptom of psychosis with arteriosclerosis.

The last of the primary symptoms is *ambivalence*. This means having contradictory feelings, attitudes, or wishes toward the same person, object, or situation. To be sure, mixed feelings and ambivalence are facts of life for most people in at least some situations, but in schizophrenia an extreme is reached. For example, one patient intensely dreaded attending group meetings because she did not want to be stared at or watched. In one meeting, however, she could not restrain herself from repeatedly running to the center of the room and shouting, "You're all looking at me!" Another example is that of an acutely psychotic young mother who leaned over rather affectionately to kiss her 3-year-old son and, instead, ground her lighted cigarette into his cheek. Another symptom (which is not associated just with schizophrenia but which is important in that disease entity) is **anxiety**. As schizophrenics decompensate and their personalities become disorganized, they develop tremendous anxiety. They suffer terribly, sometimes giving in to panic—either because they realize that they are "falling apart" or in response to the frightening nature of other symptoms, such as persecutory delusions. In addition, these patients tend to feel fearful and anxious when they attempt to do even simple things that other people would regard as purely routine.

On the foundation of these primary symptoms, such a large number of secondary symptoms may develop that schizophrenia is divided into types according to what these are. In the type called *paranoid schizophrenia,* hallucinations may be present via any or all of the senses. Thus, things that are not there may be heard, seen, smelled, tasted, felt on the skin, or perceived within the body. Combinations of hallucinations and delusions are sometimes incorporated:

Please hold my hand. I'm not real. I'm soft inside a hard shell. I'm a bug. How can you stand that rough claw and hair. I wish the buzzing would stop and the grating of the joints. I can't walk. Please take me back to the hospital.

Or:

I'm here because the F.B.I. has been persecuting me. They think I'm a spy, a rotten, dirty, filthy person. They have my phone bugged, my apartment bugged, and me buggered. J. Edgar Hoover talks to me. I keep hearing him call me a spy; even in the middle of the park.

It will be remembered that hallucinations and delusions are seen in other conditions, such as organic brain syndromes. In schizophrenia, however, there is no disorientation or memory disturbance despite the thought disorder and confusion which an acute psychosis can produce.

Sometimes patients become mute and appear to be in a trance. Their limbs become frozen in some posture or other, such that they feel almost

---

ANXIETY: an unpleasurable affect consisting of feelings of apprehension accompanied by physiological (somatic) changes (trembling, increased sweating, disturbed breathing, increased heart action, and so on); contrasted to fear in that the latter is a reaction to a specific, real, or threatened danger, while anxiety is related to less specific, more general, unknown, and sometimes unreal danger

like slightly soft wax when moved by another person. They will often stand in one spot for days, until they become physically ill unless someone takes care of them. This is called *catatonia* or the *withdrawn catatonic type* of schizophrenia. In days past, such patients would sometimes be placed at the main entrance of state hospitals, and they would stand there, immobile, holding a box of brochures or objects for sale.

A second sub-type of catatonic schizophrenia is marked by excessive, indeed fantastic, and sometimes violent motor activity. This *excited catatonic* patient is capable of clawing at a brick wall until he has torn away the first joints of his fingers or of driving himself until he dies. Mr. X. who was described at the beginning of this chapter was classified as catatonic, excited.

It should be emphasized that the types and sub-types of schizophrenia are not separate disease entities but rather clinical classifications helpful in describing symptomatology. The fact is that the secondary symptoms often change, so that a patient may appear predominantly paranoid for a time, then catatonic, and then fall under any one of eight other clinically classified types.

Let us conclude with a brief description of a chronically ill schizophrenic:

Dorothy P. was brought to the hospital because she was frightened, confused, could not sleep, and had spent the previous two days pacing the floor and mumbling. All she would say was that her trouble was nerves and that she heard awful voices. While she was clearly frightened and agitated, her facial expression resembled a wooden mask. She was 59 years old, Puerto Rican, and, to the knowledge of her relatives, had had two similar attacks of "nerves" —the first at age 18 after the loss of a fiancé, and the second at age 44 after her husband divorced her.

When she was still very young, her father disappeared, and then her mother died. Orphaned, she was brought up by various aunts who had many children and no husbands. At the age of 12, she was taken out of school and put to work behind a sewing machine. Her affairs and "marriages" brought neither children nor satisfaction.

After her second psychotic episode, she became even more quiet and withdrawn than she had been previously. She left the house rarely and lived on a disability pension granted for chronic schizophrenia. She seemed to care little for those around her, including her brother-in-law, Mr. I., who took her in to help his sister with the housework and whose indifferent lover she became. Shortly before she again became acutely ill, her brother-in-law-lover began to talk of retiring, selling his house, and moving to Puerto Rico. At the same time, his sister (the other woman in the house) had a gallbladder operation.

After the patient was admitted to the hospital, medication soon helped the hallucinations go away; but she remained quiet, fearful, withdrawn, and apathetic. Her vocabulary was poor, and she seemed to care little what was said to her. Slowly she began to take part in some hospital activities for patients, but she remained virtually mute. Her therapist (a psychiatrist in training), frustrated in his efforts to elicit any communication from the patient, finally smacked his hand on the desk and howled the only Spanish expletive he knew. A faint smile appeared on Dorothy's face. The next day she began to talk a little more, but never for more than 10 minutes. Soon, the two of them developed an odd "dialogue." She talked of going back to work, and he (feeling that this was inadvisable) talked instead about how people like her lover ought to be "told off" when they became too overbearing. It was never clear whether or not they completely understood each other.

Three months later she was out of the hospital and back behind the sewing machine. Sighing and smiling, she complained often about the hard work. She continued to see her psychiatrist periodically for three years; when he left the hospital, she was transferred to the care of a new resident. In those first three years following her discharge, she had two brief episodes of hallucinations, each of which cost her a day's work and subsided with medication.

On the day exactly eight years after her admission to the hospital, she called her previous psychiatrist for an appointment. She arrived smiling, wearing perfume, and obviously delighted to see him. She happily filled him in on her work experience, her retirement with her legal husband of two years (she and Mr. I. had gotten married), the nice house they had in Puerto Rico, how good it was to have her own money, and so on. The occasion of her return was a reappearance of the hallucinations (this occurred after she had been told that she had diabetes). Although she had been upset by their recurrence, she knew that help was possible and had flown to New York to see her therapist and to receive medication. The latter was prescribed, and she has been functioning very well since that time.

There are some important points to consider here: chronicity does not rule out the possibility of obtaining great improvement. Social class and language differences need not be barriers. Further, it must be noted that although language-words and listening comprise the backbone of treatment, something else must be at work as well. There is room for empirical variation in treatment. In this case, the psychiatrist carefully refrained from overtly encouraging the patient's going to work and, instead, focused on the expression of frustration and anger. Loss plays an important role in the precipitation of all mental illness, and schizophrenia is no exception. Note that Dorothy had lost her parents and then suffered acute schizophrenic episodes after the loss of two men. Although the precipitating events leading to her hospitalization were somewhat vague, they seemed to be the threatened loss of her lover and his sister (the two most important object relationships in her life) and the loss of her basic sources of security (the house, the people, the neighborhood). Finally, her last, brief decompensation occurred when she developed a physical illness which frightened her and aroused fears of further serious illness, disability, and death. These are also common precipitating factors in all mental illness.

Although it is true that we have come a long way from the days of medieval superstition and ignorance, the intricacies of human behavior and feelings still provoke more questions than there are answers. It is hoped that this very brief introduction to the complex world of mental illness will serve as a stimulus for further thought and study. It is further hoped that the reader will now have the background to maintain a healthy skepticism about reported "cures" or causes of such illnesses as schizophrenia and an equally strong skepticism about the "new," faster, easier approaches to psychotherapy.

Footnotes

1 *Malleus Maleficarum,* the handbook of the Inquisition, had papal (Innocent VIII) approval; civil approval from Maximilian I, King of Rome; and intellectual approval from the University of Cologne. Other quotes from this document help elucidate roots of misogyny (hatred and distrust of women) in western culture: "Woman is a temple built over a sewer. . . . Three general vices appear to have special dominion over wicked women, namely, infidelity, ambition, and lust. Therefore, they are more than others inclined towards witchcraft who more than others are given to these vices."

2 We probably would not even know his name were it not for John C. Nemiah, Professor of Psychiatry at Harvard, who discovered Pussin's role in history.

3 It is not within the scope of our discussion to pursue this complex subject. However, the interested reader who wishes to do so may find the works of Erik Erikson and Norman Cameron particularly helpful. (See references for this chapter.)

4 Because the scope of this discussion is necessarily limited, the neuroses, personality disorders, and psychosomatic illnesses are omitted even though each of them sheds additional light on personality structure and man's adaptation to society. Those wishing to pursue these topics are referred to Cameron, Brenner, and Freedman and Kaplan in the references at the end of the chapter.

5 Note that this is the old "organic vs. dynamic" question.

References

Alexander, F. and Selesnick, S. The History of Psychiatry. New York, W. W. Norton & Co., 1950.

Bleuler, E. Dementia Praecox or the Group of Schizophrenias. New York, International Universities Press, 1950.

Bockoven, J. S. Moral Treatment in American Psychiatry. New York, Springer, 1963.

Brenner, C. An Elementary Textbook of Psychoanalysis. New York, Anchor Books, 1957.

Burton, L. and Smith, H. Public Health and Community Medicine. Baltimore, Williams and Wilkins, 1970.

Cameron, N. Personality Development and Psychopathology. Boston, Houghton Mifflin, 1963.

Erikson, E. Childhood and Society. New York, W. W. Norton & Co., 1950.

Freedman, A. and Kaplan, H. Comprehensive Textbook of Psychiatry. Baltimore, Williams and Wilkins, 1967.

Nemiah, John C. Pinel and after. Mass. J. Mental Health, 1:4, 1971.

Nemiah, John C. Pinel's Superintendent. Unpublished.

Nunberg, H. Practice and Theory of Psychoanalysis, Vol. 1. New York, International Universities Press, 1961.

Rapaport, D. Organization and Pathology of Thought. New York, Columbia University Press, 1951.

Solomon, P. and Patch, V. Handbook of Psychiatry. Lange Medical Publications, 1969.

Stanton, A. and Schwartz, M. The Mental Hospital. New York, Basic Books, Inc., 1954.

Zilboorg, G. A History of Medical Psychology. New York, W. W. Norton & Co., 1941.

National Institute of Mental Health, Public Health Service, The U.S. Department of Health, Education and Welfare, Statistical Notes 1–25, December, 1971.

Psychiatric News, Volume VII, No. 8, Washington, D.C. April 19, 1972.

CHAPTER

8

The Social Environment

In this chapter we will consider some of the health problems that are directly related to the society in which we live. They include drug abuse, alcoholism, cigarette smoking, venereal disease, and even accident patterns and housing problems. In each case our system of values promotes, enhances, or at least condones the political, economic, and social conditions which sustain the growth of these widespread afflictions. This can be illustrated by even a cursory look at the general way in which drugs are handled in this country.

Although drug abuse is without doubt a health problem of major proportions, it is an open question whether it is best attacked through methods which are primarily medical in nature. The simple truth is that drug abuse is pervasive in American society, and social condemnation exists only in relation to certain kinds of drugs. The use of alcohol is condoned, expected, and indeed promoted at most adult social gatherings. It is not considered at all unusual or improper for people to use drugs to sleep, to stay awake, to elevate the mood, to soothe the nerves, to allay anxiety, to lose weight, to gain weight, to avoid constipation, to cure indigestion, and so on. Television commercials extol the virtue of proprietary drugs for headache, hayfever, colds, allergies, hemorrhoids, irregularity, "tired blood," and "the heartbreak of psoriasis." A common complaint of those who have just visited a physician is that "he didn't do anything," and what this usually means is that the doctor did not give or prescribe a drug or, better yet, several drugs. Moreover, without a prescription anyone can purchase 287 separate remedies for athlete's foot; for boils there are 42 available ointments; for dandruff, 76 different preparations; for warts, 26 removers; for chapped lips, 14 varied remedies; and for "muscular aches and pains" there are no less than 325 analgesic balms! Although the effectiveness (and sometimes even the safety) of any one of these products may be highly questionable, the public clearly provides an eager market for them, and the manufacturers provide a profitable supply.

These same people are nevertheless surprised, shocked, and angry when they learn that their children are experimenting with amphetamines, barbiturates, or perhaps heroin. The same television that extols Nytol, Sominex, and Cope as solutions to sleepless nights and the pressures of everyday life urges young people to avoid narcotic drugs because they are illegal and dangerous. Narcotics are indeed illegal and certainly dangerous, but it is of interest to reflect on the values and nature of a society which promotes the sale of proprietary drugs that do not work, while it condemns the use of drugs that work only too well—a society whose adults accept seductive ways of escaping tension, and yet admonishes its youth that to do so is "copping out."

We are still in the infant stages of determining the etiology of this problem, of diagnosing its nature, and certainly of finding ways to combat it. Not only is there an inherent contradiction in the public attitude toward drugs, not only are myriad economic and social factors implicated, but the problem is compounded by a widespread lack of knowledge about drugs in general as well as about the so-called "dangerous drugs." The following section on drug abuse focuses specifically on those "dangerous drugs" that have figured most prominently in current concern. Like each of the subsequent sections, this one is designed to be a brief introduction to the nature of the particular problem and to provide a frame of reference for the reader who wishes to explore the subject further.

Drug Abuse

The abusive use of drugs is a problem virtually as old as man himself. Although it is currently a phenomenon of particular interest, it has an old history even in the United States. In the late 1880s, for example, remedies for alcoholism were sold which frequently contained enough opium to keep the reformed drinker in a state of perpetual stupor. Indeed, it is believed that the prevalence of narcotic addiction in this country is less today than it was at the turn of the century. This is perhaps particularly surprising when one considers that the number of chronic heroin users in the United States is presently estimated to be 300,000.

A drug may be defined as any substance which is utilized to alter the physical or mental function of the human body. Aspirin, an **analgesic,** thus changes pain perception, and digitalis alters cardiac function. Abuse implies the *deliberate* misuse of a drug. The person who misreads a label misuses the drug; the housewife who takes diet pills to "pep her up" has abused that drug. Drugs which are commonly abused include many of the **over-the-counter** medicines, caffeine, alcohol, barbiturates, amphetamines, narcotics, and various hallucinogens. It has already been suggested, but it is important to emphasize again here, that drug abuse is a culturally defined problem and that drugs are subject to selective sanction. Indeed, drug abuse has been defined as "the use, usually by self-administration, of any drug in a manner which deviates from the approved medical or social patterns within a given culture."

Listed below are some of the factors that investigators have suggested led to the marked abuse of drugs in the 1960s and 1970s. The size and scope of this list attest to the fact that the etiology of drug abuse is both poorly defined and incompletely understood.

Absence of father	Family relationships
Addictive personality	Hedonism
Availability of drugs	Materialism
Boredom	Peer-group pressure
Cultural decay	Racial unrest
Curiosity	Rebellion against authority
Drug laws	Social problems
Emotional problems	Television advertising
Faddishness	War in Vietnam

Whatever the underlying causes of drug abuse may be, certain drugs have particular characteristics which increase their abuse potential. Habituation, or psychologic dependence, can occur with such drugs as marihuana and LSD, not to mention the more mundane compounds like

---

ANALGESIC: that which relieves pain
OVER-THE-COUNTER: a phrase used in medicine to indicate any drug which can be purchased without a prescription

nicotine (in cigarettes) and caffeine (in coffee and soft drinks). Habituation has occurred if the individual experiences a sense of unrest, anxiety, nervousness, or emotional distress when he is not using the particular drug. Some drugs (including alcohol, narcotics, and barbiturates) produce additional physical, or physiologic, dependence. This is an incompletely understood condition which develops after long use and high dosages of certain drugs. If the drug on which an individual is physically dependent is withdrawn, he suffers not only an emotional disturbance but a disruption in the function of various body systems. The symptoms of this withdrawal syndrome vary from drug to drug, but the syndrome is stereotyped for each drug. Withdrawal syndromes may lead to muscle pain, vomiting, diarrhea, convulsions, and even death. Frequently, the chronic drug user requires progressively larger doses of the drug in order to continue achieving the same effect. This phenomenon is known as tolerance. Although it usually accompanies physical dependence, tolerance may occur without it.

This general review will not discuss all the various drugs which are abused in the United States. Narcotic **addiction** will be described, and brief consideration given to the abuse of barbiturates, amphetamines, and marihuana. A list of commonly abused drugs and some of their characteristics appears in Table 8-1.

NARCOTIC ADDICTION

Most of the narcotic drugs abused in the United States are derivatives of the poppy plant (Fig. 8-1). The dried juice of this plant is known as opium and has been used and abused for centuries. In the early 1800s opium was modified for the first time to produce morphine. During the Civil War morphine was extensively used for analgesia, and addiction to the drug was so common that it was called the "soldier's disease." In the late 1890s diacetyl-morphine, or heroin, was produced—supposedly as a drug with the same analgesic effect as morphine but with none of its addicting qualities (see Fig. 8-2). Heroin, at this time, was commonly used in cough medicines and various elixirs; and some sources estimate that by the early 1900s one million people were addicted to heroin in this form.

If one million persons were addicted to opiates in the past, why is

---

ADDICTION: a condition of either or both psychologic dependence (habituation) or physical dependence on a particular drug

TABLE 8-1. Drug Classification

Drug	Habituation	Tolerance	Withdrawal Syndrome	Usual Method of Use
Depressants				
Opiates				
1. opium	Yes	Yes	Yes	Smoking
2. morphine	Yes	Yes	Yes	Injection
3. meperidine (Demerol)	Yes	Yes	Yes	Injection
4. heroin (junk, horse, H.)	Yes	Yes	Yes	Sniffing; injection
5. codeine	Yes	Yes	Yes	Injection; oral
6. methadone (dollies)	Yes	Yes	Yes	Oral
Alcohol	Yes	Yes	Yes	Oral
Barbiturates (goofballs, peanuts)				
1. Seconal (reds, red devils)	Yes	Yes	Yes	Oral; injection
2. Nembutal (yellow, yellow nembies, jackets)	Yes	Yes	Yes	Oral; injection
3. Tuinal (rainbows, blue heavens, bluebirds)	Yes	Yes	Yes	Oral; injection
Stimulants				
Amphetamines				
1. Benzedrine (bennies)	Yes	Yes	No (?)	Oral; injection
2. Dexedrine (dex)	Yes	Yes	No	Oral; injection
3. Methedrine (speed, bombitas)	Yes	Yes	No	Oral; injection
Cocaine (coke)	Yes	Yes	No	Oral; sniffing; injection
Caffeine (in coffee and soft drinks)	Yes	No	No	Oral
Hallucinogens				
LSD (acid)	Yes	?	No	Oral
Mescaline (peyote)	Yes	?	No	Oral
Marihuana (pot, grass)	Yes	No	No	Smoking; oral
Gasses				
1. glue	Yes	?	?	Sniffing
2. gasoline, etc.	Yes	?	?	Sniffing

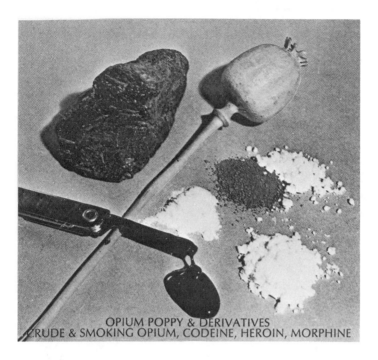

FIG. 8-1.   *Powdered heroin is the most popular opiate in the United States. (Courtesy of Bureau of Narcotics and Dangerous Drugs, U.S. Department of Justice.)*

there such concern over a possible 300,000 who are addicted now? The Harrison Act of 1914, which led to the control of opiate use in the United States, may be a partial answer to this question. The one million persons who were using heroin in the early 1900s were doing so quite legally. They were involved in an activity that was neither criminal nor socially unacceptable. We now have 300,000 persons who are in conflict with their society and its laws because they have a psychologic or physical dependence on heroin and cannot obtain it legally.

The stereotyped narcotic addict is the "junkie." He is in his twenties; he is a member of a racial minority group; he is from an economically depressed area of New York City; he is often found sick and dirty, nodding on a street corner; and he obtains the money to support his habit by mugging old ladies. Although some narcotic addicts fit this picture, the narcotic user of the 1970s is liable to be 15 years old, to live in any part of any American city or suburb, to attend school more or less regularly, and to get his money from petty thievery or from his parents and friends.

Narcotic addiction is a progressive, chronic, relapsing condition char-

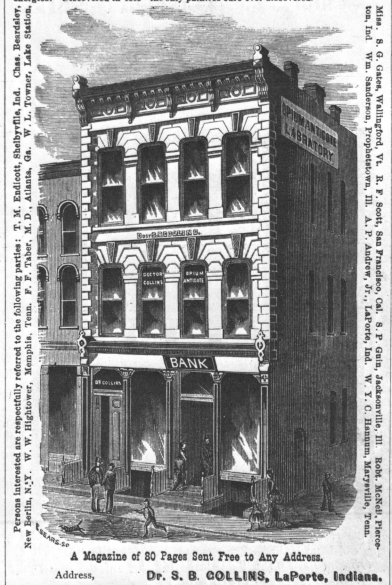

FIG. 8-2. *This 1873 advertisement from The American Medical Journal alludes to a "painless cure" by an unknown preparation. Similarly, a few years later preparations containing heroin were being sold as a cure for morphine addiction. (Courtesy of National Library of Medicine.)*

acterized by ever-increasing use of narcotics and steadily decreasing ability to function socially. The adolescent may experiment with heroin because of peer pressure and may begin by sniffing the drug into his nostrils. The effect of the heroin is to produce euphoria, or a "high," which is the desired state of consciousness prior to a party or social occasion. In order to achieve this same high or effect again, the individual often finds that he must increase the dose of heroin used or switch to a more direct method of administration (such as "mainlining," or injecting of the drug into a vein (see Fig. 8-3). The increased use and dose required results in ever-greater cost, and the individual is frequently forced into criminal activity to finance his habit. The life of the user eventually is characterized by intervals of stupor alternating with periods of criminal activity to obtain money—with little time for anything else. The adolescent who begins as an occasional user of heroin thus deteriorates into the stereotyped "junkie."

Narcotics abuse is a national health problem among younger people. A recent survey of high school students in Dallas, Texas, indicates that 3 to 4 percent have had some experience with narcotics. A similar study in Georgia estimates that 1 to 2 percent of their urban high school students have experimented with these opiates. The highest estimates we have are that 35 to 40 percent of students in certain New York City high schools

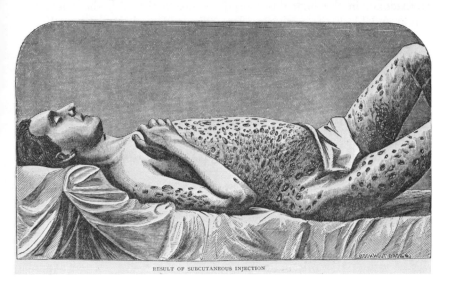

RESULT OF SUBCUTANEOUS INJECTION

FIG. 8-3.   *Abscessed and ulcered skin of a morphine addict shortly before his death in 1881. Most of the medical complications of opiate use are due to the manner of administration—in the case of this male nurse the method was subcutaneous injection or skin-popping. (Courtesy of National Library of Medicine.)*

have used narcotics. Statistics also show that narcotic-related deaths are the leading cause of mortality among persons aged 15 to 35 in New York City.

The abuse of narcotics has been a problem in New York City since the 1930s, and the present number of narcotic addicts in this city is estimated to be about 100,000. Table 8-2 shows the marked increase in narcotic-related deaths in New York City since 1960. This increase is a reflection of greater use and also probably a change in the death rate among users.

The national cost of narcotic addiction has been estimated at one billion dollars a year. This figure includes the losses due to robbery, the costs of law enforcement, penal confinement, medical care, and rehabilitation programs, as well as the economic loss of productive manpower.

Until recently, the only treatment available for the narcotic addict was confinement at a Public Health Service facility. At present, there are a dramatically increased number of facilities designed to treat addiction, although the need still exceeds the available help. Two principal modalities of treatment have gained acceptance: methadone maintenance and residential rehabilitation. Methadone maintenance involves sustaining the addicted individual on a regimen of methadone, a synthetic narcotic closely related to heroin, so that he can begin to readjust his life style. Methadone, in the high doses used, seems to diminish the craving for heroin and blocks its euphoric effect. The addict obtains the methadone at minimal or no cost from legal sources and often begins to return to a more normal level of social function.

Methadone maintenance programs are rapidly gaining popularity among those who work with drug abusers. However, methadone is only a medium to facilitate a change of life style and behavior in the heroin addict. Al-

TABLE 8-2. Narcotic-Related Deaths in New York City

Year	Number of Deaths	Percent Less than 25 Years Old
1960	199	30
1962	201	30
1964	346	32
1966	337	36
1968	654	32
1969	1,006	43
1970	1,100	50
1971	1,259	50

though this modality of therapy has the best record for holding the individual in treatment and reducing his antisocial behavior, it is probably applicable only to a selected group of addicted persons—particularly those who are older, who have been addicted for a considerable period of time, and who have been in other treatment programs. Methadone maintenance is relatively unsuccessful with the younger addict, who tends to be less motivated to change his life style or has not reached a state of physical and mental exhaustion from his habit.

Residential rehabilitation centers such as Synanon, Phoenix House, Daytop, Teen Challenge, and so on attempt to readjust the individual's life style within the drug-abstinent environment of a treatment house. A structured and disciplined milieu is provided in which the individual examines his behavior; and through the positive group pressure within the residential facility, he begins—over a year or more—to return to an acceptable level of functioning. Many other forms of treatment exist which are based on the residential-rehabilitation model or on case counseling.

It is not our purpose here to explore the many theories about drug abuse nor to review the numerous suggestions on how to treat and control it. However, it seems clear that a combination of many approaches—legal, chemical, psychologic, and cultural—will be necessary to alter this major health problem.

BARBITURATE ABUSE

Like the opiate drugs, barbiturates have a depressant effect on the central nervous system (Fig. 8-4). Abusive use of these drugs causes a progressive decrease in brain function, and in an overdose they produce coma and death by respiratory depression. The barbiturate abuser tends to be the housewife who uses the barbiturate as a tranquilizer, or the young person who uses the pills for "kicks." Narcotic addicts also use barbiturates to enhance their "highs" or when narcotics are not available.

As sedatives, barbiturates can produce a feeling of well-being and allow a person to escape anxiety. The reasons for barbiturate abuse are related to these effects as well as to the availability of the drugs, which in the United States are widely and freely prescribed for a number of symptoms. Indeed, they are generally over-prescribed and thus misused not only by patients but by physicians as well. Many young people obtain their barbiturates from their parents' supply of sleeping pills and tranquilizers.

Each year about 3,000 Americans die of barbiturate overdose. These drugs are often used in suicides, and, in addition, many accidental deaths

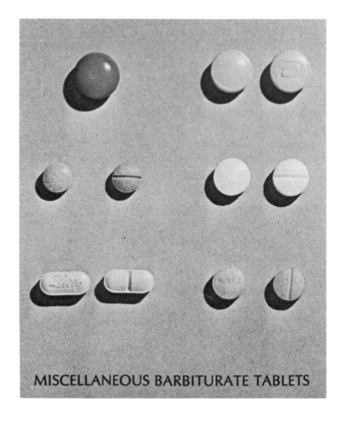

MISCELLANEOUS BARBITURATE TABLETS

Fig. 8-4.   *Barbiturate comes packaged in many shapes and colors. It is one of the most extensively abused drugs. (Courtesy of Bureau of Narcotics and Dangerous Drugs, U.S. Department of Justice.)*

occur when barbiturates are used with alcohol. The effects of each are intensified, and this dangerous combination is especially likely to result in death secondary to respiratory depression. The withdrawal syndrome in barbiturate addiction is one of the most serious, particularly because of the great danger of convulsions which can be fatal.

The only treatment presently available is hospitalization followed by residential rehabilitation or a similar therapeutic arrangement. There is no maintenance drug for barbiturate addiction. Moreover, the pressure for treatment of barbiturate addicts is relatively slight, since their habit usually does not necessitate the antisocial activity seen with narcotic addicts.

AMPHETAMINE ABUSE

Amphetamines are drugs which have an effect opposite to that of barbiturates (Fig. 8-5). The use of amphetamines excites the central nervous system and produces a state of hyperfunction in which there is increased alertness and wakefulness as well as heightened feeling of initiative and ability. Conversely, when the drug is stopped or the stimulating effect has worn off, the person is often left in a state of marked depression.

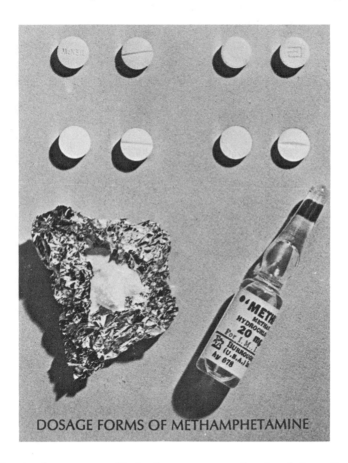

DOSAGE FORMS OF METHAMPHETAMINE

FIG. 8-5.   *Amphetamine in pills is the most commonly abused form. Powder or liquid amphetamine is used by the "speed freak." (Courtesy of Bureau of Narcotics and Dangerous Drugs, U.S. Department of Justice.)*

In situations where there has been heavy use, the depression may be so severe as to lead to suicidal behavior.

Amphetamines are usually taken orally. However, some individuals (known as "speed freaks") inject the drug intravenously. This can result in such extreme overstimulation that the user is unable to eat or sleep, and frequently becomes severely debilitated. In addition, any excessive use of amphetamines can produce a psychotic state in which bizarre, paranoid, and violent behavior is not uncommon. Fortunately, this condition is generally limited to the period during which the drug is being used.

The groups of people who abuse amphetamines tend to be similar to those who abuse barbiturates. Amphetamines depress the appetite, and

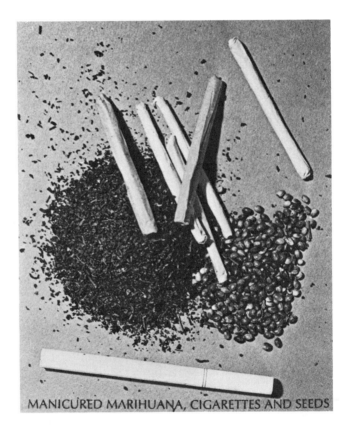

MANICURED MARIHUANA, CIGARETTES AND SEEDS

FIG. 8-6. *"Rolling your own" is the common method of preparing a joint of marihuana. The regular cigarette looks very professional by comparison. In terms of human health, the cigarette is perhaps a greater threat than the joint. (Courtesy of Bureau of Narcotics and Dangerous Drugs, U.S. Department of Justice.)*

these drugs are therefore prescribed by some physicians for weight reduction. Many women become amphetamine abusers after the drug has been so prescribed. When it is stopped, not only do these women tend to regain their lost weight, but they lose the feeling of energy and "pep" generated by the drug, and so they return for more pills.

Although a tolerance develops to amphetamines, and the psychologic effects of withdrawal can be severe, there is no easily demonstrable physical withdrawal syndrome. Treatment for amphetamine abuse, like that for barbiturate addiction, usually requires hospitalization and a follow-up period of residential rehabilitation or other similar care.

MARIHUANA ABUSE

Marihuana is a drug which has been used for various purposes for many centuries (see Figs. 8-6 and 8-7). An ancient Chinese volume lists the drug as effective for gout, rheumatism, malaria, constipation, and absent-mindedness. Marihuana is used presently in many forms in various countries throughout the world; in recent years the use of marihuana in the United States has increased markedly.

Marihuana is derived from the female *Cannabis sativa* plant; hashish is the resin from this same plant. The active ingredient, tetrahydrocannabinol (THC), has been extracted, and experimental work with THC indicates that it belongs to the hallucinogen class of drugs but produces hallucinations only in high doses. Tolerance to THC does not seem to develop readily, nor is there a withdrawal syndrome. High doses of THC will sometimes produce a psychotic episode, but it has been impossible to identify any long-term effects from occasional use. The effects of chronic heavy use of the drug are largely unknown.

Reactions to marihuana are highly subjective. Euphoria, alteration in time sense, visual distortion, and difficulty in concentrating are frequent effects of moderate doses. In 1967, surveys of college and high school students revealed that the prevalence of marihuana use was highest in large urban universities and lowest in smaller colleges located in rural areas. Among high school students a similar pattern emerged, i.e., use was far more common in large urban high schools than in smaller rural ones. Additional surveys indicate that after a rapid and sustained rise in use during the early and middle sixties, there has been a general leveling off in use among students since 1969.

Chronic heavy use of marihuana can lead to a severe habituation which changes the life style of the user. The individual becomes lethargic and withdrawn, using much of his time in consumption of marihuana. Treat-

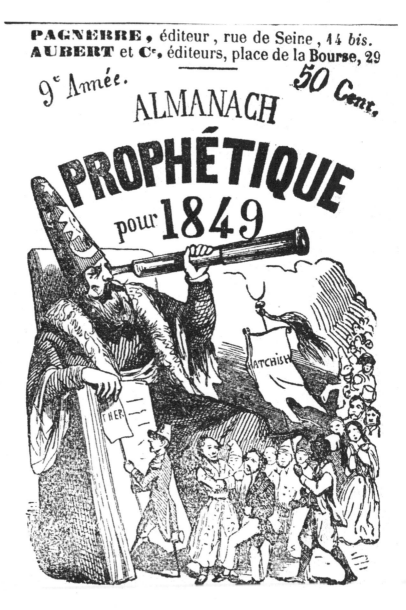

FIG. 8-7.   *An 1849 French almanac shows a great wizard peering into the future while a line of 19th century "hippies" march to proclaim the value of the drugs ether and marihuana. One wonders whether the seer could have possibly prophesied today's drug scene. (Courtesy of National Library of Medicine.)*

ment for this situation usually requires a residential rehabilitation program. Until recently, marihuana was classified as a narcotic, with severe penalties for use. The federal government has now reclassified this drug as an hallucinogen, and many state governments are following suit.

Alcoholism

Alcohol is one of the oldest drugs known to man, and its abuse is one of the western world's most common medical and social problems. Throughout the ages alcohol has enjoyed varying degrees of popularity. When the distillation process was introduced to Europe from the Middle East, alcohol was viewed as the salvation of all medieval man's physical problems. (In fact, the term *whiskey* derives from a Gaelic

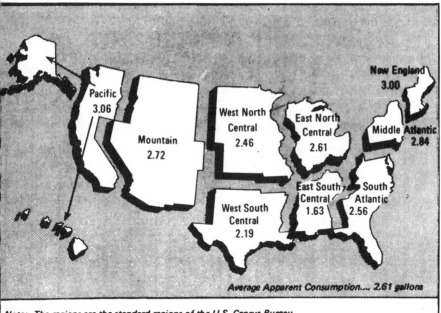

Note: *The regions are the standard regions of the U.S. Census Bureau.*

For comparative purposes only. Amounts calculated according to tax-paid withdrawals.

**Age 15+*

FIG. 8-8A.   *Apparent consumption* * *of absolute alcohol, in U.S. gallons per person in the drinking-age population* ** *by region, U.S.A., 1970. The Pacific and New England regions consume the greatest amounts of alcohol, while the South Central regions consume the least.*

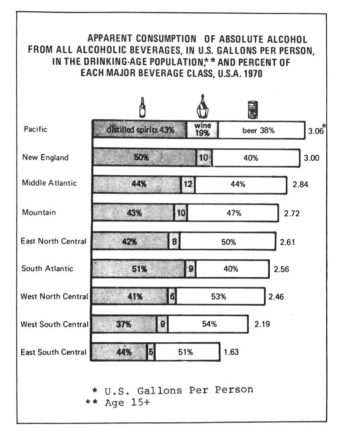

FIG. 8-8B.   *The West South Central region consumes only 37% of absolute alcohol from spirits and 54% from beer, while South Atlantic States consume 51% from spirits and 40% from beer. The Pacific region stands out by taking 19% of its alcohol in the form of wine. (From* First Special Report to the U.S. Congress on Alcohol and Health, National Institute on Alcohol Abuse and Alcoholism, Department of Health, Education and Welfare, December 1971.)

word meaning "water of life.") In contrast, at other times in human history entire societies have outlawed the consumption of alcohol.

The abuse of alcohol is said to be the fourth most prevalent health problem in the United States today. And yet alcohol is the only one of the intoxicating drugs whose self-administration is socially acceptable and at times even encouraged. Experts in the field agree that the use and abuse of alcohol is more of a problem than all other drugs combined. In a recent year, alcohol consumption in the United States averaged 253 cans of beer, 15 bottles of wine, and 13 bottles of hard liquor for every man and woman over the age of 15. This represents 2.6 gallons of pure alcohol per person; and its consumption generates 10 billion dollars worth of business annually and supports one of the largest industries in the country, with untold revenues expended in the media to encourage further consumption (see Fig. 8-8A and B).

The drinking population of the United States is in excess of 70 million. Of these there are 6 to 9 million Americans (approximately 6 percent of the adult population) with a severe drinking problem (see Fig. 8-9). The national cost of this problem is said to range from two to eight billion dollars—a figure which does not include the costs of compensation for industrial and other accidents secondary to alcohol abuse. Problem drinkers comprise 3 percent of the total work force, and they average over two days more of work loss annually than other workers; the total of 352 million working hours lost by this population is estimated to be half of the total dollar loss from drinking (see Fig. 8-10). The other half is expended in the care of alcoholic patients (a cost estimated to be 20 percent of New York City's hospital budget), in correctional costs (alcohol is the largest cause of arrest in the United States), and in support of the families of problem drinkers.

The human costs associated with alcohol are astronomical. Alcohol has been implicated in 30 percent of all violent deaths in the United States. A Philadelphia study showed that alcohol was a factor in 64 percent of all homicides. One-quarter of all suicides occur in alcoholics. One-half of all fatal highway accidents involve the use of alcohol, and 75 percent of these accidents involve problem drinkers. Thirty percent of pedestrians killed in automobile accidents are under the influence of alcohol. Other studies indicate that 30 percent of men admitted to prison have a severe drinking problem. Alcohol plays a central role in the genesis of home accidents and has been implicated in 24 percent of all nonindustrial and nontraffic accidents. Twenty percent of all divorces are attributable to drinking, and two-thirds of all alcoholic husbands have been physically abusive to their wives.

The offending agent in alcoholic beverages is ethanol. Also known as ethyl alcohol, ethanol is a simple hydrocarbon with the formula C_2H_5OH. In addition to its role as our culture's major agent of socialization, it kills germs on the skin on contact and is a good paint remover. Ethanol is produced in the process of fermentation of grapes (wine), the fermentation of hops and barley and corn (beer), and the distillation of fermented mash and malted cereal grain (whiskey). The alcoholic content of a beverage is expressed by the term *proof*. The proof of a beverage is twice the

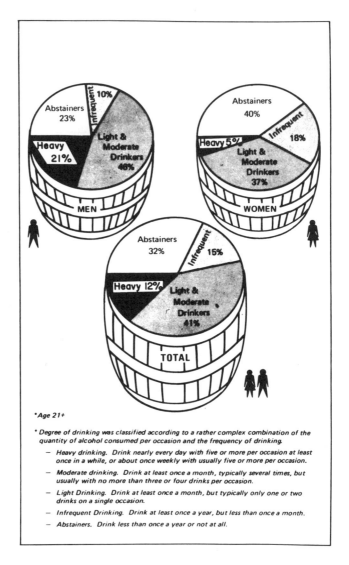

FIG. 8-9. *This figure shows that 12% of all adults are classified as heavy drinkers with 21% of all men and 5% of all women in this classification. (From First Special Report to the U.S. Congress on Alcohol and Health, National Institute on Alcohol Abuse and Alcoholism, Department of Health, Education and Welfare, December 1971.)*

percentage alcohol composition by volume, e.g., 86 proof whiskey is 43 percent ethanol; beer is 24 proof.

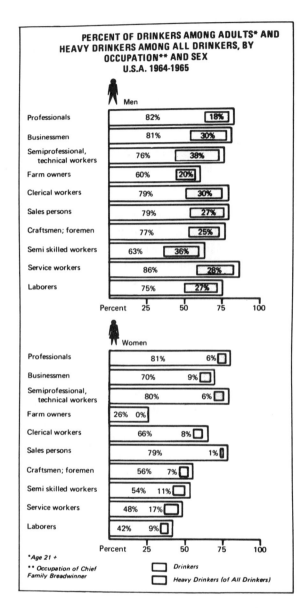

FIG. 8-10.   *Farm owners have the lowest percentage of drinkers and heavy drinkers. Of the men who drink, semiprofessionals have the highest proportion of heavy drinkers (38%), while service workers have the highest proportion of female heavy drinkers (17%).(From* First Special Report to the U.S. Congress on Alcohol and Health, *National Institute on Alcohol Abuse and Alcoholism, Department of Health, Education and Welfare, December 1971.)*

Cherished for its euphoric effects, alcohol is actually a depressant of the central nervous system and a general anesthetic. Before the advent of ether, alcohol was in fact widely used for surgical anesthesia. This is no longer the case because of (1) the length of time necessary to induce levels of anesthesia sufficient for pain relief; (2) the length of time required for recovery from the anesthesia (alcohol's slow metabolic rate); and (3) the slim margin of dosage between pain relief and respiratory and circulatory failure.

The euphoric effect of alcohol is pleasant but short-lived. It is accomplished primarily by a depressant effect on centers in the brain stem which are responsible for monitoring and controlling behavior. With these inhibitory centers depressed, behavior becomes voluble and provocative. Freed of inhibitions, the drinker at first feels at ease with his surroundings but soon may find himself saying or doing things he later sorely regrets. As the dose of alcohol increases, depression of the central nervous system spreads. Thoughts become clouded, speech becomes slurred, and activity is slowed. Sleep readily ensues or, if the dosage is high enough, the individual may pass into unconsciousness. A sufficiently high dosage consumed at one time can result in coma, with respiratory and circulatory collapse, and often death.

These effects of alcohol are directly related to the concentration of ethanol in the blood. The average person can metabolize about one ounce of whiskey and eight ounces of beer per hour. Alcohol intake in excess of these amounts raises the levels of alcohol in the blood to a point where the effects of the drug ensue. For medicolegal purposes, a blood ethanol level of 150 mg % (150 mg of alcohol per 100 cc of blood) is defined as the level at and above which an individual is "under the influence" of alcohol; a person with a blood level under 50 mg % is considered not under the influence; and a blood level between these two can be interpreted either way, depending on the person's behavior. A level of 200 implies mild to moderate intoxication; and a level of 250, moderate to marked. Taken on an empty stomach, four ounces of whiskey will raise the blood alcohol level of the average person to a range of 67 to 92 mg %; after a meal, this intakes raises the level to between 30 and 53 mg %. The same amount of alcohol consumed as beer will produce levels of 41 to 49 mg % and 23 to 29 %, respectively.

It takes the average person five to six hours to metabolize the alcohol consumed at a social function. For five to ten hours after that he will experience a period of unpleasantness. This period is known to all as a "hangover"; it is, in fact, a state of withdrawal. Although the hangover is not widely recognized as a withdrawal state, its true nature is attested to by the tendency of even moderate social drinkers to have some alcohol in a breakfast drink after a night of partying. Volumes have been written on how to cure the hangover. However, other than specific symptomatic therapy—hydration, antacids, and analgesics for headache—not much can be done beyond "waiting it out."

The withdrawal state presents a much more serious problem for the problem drinker. Only a few hours after his last drink and the falling of the blood level to zero, severe anxiety, perspiration, and nausea begin. The sufferer pleads for a drink of alcohol in any form; and at this stage the alcoholic will frequently drink alcohol-containing fluids intended only for industrial or commercial use—an action which is often fatal. His state of awareness may deteriorate to the point of gross disorientation. Indeed, the chronic drinker may start hallucinating, with visions of crawling insects and other animals figuring prominently in these hallucinations. Occasionally, however, the early symptoms and signs in the withdrawal state may be so mild as to pass unnoticed until the third or fourth day, when a state of frank delirium with seizures may set in. This rampant delirium, the "D.T.s" (delirium tremens), does not augur well for the patient, the mortality from this condition being 15 to 20 percent. D.T.s in a postoperative patient carries a mortality of 50 percent. It is not unusual for a victim of an automobile or other accident to undergo major life-saving surgery, to begin a favorable postoperative course, and, when seemingly out of danger, to slide into a fatal case of the D.T.s.

The widespread social inducement to consume alcohol, the short-lived sense of well-being it produces, and the existence of the withdrawal syndrome combine to beget and exacerbate the problem of alcohol abuse. The feeling of well-being from alcohol can be for some the only solace they enjoy. The effect of the alcohol creates a transient sense of security and a temporary escape from daily problems. Initially experiencing these feelings in a social setting on a specific occasion, the individual attempts to incorporate them more regularly into his daily life. Drinking at lunch begins and grows heavier; drinking before and after meals becomes more frequent, and the quantities consumed increase. In time, the cessation of drinking is associated with a feeling of anxiety and emotional tension, and a condition of psychologic dependence results. The continued use of alcohol soon produces a state of physical dependence, such that the falling of the blood alcohol level results in a withdrawal syndrome so severe that the person is almost literally driven to drink for survival. This drive to drink remains inexorable, and a full-blown addict is thus created. Some tolerance to alcohol develops along the way, but an upward limit of this tolerance is reached rapidly and remains fixed.

The path to addiction is highly individual, and it is of note that only one in five heavy drinkers becomes physically addicted to alcohol. Some addicts report that from the very first taste they could not stop drinking, and that every time they are confronted with alcohol they drink until they drop. Others take years to develop addiction. In one study of alcoholics, the average subject reported that he began drinking at age 18, became a heavy drinker at age 29, and was an alcoholic at age 36.

The literature on the abuse of alcohol is complicated by a failure to define terms and a lack of agreement on terms when they are defined. According to the World Health Organization, alcoholism is a chronic behavioral disorder that is manifested by repeated drinking of alcoholic beverages—in excess of the dietary and social standards of the community and to an extent that the drinking interferes with the person's health or his social or economic functioning. With minor modifications, this definition is fairly widely accepted. Such is not the case with the term *alcoholic*. There is no dispute that the drinker in a state of physical dependence on alcohol is an alcoholic. However, some exclude from this definition of alcoholic those with a psychologic dependence on the drug; others go so far as to include those with a pattern of heavy social drinking. Some have dropped the term *alcoholic* completely, in favor of terms such as infrequent, moderate, or severe problem drinker (see Fig. 8-9). In view of the traditional neglect of the problem, the need to increase the public's awareness of it, and the need to implement public and private health programs to combat alcoholism, the broadest interpretation of the term *alcoholic* is probably the best. Only with the earliest recognition of the signs of alcoholism can one hope to intervene and avert the consequences.

Who becomes an alcoholic? Increasingly, alcoholism is viewed as an inadequate adjustment to social pressures and personal tensions. The poor are more susceptible than the rich; men more than women; blacks more than whites. Black women in urban settings are especially liable. Single men and widowers are more susceptible than married men, with widowers in one New York town having a prevalence rate of 105 per 1,000. The French traditionally have been reknowned for their alcoholism, while the Italians have a low rate of alcohol-related problems (Fig. 8-11). In the United States the drinking prevalence among the American Indians is disastrously high. It is also common among Americans of Irish and Swedish backgrounds. Ninety percent of the Jews in the United States drink, but less than 1 percent are alcoholics.

Although secular studies have shown that individuals with a low image of themselves and their ability to succeed develop the highest prevalence of alcoholism, no single personality type is particularly characteristic of the alcoholic. A concurrence of alcoholism and schizophrenia is repeatedly noted in the medical literature, but it is not known to what extent schizophrenia is a cause or an effect of alcoholism. Alcoholism has been as-

APPARENT CONSUMPTION, IN 20 COUNTRIES, OF EACH MAJOR BEVERAGE CLASS, AND OF ABSOLUTE ALCOHOL FROM EACH CLASS, IN U.S. GALLONS PER PERSON IN THE DRINKING-AGE POPULATION *
(listed in descending order of total)

Country	Year**	Distilled Spirits	Absolute Alcohol	Wine	Absolute Alcohol	Beer	Absolute Alcohol	TOTAL Absolute Alcohol
1. France	1966	2.35	1.18	43.03	4.52	20.10[a]	0.83	6.53
2. Italy	1968	[1.11]	0.55	41.29	3.30	3.54	0.16	4.01
3. Switzerland	1966	1.53	0.61	13.61	1.43	29.73[a]	1.35	3.39
4. West Germany	1968	[2.35]	0.89	4.04	0.40	44.65	1.97	3.26
5. Australia	1966	0.54	0.31	2.58	0.44	42.86	2.14	2.89
6. Belgium	1967	0.67	0.33	3.14	0.44	42.07[a]	2.10	2.87
7. U.S.A.	1970	2.56	1.15	1.84	0.29	25.95	1.17	2.61
8. New Zealand	1964	0.79	0.45	0.98	0.17	39.28	1.96	2.58
9. Czechoslovakia	1968	[0.83]	[0.42]	[3.51]	[0.49]	[30.91]	[1.54]	2.45
10. Canada	1967	[1.86]	0.75	[1.12]	0.18	[25.47]	1.27	2.20
11. Denmark	1968	0.78	0.34	1.53	0.22	29.03	1.38	1.94
12. United Kingdom	1966	0.51	0.29	1.08	0.18	31.77	1.43	1.90
13. Sweden	1968	2.13	0.85	1.77	0.24	15.57	0.65	1.74
14. Japan	1968	[1.10]	0.35	[5.10][b]	0.81	8.22	0.37	1.53
15. The Netherlands	1968	[1.38]	[0.69]	[0.86]	[0.15]	[15.38]	[0.69]	1.53
16. Ireland	1966	0.70	0.40	0.56	0.09	22.26	1.00	1.49
17. Norway	1968	1.20	0.52	0.70	0.10	10.82	0.51	1.13
18. Finland	1968	1.33	0 92	1.06	0.17	6.85	0.34	1.03
19. Iceland	1966	2.11	0.73	0.62	0.08	4.26	0.15	0.96
20. Israel	1968	0.89	0.44	1.66	0.20	3.58	0.18	0.82

NOTES: (a) Includes cider.   (b) Includes saké.   [ ] Bracketed data converted from source terms.

* Age 15+

** Latest available year for each country.

FIG. 8-11.   *This data cautions us against simplistic explanations of alcohol problems. The Italians rank second among nations in alcohol consumption. Yet Italy has a relatively low rate of alcohol problems compared to several countries with substantially lower alcohol consumption. Also surprising is the low rank of Irish consumption in view of the high rate attributed to Irish Americans. (From* First Special Report to the U.S. Congress on Alcohol and Health, *National Institute on Alcohol and Alcoholism, Department of Health, Education and Welfare, December 1971.)*

sociated with maternal deprivation, with a personal and familial history of antisocial behavior, and with being the youngest child in a family. In one study of alcoholics, 40 percent of their fathers and 6 percent of their mothers were alcoholics. Alcoholism runs in families to such an extent that researchers have looked for genetically determined metabolic patterns that might make an individual more susceptible to intoxication by alcohol. When compared with the wives of nonalcoholics, those of alcoholics are more likely to have an alcoholic father or alcoholic siblings.

Alcoholics are commonly imagined to be Skid Row or Bowery "bums." Actually, this group accounts for only 5 percent of the country's alcoholics. Many alcoholics not only do not deteriorate to this social level but continue to function for years in their own social setting. Moreover, studies have shown that, in a given three-year period, 6 percent of serious problem drinkers will spontaneously control their drinking without specific treatment.

In addition to intoxication and withdrawal, alcohol produces a number of other important effects on the body. Chronic usage has been associated with an increased prevalence of carcinoma of the mouth, pharynx, esophagus, stomach, and pancreas. Ethanol irritates the lining of the stomach and produces gastritis, which can bleed, become chronic, and lead to pernicious anemia. It also causes increased gastric acidity and results in ulcers. Individuals with ulcers should not drink, and sudden death from the perforation and bleeding of an ulcer in an alcoholic is not uncommon. Ethanol causes pancreatitis which can become chronic and lead to diabetes. It is also associated with the accumulation of fatty material in the muscle of the heart. Although it is reversible if drinking stops, this condition can cause permanent cardiac damage.

Long-term consumption of alcohol can result in fatty infiltration in the liver (even in doses associated with social drinking). This, in turn, can produce disturbed liver function and, in 15 percent of chronic users, cirrhosis. Cirrhosis is a disease characterized by the gradual scarring and contraction of the liver and a resulting decline in this vital organ's ability to function normally. One consequence of cirrhosis is an alteration of the venous circulation around the stomach and esophagus, and the severe alcoholic with cirrhosis lives under a constant threat of rapidly fatal hemorrhage. Operations to correct this condition are risky and not always successful. Although cirrhosis death rates vary somewhat from year to year, this disease usually ranks about tenth as a killer in the United States; most cirrhosis is preceded by regular and prolonged alcohol intake. Alcohol abuse is also associated with injury to the peripheral nerves, which often results in wasted muscles and painful extremities. Furthermore, it is not uncommon for alcoholics to suffer cerebral deterioration which leads to difficulty in maintaining balance, as well as to a form of psychosis involving lack of memory and fabrication of events.

The abuse of alcohol traditionally has gone hand in hand with poor nutrition. Paradoxically, ethanol is one of the most potent sources of energy available for human consumption. Ethanol contains seven calories per gram, as opposed to five calories per gram of carbohydrate. Alcoholic beverages, however, lack vitamins and (with the exception of beer) protein. Alcohol depresses the appetite, and chronic users consume little else. This neglect of proper nutrition is so widespread and so extreme among chronic alcoholics that medical researchers are beginning to feel that many changes in the liver, central nervous system, and peripheral nerves of the alcoholic are due more to vitamin deficiency than the direct effect of alcohol. In addition, the severe nutritional deprivation of alcoholics has been partly responsible for their susceptibility to tuberculosis, vulnerability to pneumonia, and poor response to withdrawal; yet efforts by members of the medical profession to have small amounts of vitamins added to alcoholic beverages have been consistently ignored.

Another effect of alcohol is its action as a **diuretic**, an action which at one time or another has produced a social emergency for most alcohol consumers. Ethanol blocks the secretion of an antidiuretic hormone (ADH) from the brain stem. This **hormone** acts to help the kidney resorb large amounts of water and thus decreases the flow of urine. In the absence of this hormone, the kidney excretes copious amounts of urine—far over that amount due to the ingestion of the alcoholic beverage alone. This also results in a state of mild dehydration which contributes to the unpleasantness of the withdrawal period.

With the end results so dismal and the social costs so high, what can be done for the victim of America's fourth most common disease? For centuries, the alcoholic was regarded both by society and organized medicine as a moral derelict in a state of sin, and efforts to treat the alcoholic have been marred by a widespread persistence of this moralistic attitude. Alcoholism has thus been a problem resistant to solution and particularly frustrating to the medical professional, who has often preferred to avoid dealing with it directly. However, this situation is changing. The early and continuous efforts of Alcoholics Anonymous, and the more recently enlightened views of medicine, have gone far to convince the public that alcoholism is not a condition of moral weakness but a disease to be treated by professionals and overcome by individual and group effort. Specialists in alcohol therapy are emerging, hospitals are devoting facilities to the problem, research is being funded, and the National Institute on Alcohol and Alcoholism has been created by the federal government. In addition, a new approach has been taken recently which seems to be gaining acceptance. Advocates of this approach argue that alcoholism is in fact not a disease with specific and immutable biologic lesions but

---

DIURETIC: a drug which induces urination
HORMONE: a chemical produced by a body organ and having an effect on an organ
        other than that which produced it, i.e., ADH is produced in the brain
        stem but has its effect on the kidney

rather a neurosis characterized by a lack of successful adaptation to social pressures. This view has significant implications for the future treatment of alcoholics. For the present, a number of therapeutic modalities are in common practice, and they will be discussed briefly.

1. *Detoxification Centers.* Centers have been established across the country to hospitalize the alcoholic and allow withdrawal to take place under proper medical supervision. These detoxification centers may be wards in hospitals, adjuncts to emergency rooms, or independent institutions. Length of stay in the centers is generally under a week. Sobriety is established, and the patient is discharged to a therapeutic setting for follow-up care.

2. *Halfway Houses.* These houses are growing in number throughout the United States. They enable the alcoholic to continue in a supervised environment that offers medical treatment, group therapy, and psychotherapy while he resumes a job, begins a new one, or learns a new trade. The length of stay at these halfway houses is flexible—from three to six months—and allows each individual to develop at his own rate. A successful program in one of these houses, as in all phases of treatment of the alcoholic, involves the cooperative effort of professionals from a multitude of health careers. Upon discharge from a halfway house, the rehabilitated alcoholic can continue to participate in its programs as an outpatient. If this is not feasible, he is encouraged to pursue some other ongoing therapy.

3. *Alcoholics Anonymous* (A.A.). Founded in 1934 (in Ohio) by two once-successful but virtually ruined alcoholics, A.A. was really the first treatment modality directed to the needs of the alcoholic; in essence, it brought the treatment of alcoholism out of the Middle Ages. Much of the attention medicine has directed to this problem stems from the leads begun by Alcoholics Anonymous. As its name implies, it is a heterogeneous group of former alcoholics gathered together to reinforce each other's sobriety and help others not so fortunate. A.A. makes itself available to other treatment modalities. If an alcoholic is referred to them directly, two members of the organization immediately meet him personally, explain the program, and, if he is interested, personally conduct him to early meetings. A.A. requires a new member to make a personal decision for sobriety, to pledge never to touch alcohol again, to admit that he has lost control over his life, to redress any wrongs done, and to acknowledge the importance of a "higher power" (defined as each member desires) in the future restructuring of his life. A.A. has been criticized for its stress on this last concept but insists that such a commitment is necessary for survival. It is felt that A.A.s approach—in some respects similar to that of group therapy—is most successful with middle-class alcoholics who have

some strengths in their backgrounds. A recent study revealed that 40 percent of new members achieved sobriety immediately, 25 percent did so within a year, and 15 percent reached eventual sobriety.

4. *Psychotherapy.* It had long been thought that the behavioral disorder of the alcoholic did not lend itself to psychotherapy. However, contrary to previous skepticism, a significant advance during the last decade was the demonstration that psychotherapy—alone or as an adjunct to other therapies—can be extremely effective in helping the alcoholic. The success of this methodology reinforces the view that alcoholism is a social rather than a biologic disease. Although individual and group therapy are being used increasingly, the availability of such treatment is still limited by the relatively small number of trained therapists.

5. *Antabuse.* Antabuse (disulfuran) can be used as the sole therapeutic modality or in combination with other therapeutic measures. Taken regularly in pill form, antabuse itself has no effect on the reformed drinker. However, if he drinks an alcoholic beverage, alcohol combines with antabuse in the body to produce a syndrome of flushing, shakes, chills, nausea, and vomiting. Although these symptoms last for only a short period, the alcoholic is made so miserable that, in time, he is conditioned to avoid further drinking by the memory of its consequences. This drastic therapy has had some success in helping the individual who has great difficulty resisting "just one drink"; however, its effectiveness is compromised by the fact that it is often easier to avoid antabuse than alcohol.

The best way to treat alcoholism is to prevent it. To this end, some argue for stricter controls on the availability of alcohol. Alcoholism is more common where liquor is easier to obtain; full-scale prohibition, however, has been shown to be a monumental failure. Some religions call for alcohol abstinence, but studies indicate that those who follow such dictates are motivated more by their social and familial settings than by religious zeal.

The medical literature reveals a growing clamor for the reformation of social attitudes toward the acceptability of alcohol intoxication. Some of the writers ask that each of us publicly chastise any associate who may be tempted to drink to excess. This suggestion not only has some of the old moralistic overtones but offers little hope as a viable way of preventing alcoholism. However, it is important that many of our societal values in relation to alcoholism be reexamined, e.g., the tendency to associate masculinity with an ability to consume large amounts of liquor; and, in this connection, we will have to reevaluate the role of advertising in the beverage industry.

In an article on alcoholism, J. H. Masserman goes beyond the area of social change and suggests a root attack on the genesis of the problem: "We must exercise every effort and employ every modality to prevent or reduce individual conflicts, and modify or control the social stresses which precipitate episodes of alcoholism in order to counter their growing threat to individual and social welfare." It is perhaps by this broadest of approaches that we will achieve our soundest results.

Venereal Disease

In the United States there are five communicable diseases that are grouped together as the venereal diseases. They are alike in that they are transmitted almost exclusively through sexual relations, either heterosexual or homosexual. Further, they are classic examples of how in-

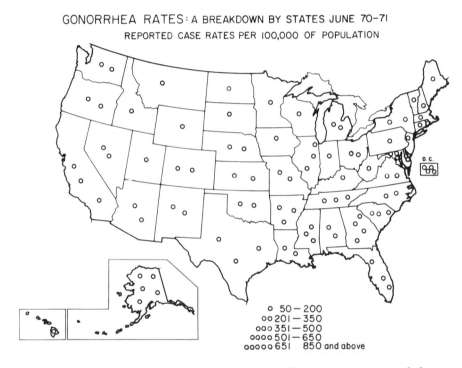

GONORRHEA RATES: A BREAKDOWN BY STATES JUNE 70-71
REPORTED CASE RATES PER 100,000 OF POPULATION

o   50 − 200
oo   201 − 350
ooo   351 − 500
oooo   501 − 650
ooooo 651   850 and above

FIG. 8-12A, B.   *These two figures illustrate the differing rates of venereal disease from state to state. A high rate, such as syphilis in Florida, may mean excellent case reporting or an extraordinarily great number of cases. Similarly, the low rate for Wyoming, Utah and Colorado may mean poor reporting rather than fewer actual cases. (Adapted from Statistics Department of American Social Health Association.)*

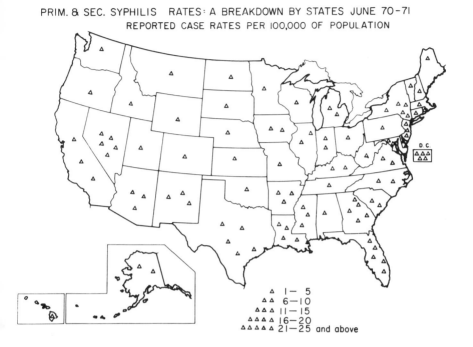

PRIM. & SEC. SYPHILIS   RATES: A BREAKDOWN BY STATES JUNE 70-71
REPORTED CASE RATES PER 100,000 OF POPULATION

△   1— 5
△ △   6—10
△ △ △   11—15
△ △ △ △ 16—20
△ △ △ △ △ 21—25 and above

FIG. 8-12B.

fectious disease is transmitted 'from person to person through skin-to-skin contact. This group includes syphilis, gonorrhea, chancroid, granuloma inguinale, and lymphogranuloma venereum. Syphilis and gonorrhea are widespread and are major problems, whereas the other are of minor importance and comprise only a small number of the reported cases of venereal disease.

Although physicians, clinics, and hospitals in all 50 states are required by law to report cases of venereal disease to the local health departments, many cases do not get reported because of the sensitive issues involved with this group of diseases (see Fig. 8-12A, B). Nonetheless, as Figure 8-13 indicates, venereal diseases account for the largest number of all the reported cases of communicable diseases. Table 8-3 gives an estimate of the total number of cases of gonorrhea and syphilis treated in the year 1968, and the total number of cases treated but not reported.

Why is this failure to report cases a serious problem? Syphilis and gonorrhea represent a paradox of modern medicine. They are communicable diseases for which the cause, method of diagnosis, mode of spread, and treatment are known. Yet they are still with us, in some areas in

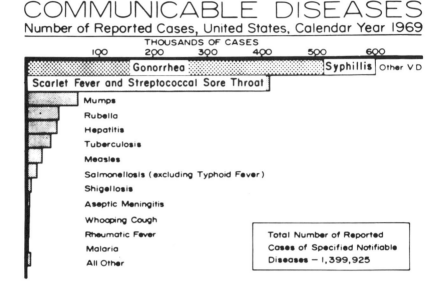

FIG. 8-13. *(Courtesy of American Social Health Association.)*

epidemic proportions. Failure to report cases to health officials often prevents and certainly hinders epidemiologic follow-up of contacts. This follow-up process traces chains of infection and insures proper treatment for all persons who are involved and located. Unchecked in this fashion, either disease can spread from any infected person to another person

TABLE 8-3. Estimated Total Syphilis and Gonorrhea Cases Treated
(Fiscal 1968)

	Infectious Syphilis	"Other" Syphilis	Gonorrhea
Number of cases treated and reported by public sources	12,953	32,714	307,624
Number of cases treated and reported by private physicians	7,229	45,299	123,756
Number of cases treated but not reported by private physicians (total estimated treated less total reported by them)	55,025*	93,931*	1,018,201*
Estimated total number of cases treated during fiscal 1968 by all sources	75,207*	171,944*	1,449,581*

Projected from results of 1968 National Survey of Venereal Disease Incidence, conducted by the American Social Health Association.

who, in turn, can spread it to others; and soon a great number of people have been infected. Though curable, syphilis is still the primary cause of death for at least 3,000 persons a year in the United States. As shown in Figure 8-14A and B syphilis and gonorrhea are primarily diseases of adolescents and young adults.

SYPHILIS

Syphilis is caused by a spirochcte, *Treponema pallidum.* This is a very fragile corkscrew-like organism which can survive only briefly outside the human body and is rapidly killed by heat, drying, or antiseptic solution. As a result, syphilis can usually be contracted only through intimate sexual contact with a person in an infectious stage of the disease. The organism enters the body at the point of contact through the genital skin or mucous membranes. The incubation period is about three weeks.

Although the progression of the disease is in reality a continuum, syphilis is usually described in stages which correspond to clinical manifestations. These stages are (1) primary, (2) secondary, (3) latent, and (4) late symptomatic.

After the three-week incubation period, the first sign of thc disease appears as a solitary lesion called a chancre, which occurs at the site of contact. The chancre starts as an asymptomatic **papule** that feels like a bump under the skin surface. The surface soon erodes, and a solitary painless ulcer is formed. Lymph nodes in the area usually enlarge at this time, and these are also painless. The lesion most commonly occurs in the genital area, although it may be at any site of inoculation. Since the penis most usually is infected, symptoms generally are obvious in the male. In the female, however, the vagina or cervix may be involved, and there may be no visible symptoms; the woman, therefore, may be infected without realizing it.

In this primary stage the ulcer contains large numbers of spirochetes, and the lesion is highly infectious. Even without treatment, however, the chancre will heal spontaneously in a few weeks, and the lymph nodes will regress. The disease continues within the host but gives no evidence of the damage it is causing.

Several weeks to several months after infection—and usually after the

---

PAPULE: a round, solid, raised skin lesion; a bump

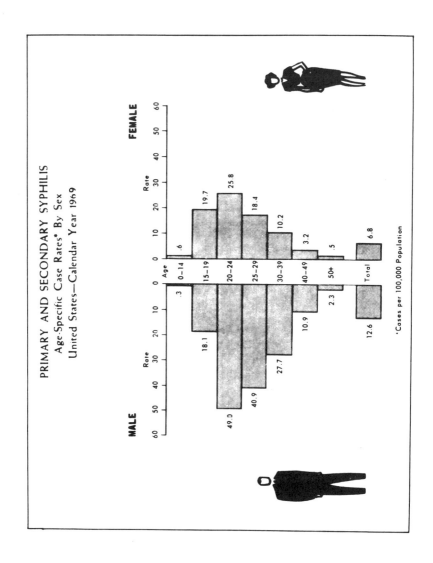

PRIMARY AND SECONDARY SYPHILIS
Age-Specific Case Rates* By Sex
United States—Calendar Year 1969

*Cases per 100,000 Population

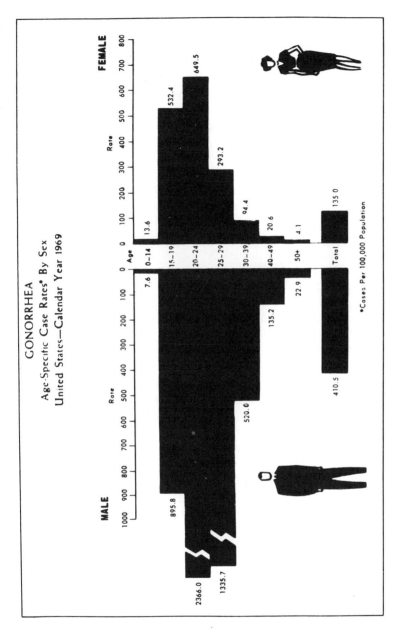

FIG. 8-14A, B. (After Millar, The Veneral Disease Problem in the United States, Center for Disease Control, Public Health Service, November 1, 1971.)

255

chancre has disappeared—a new set of signs and symptoms appear. They represent the secondary stage of the disease. Different people manifest different signs, although the most common sign of this stage is a symmetrical skin rash that may take on many characteristics and vary from a few small lesions to a generalized eruption. This rash is usually not **pruritic** and may manifest itself in any form from a dry crusty area to a frank **pustule**. At the same time, generalized symptoms such as low-grade fever, sore throat, and **malaise** may occur. A patchy loss of hair from the scalp and eyebrows is characteristic of this stage, as is painless enlargement of the lymph nodes throughout the body. Any one or a combination of these symptoms may occur. Secondary lesions of the skin or mucous membranes often contain organisms and are therefore infectious. Once again, as was true of the primary stage, these symptoms will disappear over time without any therapy.

Following the primary and secondary stages, untreated syphilis enters a latent, or hidden, period which may last for many years. During this time, the disease cannot be recognized on physical examination, and a special blood test (discussed later in this section) must be carried out to establish a diagnosis. The skin lesions of the secondary stage may reappear in this first few years of the latent stage. When these lesions do appear in an otherwise latent case, the patient is capable of transmitting the disease.

Syphilis may manifest itself as a chronic disease any time from the onset of the latent period to as long as 20 years later. Signs and symptoms will depend on what body system has been attacked by the spirochetes. Involvement of the cardiovascular system may lead to diseased heart valves and consequent heart failure; sometimes, an aneurysm develops in the aorta. Involvement of the central nervous system may result in blindness and insanity. By the time these symptoms appear, the damage that has occurred is not reversible. Spirochetes are not found at this stage, and the disease at this time is not infectious. It is a threat only to its victim—the untreated syphilitic.

Unlike gonorrhea, which can make females sterile, syphilis is rarely a cause of sterility; and a pregnant woman who is in the primary, secondary, or early stages of the latent phase can transmit the disease to her unborn child. This may result in early miscarriage, stillbirth, premature delivery, or a spectrum of diseases in the fetus (including changes which appear in

---

PRURITIC: derived from pruritis; itching
PUSTULE: a rounded, raised skin lesion filled with pus
MALAISE: a term referring to a general feeling of indisposition or discomfort

the developing child after the neonatal period). Congenital syphilis is completely preventable through treatment of the mother, especially in the first 18 weeks of pregnancy. For this reason, most states have laws requiring **serologic** blood tests for syphilis in pregnant women. In New York City this has resulted in a drop of reported cases of congenital syphilis—from 1,139 in 1940 to 42 in 1970.

Syphilis can be diagnosed by history, physical examination, and laboratory tests. The diagnosis of primary and secondary syphilis may be made by obtaining liquid material from the lesions and examining it for spirochetes. This is done by a special microscopic technique called dark-field examination. One to three weeks after the appearance of the primary lesion, i.e., four to six weeks after contraction of the disease, blood tests become positive. Although it is not used very often today, the most well-known of these is the Wassermann test. The S.T.S. (Standard Test for Syphilis) and the V.D.R.L. (Venereal Disease Research Laboratories) are nonspecific, commonly administered tests that are cheap and efficient for screening. When false-positives occur, more specific tests are used to clarify the diagnosis. Cerebrospinal fluid must be examined to diagnose syphilis of the central nervous system, while x-ray examination is often helpful in diagnosing tertiary and congenital syphilis.

Syphilis responds to antibiotic therapy. Penicillin is the drug of choice, while other antibiotics are used when the patient is allergic to penicillin. Prompt treatment is curative in the early stages. In the tertiary stage, when permanent damage has already occurred, treatment is aimed at stopping further destruction. After treatment, it is important that repeated serologic tests be performed, at least monthly, to confirm the cure. The United States Public Health Service, which recommends preventive treatment of any person known to have been exposed to syphilis, states that "It is a fallacy to wait for the disease to develop to the clinical or reactive serologic stage, meanwhile allowing reinfection of treated patients and the infection of additional persons."

GONORRHEA

Gonorrhea is caused by a bacterium, *Neisseria gonorrhoeae.* Like the organism that causes syphilis, it is extremely fastidious and will not live outside the body for any period of time, except in special culture media. Unlike syphilis, the incubation period of gonorrhea is extremely

---

SEROLOGIC: referring to serum

short—only two to five days. For this reason, contacts should be treated immediately and on the basis of history alone.

The symptoms of gonorrhea in men and women often differ. In the male the common early symptoms, acute and noticeable, are a usually **purulent** urethral discharge and a severe burning on urination. In the female there may be no early symptoms. Symptoms, when they occur, vary from minimal to severe. Minimally, there may be an uncomfortable inflammation of the urethra or a painless discharge. In severe cases, pelvic peritonitis may develop and produce high fever and severe pain. Because symptoms are often slight or nonexistent, the infected female may be unaware of her disease; and having no reason to seek treatment, she thus can become a carrier who spreads infection to her male sexual partners. In addition, untreated gonorrhea often leads to later complications, especially sterility.

While the spirochete of syphilis invades the bloodstream immediately, the gonococcus usually confines its damage to the genitourinary system. However, a systemic form of gonorrhea sometimes occurs, with arthritis and endocarditis as common complications. The eyes of the newborn may be infected if he passes through an infected birth canal. This eye disease, gonorrhea ophthalmia neonatus, is rarely seen today because most states require that newborns be treated **prophylactically**, at birth, with either silver nitrate drops or penicillin.

The gonococcal organism presents a classic pattern in smears made from secretions and stained by the gram-stain technique. The organism is located within white blood cells and resembles a pair of kidney-shaped beans. Initial identification is only presumptive, however, since other organisms occasionally may mimic the gonococcus. Definitive diagnosis can be made by culture and special tests to separate this organism from others. Thayer and Martin devised a culture medium which allows the fragile gonococcus to survive and grow; if this selective medium is used, it has been found that the organism can be demonstrated in a high percentage of female contacts of males with urethritis from any cause. The cervix is the most productive source for positive cultures in the female, especially the asymptomatic woman. At present, there are no serologic tests for gonorrhea. For this reason, screening is practical only when symptoms occur in the male or female patient or when a routine pelvic examination is being done on the asymptomatic female.

Although there has been a recent increase in the emergence of peni-

---

PURULENT: referring to pus
PROPHYLAXIS: disease prevention

cillin-resistant strains of gonococcus, penicillin is still the drug of choice for the treatment of gonorrhea. The United States Public Health Service suggests the use of large doses of the drug to achieve high blood levels. Gonococcal strains resistant to penicillin are treated with other antibiotics or combinations of antibiotics. It is also recommended that all patients treated for gonorrhea have a series of serologic tests for syphilis. Fortunately, penicillin will cure the gonorrhea infection, and, if the drug is taken over a longer period, a possible syphilitic infection as well. Follow-up cultures are necessary to confirm that the organism has been eradicated completely.

CHANCROID

Chancroid is caused by a bacterium called *Hemophilius ducrey;* and granuloma inguinale is caused by the Donovan body, or *Donovania granulomatis.* Lymphogranuloma venereum is caused by a filterable virus. While each of these diseases may cause severe complications, better sanitation and hygiene have eliminated them as major public health problems in most parts of the United States.

LESS COMMON VENEREAL DISEASES

The control of venereal disease rests with increased screening, accurate reporting of infected persons, and diligent tracing of their sexual contacts. As part of the National Syphilis Eradication Program, the federal government has instituted training to develop a corps of casework epidemiologists. These people are highly skilled in interview techniques and exhaustively question each individual with a reported case of syphilis. At present there is no such program for gonorrhea control.

Studies show that the average patient with infectious syphilis will have had sexual contact with approximately five people during the incubation period. In the example shown in Figure 8-15, the index case led to 48 other people, 12 of whom were found to be positive. In the great majority of cases, unfortunately, feelings of guilt and fear of involving others (as well as a tragically false sense of protecting them) prevent the infected person from revealing the identity or even acknowledging the existence of sexual partners.

About 40 percent of people with untreated syphilis will develop serious complications. One out of 15 will develop heart disease; 1 in 25 will

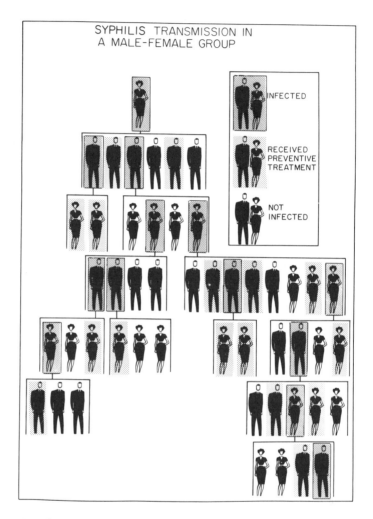

FIG. 8-15. *The single case of syphilis at the top of the figure leads to a chain of contacts involving 48 other people. Note that some contacts are not infected (about 40%) and that, as one might expect, transmission occurs as a result of homosexual as well as heterosexual exposure. Note that many of those treated with antibiotics may have been infected but that is unknown.*

become crippled or incapacitated; 1 in 50 will develop syphilitic insanity; and 1 in 200 will become blind. Twenty-three percent of the entire group can be expected to die primarily as a result of syphilis.

Data on the long-range effects of untreated gonorrhea is not as accurate as for syphilis. However, it is known that severe complications can occur, and many operations for chronic pelvic disability in females result from untreated gonorrhea. Sterility in both males and females is not uncommon. The relative paucity of symptoms in the early stages of gonorrhea in the female makes treatment less likely and later complications more likely than is the case with males. In order to locate this asymptomatic reservoir of disease in female patients, it has been suggested that routine testing for gonorrhea be part of every gynecological examination—just as a routine serology has become part of most medical examinations.

Large-scale screening programs for venereal disease are expensive. In comparison to the damage done to human life, however, the cost is slight. In the middle 1960s, the National Center for Health Statistics estimated that over 49 million dollars was spent in the United States to maintain people with syphilitic psychosis and blindness. It was also estimated that national loss of income due to syphilis alone was 33 million dollars. Less than one-quarter of the total expended or lost that year was spent on control programs, although it is particularly true of venereal disease that "an ounce of prevention is worth a pound of cure." In the long run, the best hope for eliminating these diseases lies in a public educated to the nature of venereal disease and to the nature of human sexuality itself.

Cigarette Smoking

No discussion of the relationship between health and the social environment would be complete without a consideration of cigarette smoking. During the first 50 years of this century, cigarette smoking gradually became a national activity whose extent is now rivaled only by that of alcohol consumption. Over the past 20 years, still-mounting evidence has established beyond challenge the harmful effects of cigarettes. The

TABLE 8-4. Cigarette Smoking and Mortality Ratios
for Selected Causes of Death

Cause of Death	Cigarettes per day		Former Smoker
	10–20	21–30	
Cancer of lung	9.05	16.93	4.71
Cancer of larynx	8.33	13.26	7.22
Cancer of bladder	2.29	3.15	1.60
Bronchitis	4.34	4.01	3.06
Arteriosclerotic heart disease	1.64	1.82	1.21

relationship between smoking and various diseases is clear-cut and un-equivocal. Table 8-4 presents mortality ratios for causes of death related to smoking. This ratio is simply the mortality rate among smokers divided by the mortality rate among nonsmokers. With respect to lung cancer, the ratio among persons smoking 10 to 20 cigarettes daily is 9.05, i.e., among such smokers, the mortality rate from lung cancer is 9.05 times as high as the mortality rate among nonsmokers. It should be noted that those who stop smoking and "join the unhooked generation" not only usually enjoy a relief from some of smoking's more obvious effects (such as a cough) but have lower mortality rates than those who continue to smoke.

The now obvious relationship between cigarettes and various diseases has stimulated considerable research into exactly how cigarettes lead to these deleterious effects. At this point, knowledge of the mechanism is fragmentary; however, with regard to arteriosclerotic heart disease, it is believed that the offending agent is nicotine, which increases the blood pressure and pulse rate while constricting the blood supply to the skin. In addition to other noxious agents, cigarette smoke also contains multiple tarlike substances composed of various chemicals, some of which are carcinogenic and are believed to play a leading role in the etiology of lung cancer and other carcinomas. Cigarettes are also linked to bronchitis and emphysema; in fact, the earliest effects of smoking are a decrease in pulmonary function and the subsequent development of a cough.

Studies conducted in the late 1960s found that cigarette smokers comprised half the total adult population and these studies tried to delineate some basic characteristics of smokers (Fig. 8-16). More recently, there have been efforts to publicize the ill effects of smoking; cigarette commercials have been banned from television; and there is a growing tendency for state legislatures to generate additional revenue by increasing the tax on cigarettes (Fig. 8-17). These measures seem to be having an impact on younger people, who appear to be less than enthusiastic about taking up the habit. In view of the fact that excess mortality from smoking is greatest in those who begin to smoke before the age of 20, this trend deserves to be encouraged.

Accidents

Accidents are here defined as sudden, unexpected events which result in individual or collective bodily injury. While they occur in all human societies, the nature of such accidents (as of most health

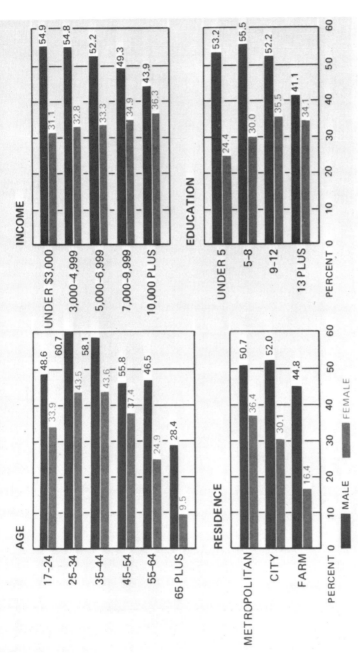

CHARACTERISTICS OF PRESENT SMOKERS

Fig. 8-16. *These statistics are based on a 1965 study of the U.S.A. civilian population. Note that among men the percentage of smokers declines with rising income, higher levels of education, and advancing age. With regard to the latter, it is interesting to ponder whether the low percentage of smokers above the age 65 is a reflection of the high mortality of smokers in the younger age groups. (From Chart Book on Smoking, Tobacco and Health, Public Health Service Publication No. 1937, June 1969.)*

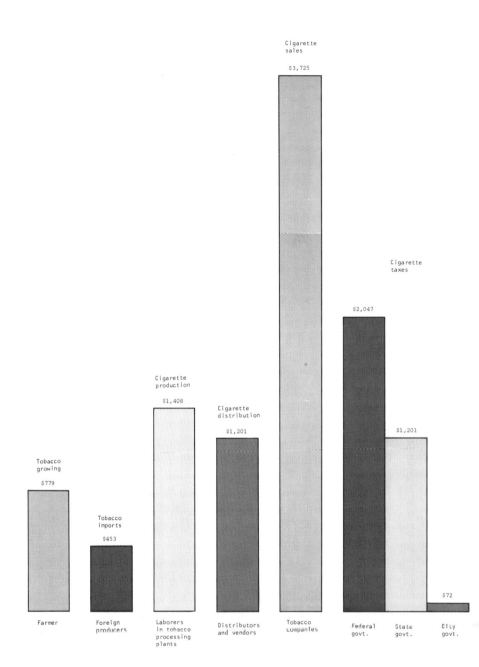

Who Profits

FIG. 8-17. *(Legend on page 265.)*

264

problems) is largely determined by the technology and mores of the society in which they happen. No doubt, accidents pose a problem of some import for the primitive tribes of New Guinea, but we can state with virtual certainty that motor vehicles are not an important cause of accidents in that society, nor are airplane crashes or accidental injury resulting from firearms. In contrast, cars, aircraft, and guns are major accident hazards in the United States and most other industrialized nations.

Accidents are the fourth leading cause of death in this country. Among people aged 1 to 34, accidents are the leading cause of death. Statistics for the year 1970 are typical of most years in the last decade; and, in that year, about 50 million accidents were reported—resulting in roughly 115,000 deaths and the impairment of 400,000 people. Accident mortality in young people and the elderly deserves special emphasis. For children between 1 and 14 years of age, accidents account for more deaths than the next six leading causes put together. Among persons aged 15 to 24, accidents claim more lives than all other causes combined. Accidental poisonings in young children was discussed in Chapter 6, as was the high prevalence of accidents among the aged. When one considers wages lost, medical expenses, property damage, and insurance claims, it should come as no surprise that the total cost of accidents is more than 27 billion dollars a year. Accident-fatality rates have been rising even though the rate at which accidents occur has declined almost 40 percent since 1910.

Essentially, injuries associated with accidents occur in any of six different ways. These are outlined in Table 8-5. Mechanical, thermal, and those accidents depriving the victim of oxygen are most common, but chemical agents are significantly involved in accidents among preschool children. Burns may result from electricity as well as from an open flame. Injuries from oxygen deprivation and from chemicals also overlap. Carbon monoxide (CO), a tasteless, odorless, and lethal gas that is a major con-

---

FIG. 8-17. *Some of the income from the production of cigarettes, U.S. 1963 (in millions of dollars). While it is true that cigarettes have been causally associated with lung cancer, heart disease, and several other conditions, it is also true that cigarettes represent a multi-billion-dollar-a-year business. Much of this vast amount finds its way into the hands of federal, state, and city governments (3.3 billion dollars in 1963). An outright ban on cigarettes or, what is the same thing, an extremely high taxation rate would deny revenue to the government and curtail the income of farmers, wage-earners, and companies whose livelihood is derived largely from tobacco products. To date, the society has opted to approach the problem on an individual basis. This approach is similar to that used with regard to alcohol. Note the totally different societal attitude toward "hard drugs" such as heroin. (Adapted from Smoking, Tobacco and Health, Public Health Service, Publication No. 1937, June 1969.)*

TABLE 8-5. Types of Injuries Associated with Accidents*

Mechanism of Injury	Type of Injury	Example
Mechanical	Breaking, tearing, crushing, etc.	Bullets, knives, falling objects, autos, aircraft, falls
Thermal	Burns, freezing, failure of body's heat-regulating mechanism	Fires, exposure to sunstroke
Electrical	Compromise of normal neuro-muscular function; also burns	Electrocution
Radiation	Compromise of normal cellular function	Fallout, over-exposure to x-ray or other sources of radiation
Chemical	Varies with chemical involved	Plant, animal, and micro-biologic toxins; noxious agents such as lye, strong acids, etc.
Compromise of oxygen exchange	Suffocation	Drowning, choking, etc.

Modified after Haddon, W. The prevention of accidents. In Clark, D. and MacMahon, B., Eds. Preventive Medicine. Boston, Little, Brown, and Co., 1967.

stituent of automobile exhausts, combines readily with hemoglobin and thereby deprives the body of its oxygen-transport system. CO causes suffocation just as effectively as does drowning.

Accidents are usually categorized according to where they occur, namely, in the home, in public places, at work, and in motor vehicles. Although the home is the most common site of accidents and produces the most devastating injuries, motor vehicles lead in terms of accident deaths and are responsible for nearly half of all such fatalities. Men have more accidents than women, and account for 70 percent of all accident deaths. Death rates are higher for blacks than for whites and higher in mountain states than in other regions of the country. Rural areas are far more dangerous than cities. The summer months (June, July, and August) account for more accidents than any other season of the year.

The high incidence of home accidents is ironic in view of the popular notion that the home is a secure fortress against the dangers of an unpredictable outside world. Most susceptible to home accidents are children under 5 and persons over age 65. Seventy percent of all accidents in young children occur at home, where the youngster spends virtually all of his time. Among the aged, fully half of all accidental deaths involve home accidents. The latter most commonly occur in the bedroom and, in descending order, the kitchen, on the stairs, in the living room, and in the basement. Fifty percent of the fatalities resulting from these accidents are due to falls, with burns, suffocation, poisoning, firearms, and gas inhalation accounting for the remainder. Burns due to general household conflagration, as well as those resulting from specific episodes such as the spilling of scalding hot liquids, are most common in the very young and the very old. Suffocation is peculiar to childhood and too frequently is the result of a youngster's fatal attraction to plastic bags or discarded refrigerators. Gas inhalation is a particular hazard for the aged, who often forget to shut off the gas stove. In these deaths, CO is most commonly the offending agent. Although accidents involving firearms are often equated with hunting mishaps, 50 percent of firearm deaths occur at home, and such deaths are becoming increasingly common. They are especially frequent in children 5 to 14 years of age.

Accidents which occur at places of work are categorized as either industrial or agricultural. Although there are more accidents in industry, more accidental deaths occur in an agricultural setting. In the past 40 years, much has been done to improve the safety of working conditions in industry. This trend was greatly stimulated by the passage of workmen's compensation laws in all states. These laws make it mandatory for the employer to compensate workers for job-related injuries regardless of fault. Although the provisions of these laws vary considerably from state to state, the net effect has been a major decline in industrial accident rates, primarily because the employer has been encouraged, by his liability, to install safety equipment and encourage safe working conditions. Vehicular accidents account for most deaths and permanent disability, but accidents involved with lifting and moving heavy objects cause most industrial work injuries. Other important causes of injury are falls, falling objects, and machinery. Studies have shown that injuries occur with greater frequency as the number of hours worked per week increases, and that most accidents occur in the first half of an eight-hour working day.

Except for those in the construction and mining industries, agricultural accidents more often end fatally than those in industry. The higher death rates from agricultural accidents are attributable to the remoteness of many farms from a source of medical care, the failure of most workmen's compensation laws to provide adequate coverage for agricultural workers, and the exemption of agriculture from laws regulating the conditions under which children can work. Twenty-five percent of all agricultural deaths occur in persons under 19 years of age. As is true of accidents generally and of industrial accidents as well, motor vehicles are the leading cause of fatalities in farm accidents.

Accidents in public places comprise those which happen away from home and work but which do not involve motor vehicles. Falls and drowning are the leading killers in this category, followed by accident fatalities due to firearms, transportation, and fires. Drowning is most common in children and young adults; and falls, as we know, are most frequent

TABLE 8-6. Some Statistics Related to Principal Classes of Accident, 1970*

Class	Deaths	Percent of All Deaths	Disabling Injuries	Percent of All Injuries
Motor vehicle	54,800	47	2,000,000	18
Work**	14,200	12	2,200,000	20
Home	26,500	23	4,000,000	37
Public	22,000	18	2,700,000	25
TOTAL	117,500	100	10,000,000	100

*Modified after Accident Deaths. Chicago, National Safety Council, 1971.

**Seventy-seven percent of these deaths involve motor vehicles in an industrial or agricultural setting.

among the aged. Firearm fatalities in the public-places category most often refer to hunting accidents, the usual victim being a young person between the ages of 15 and 20.

Deaths resulting from transportation accidents involve private, commercial, or military aircraft in one-third of cases. Another third is accounted for by water transportation, almost always involving small boats. Rail accidents make up most of the remainder, with bicycles, busses, and elevators contributing a small fraction. Table 8-6 compares the principal classes of accident. The most casual glance at this table will leave the reader impressed with the extent to which motor vehicle accidents dominate all other types of accidents as a cause of death. The motor vehicle death rate per 100,000 population is lower today than it was 35 or 40 years ago, but the actual number of people killed each year has risen more or less steadily since 1925. The lower death rate is explained by the fact that although the number of yearly fatalities has increased, this increase is less than the growth of the population.

Two-thirds of all auto fatalities occur in rural areas. In cities, almost 40 percent of fatalities involve pedestrians, while this is true only about 10 percent of the time in rural areas. Fatal accidents are somewhat more common at night than during the day, although this difference is less striking than may be supposed (53 percent, night; 47 percent, day). Saturday night is the most dangerous time of the week, October the most dangerous month of the year. Young people below the age of 25 account for 21 percent of all drivers but have 34 percent of the fatal accidents (Fig. 8-18). Males have higher fatality rates than females, but this may be largely due to very particular circumstances. Males, for example, are more likely

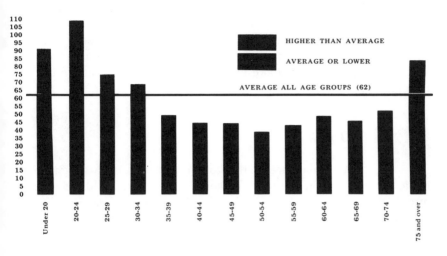

NUMBER OF DRIVERS IN FATAL ACCIDENTS

PER 100,000 DRIVERS IN EACH AGE GROUP IN 1970

FIG. 8-18.   *Accident fatalities are highest in young drivers and in very old ones.*
This fact is reflected in astronomical insurance rates in young drivers.
The very old driver is less of a problem because of his relative scarcity.
(From Aide Magazine, *Vol. 3, No. 11, Winter, 1972. Courtesy of United*
Services Automobile Association.)

than females to drive motorcycles; and the motorcycle fatality rate is five
times higher than that involving autos.

Speeding is more often a factor in rural deaths, 73 percent of which
occur at speeds in excess of 40 miles per hour. In urban areas, 52 percent
of vehicular deaths involves speeds below 30 miles per hour, although
this figure no doubt is heavily influenced by the high proportion of pedestrian victims. Driving is three times safer on divided limited-access highways, such as the interstate systems, than on ordinary roads. More than
half of all auto fatalities involve the use of alcohol by driver or pedestrian
or both.

Several years ago, seat belts became mandatory equipment for automobiles, and this was hailed as the beginning of an era of declining motor
vehicle fatalities. Today, almost 90 percent of cars are equipped with
seat belts, and most of these with shoulder straps as well. Many studies
have concluded that about 9,000 lives would be saved annually if the
belts were used all the time. Unfortunately, seat belts are used only about
40 percent of the time; it is thus only about one driver in three who, at
any given moment, is "buckled up for safety."

One of the most remarkable observations to be made about accidents in general and auto accidents in particular is the extent to which they are accepted by the public as largely unavoidable. Unfortunately, they will remain high on our list of problems because the leading accident hazard, the automobile, is an indispensable component of American life. Nevertheless, it is entirely possible to lower the number of accident deaths by such measures as extending safety regulations in agriculture, improving auto design, constructing more interstate-type roads, and increasing educational programs for young drivers.

Housing

An ambulance at the bottom of a cliff is always more dramatic than a fence at the top. Workers in the allied health sciences are usually associated with the ambulance rather than the fence, and it often comes as a surprise that how people live, where they live, and what they live in may have more to do with solving or aggravating health problems than do doctors, nurses, x-ray machines, hospitals, and all the other accouterments of modern medical technology. The following discussion will consider the way in which shelter, or housing, relates to the individual and to his health. The perspective for this discussion is that illness and disability are indicators of the way in which a human community interacts with its environment.

A family's house is its castle, whether the place be a tenement apartment in the slums of Harlem, an estate in suburbia, a shanty-town in the barrios of Brazil, or a Bedouin tent in the Sinai desert. The obvious contrasts in these environments underscore the fallacy of generalizations about housing adequacy. In suburbia, the provident home-owner knows a little about plumbing; in the big cities, the tenant is well-advised to find an apartment building which has a superintendent who knows about plumbing; in the barrio districts of Latin America, the recent and usually impoverished migrant from the countryside is fortunate if he can erect his shack near a source of water.

Housing and health are related to each other. Ideally, a shelter protects people from undesirable characteristics of the environments and has connections, either via structural or service arrangements, to life-sustaining water and heat supplies, electrical power, and a system of sewage disposal. In the slums of Harlem, "healthful" means, above all, the supply of heat and hot water needed to protect people from a cold New York winter. In the Sinai desert, healthful housing (here, shelter is a more appropriate term) means, among other things, a strong and enclosed tent to protect the Bedouin from the heat and sands of the desert. Quite obviously, there is no such thing as a universal **housing code.** Equally important, there are complex interrelationships between types of housing and cultural modes of behavior. The annals of public works are filled with stories of housing projects conceived to meet the needs of a particular community and its environment and then superimposed on a different community. The results sometimes have been catastrophic and occasionally comic. In essence, the story of poor miners using bathtubs to store coal in their new homes has been replicated innumerable times the world over. In the inner cities of the United States, newly built housing projects are designed in accordance with all the currently mandated standards for health and safety. Rarely, however, do the planners of such projects consider the recreational and social service needs of the residents, the problems associated with educating people to live in cities, or the projected economics of maintenance and repair.

Much has been written about how housing and health are related. Studies repeatedly have linked poor housing conditions with poor health. Infections, gastrointestinal disorders, and accidents are more common among children living in slum housing than they are among youngsters living under better conditions. The incidence of adult illnesses requiring medical care and activity limitation is also influenced by inferior housing. Infant mortality, venereal disease, tuberculosis, and mental illness have been described as being more prevalent in areas characterized by poor housing. However, the thoughtful reader will recognize that there are problems of interpretation concerning the relationship between housing and health. Sometimes, "poor housing" is a shorthand way of describing the living conditions of poor people. The poor include the aged, deprived ethnic minority groups, the infirmed, and families headed by unemployed women. In other words, the people most at risk for illness often live in inferior housing. Therefore, it is a matter of conjecture whether many people live in poor housing because they are sick or are sick because they live in poor housing (Table 8-7).

It would seem clear that the advisability of isolating an abstractly defined independent variable called "housing" and simplistically relating it to another abstract variable called "health" is dubious. Nevertheless, we can sometimes make sound empirical observations about housing and

---

HOUSING CODE: a set of regulations governing the construction and use of buildings and usually administered by the local health department. A typical housing code covers such things as ventilation, electrical standards, plumbing requirements, duties of owners and tenants, and so on.

TABLE 8-7. Tenement Preventive Maintenance and Environmental Control—Selected Health and Safety Benefits

Environmental Health and/or Safety Problem	Population Most Affected	Services Required			
		Recurring	Skill Level*	Nonrecurring	Skill Level*
Respiratory infections; pneumonia-like illnesses; extreme discomfort	Very young and very old	Boiler maintenance; assuring room humidification	(1) (3)	Major boiler repair; repair of broken windows and leaks	(1), (2) (1), (2)
Rat-bites; rat-borne infections; flea bites; salmonellosis	Very young	Vector control; garbage removal; stoppage; extermination; education and training	(1), (2) (1), (3) (1) (1), (2) (1), (2) (3)	Stoppage	(1)
Accidents, injuries, falls	All age groups primarily children and teenagers	Light bulbs in hallways, corridors	(1)	Installing window guards; repairing broken windows; repairing stair railings; repairing holes in floors	(1) (1) (1) (1)
Burns from fires	All age groups	Training; drills; education	(1), (2)	Installation of extinguishers; fire-proofing; fire retardant for high-risk areas; electrical repairs	(1) (1), (2) (1), (2) (1), (2)
Carbon monoxide poisoning	All age groups	Boiler maintnenace	(1), (3)	Boiler repair	(1), (2)
Lead poisoning	Preschool age	Removing peeling paint; plumbing repair; education; Case finding and follow-up	(1), (3) (1), (2) (3) (1) ?	Wall-covering up to 5 feet; scraping above 5 feet; plumbing repair	(1) (1)
Skin infections from insect bites; poor indoor sanitation practices	Mostly children	Drainage of pools in yards, cellars; education	(1), (2) (1), (3)		

TABLE 8-7. (Continued)

Environmental Health and/or Safety Problem	Population Most Affected	Services Required			
		Recurring	Skill Level*	Nonrecurring	Skill Level*
Asthma from dust, mites, rodent dander	All age groups	Vector and pest control; cockroach control; education; mopping and scrubbing or corridors	(1), (2) (1), (3) (1), (3) (1), (3)		
Waterborne illnesses—diarrhea, including amebic dysentery	All age groups	Plumbing repairs	(1), (2)	Major plumbing repairs	(2)
Animal bites (dogs)	All age groups			Registration	(1), (3)
Physical injuries from violent assaults	All residents	Presence/availability of someone on or near premises with access to police	(1), (3)		
Insecticides—illness from indiscriminate use?	All residents	Education	(3)		

Legend: (1) Service performed by trained maintenance personnel.

(2) Service probably requires assistance and/or work performed by back-up contracting, municipal, or specialist service.

(3) Service has education and training component for tenants. Tenants may perform certain services.

health. The fact that we cannot readily demonstrate a causal relationship between the two in purely scientific terms does not contradict the fact that there are certain specific ways in which housing quite obviously has implications for health. When a tenement boiler breaks down in the middle of winter in Harlem, the very old and the very young are most apt to suffer from respiratory and cardiovascular difficulties; in the barrios of Rio de Janeiro, the occurrence of diarrheal and skin diseases of newborns and infants is almost certainly worsened by the absence of a public water supply and sewage disposal system.

Each community differs from the next; each building, like each patient, has its own personality and problems. Above all, the community health worker should be aware that it is a fallacy to measure housing's impact on health exclusively in terms of the time-honored indices of public health, such as infant mortality, tuberculosis, and venereal disease rates. These may be correlated to poor housing, but they also may be unrelated. Furthermore, attention may be diverted from the ways in which housing truly influences health: How many falls from windows lacking window guards? How many cases of lead poisoning from buildings with peeling leaded paint? How many fires and cases of carbon monoxide poisoning? How many days of school absence among children living in unheated buildings? How much asthma from buildings with unmopped hallways? And so on.

In the days when communicable diseases were the major concern in Europe and the United States, there was much concern about crowding (usually measured in terms of persons per square mile, persons per dwelling unit, or, preferably, persons per room) and its impact on health. Excessive crowding within a dwelling unit obviously promotes person-to-person spread of various communicable diseases, either by the airborne or the fecal-oral route. However, cultural differences in the way people adapt to crowding—be it within an individual home, an apartment building in New York City, or on the sidewalks of Calcutta (see Fig. 8-19)— modify its relationship to health, especially in those societies where the classical communicable diseases are no longer the big killers. Crowding, depending on the circumstances, can contribute to social cohesiveness and a sense of cooperation within a human community and thus actually promote both physical and mental health. This is frequently the case in military barracks, summer camps, and, incredibly, even in prisons and concentration camps. On the other hand, crowding can help to push an already disorganized community into physical and social decay, as so often occurs in the refugee camps that blot the modern political landscape. An appraisal of the effects of crowding in any given community thus must consider specifically what would happen within that community

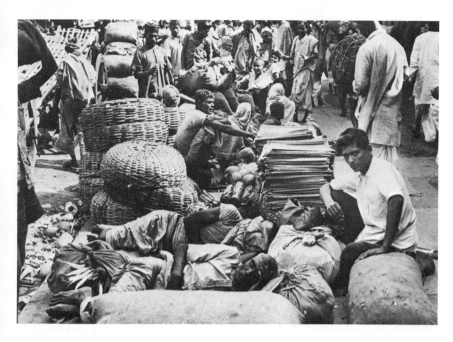

FIG. 8-19. *In most of the United States the problem is inadequate housing. In Calcutta, the problem is no housing whatever. (Courtesy of Sidney Schanberg, The New York Times.)*

if it became more or less crowded. Comparisons with other, different communities are often senseless. It is noteworthy that in New York City the accelerating trend of inner-city devastation and housing abandonment by building owners started in the mid 1960s, a period when slum crowding (as measured by the number of persons per room per *occupied* dwelling unit) was in significant decline.

DIAGNOSING THE LOCUS OF URBAN
ENVIRONMENTAL NEEDS

Outside of western Europe, North America, and Australia, much of the rest of the world has experienced enormous increases in the population of its cities. In Asia, Africa, and Latin America this has been characterized by rapid and chaotic growth of huge shanty-towns; and makeshift huts, often ingeniously patched together with wood, tin, bits and pieces of scrap, and corrugated cardboard, are now an integral part of the newly industrialized urban landscape. Contrary to popular impression, the shanties themselves are sometimes fairly livable environments, reflecting, in so far as possible, the wants and needs of the families which have built them. Indeed, the history of these shanty-towns is often one of gradually improved construction, with wood, adobe, and brick replacing the original scrap. The locus of housing and health problems in these communities lies in the fact that basic public services such as potable water, sewerage systems, electricity, and waste disposal arrangements are virtually nonexistent. Whether such towns will survive as viable communities or degenerate into foci of despair and disease will depend largely on whether the authorities can be pressured into providing the critically needed public services. Over the years, practical experience has indicated that the social and economic problems linked to making such services available may be formidable, but they are not insurmountable.

In the great cities of North America and western Europe, the problems are different. The basic public services, though at times faulty, are provided. With a few exceptions, tenants of the poorest, most devastated areas of Harlem drink the water of the same quality as do the inhabitants of Park Avenue's penthouses. Yet, New York City has equally severe housing and health problems, in certain ways more intractable than those of cities in the Orient, Africa, and South America. These are the problems of an established but aging city. Seventy percent of its buildings demolished as "unsafe" are structually sound; the problem is that they are inadequately *maintained*. The locus of breakdown is not public and not private but somewhere in between—the semipublic sector. The barrios of Rio de Janeiro need a water pipeline; but the residents of a Harlem tenement need a building superintendent.

In part, the "housing problem" has been based on the failure to recognize that housing implies not only the construction of a building but the ongoing provision of many maintenance and repair services for the inhabitants of that building. Table 8-7 summarizes some of the health and safety problems associated with the breakdown of semipublic housing services in the slums of big cities. A careful study of this list would indicate that a trained, dedicated, and competent superintendent may do more for the health of his building's inhabitants than a team of doctors and nurses. Further study would reveal that such problems as childhood lead poisoning, rat bites, and fires are all categorical manifestations of the collapse of housing-maintenance services in the inner cities of the United States.

It is presently fashionable to emphasize the hopelessness of inner-city housing problems. Yet, on a small scale, promising programs with a demonstrated potential for applicability have been initiated; and they have produced results which suggest that the trend toward decay and abandonment in the great cities can be reversed. In New York City, for example, a coalition of inner-city neighborhood housing groups, job-training organizations, tenants, owners, municipal agencies, and the Department of Community Medicine of the Mount Sinai School of Medicine have implemented an urban equivalent of the agricultural extension services. Through training and field services in preventive medicine, environmental health and safety, fire prevention, and community education, this program is redefining the role of superintendent as an environmental extension agent. It thus seeks to reverse the accelerating breakdown of the tenement houses and neighborhood environments and to eliminate the environmental health and safety problems linked to this trend. The concept is to preserve structurally sound housing and, at the same time, stimulate efforts in community organization and local economic development. This program, which has implications in housing, job-training, neighborhood development, and public health, serves as a working prototype of practical and effective approaches which can be evolved. In addition, a new type of health worker—the environmental extension agent—has emerged as a possible answer to the health and housing problems of inner city.

The United States has entered a postindustrial age in which increasing numbers of people are providers of services rather than of manufactured goods. As we have already emphasized, housing is now part of this service economy, which, experts are quick to point out, faces problems not seen in the production sector of the economy. The main problem is that technology has not been harnessed to increase productivity in the service occupations. Thanks to technology, a worker on the auto assembly line is more productive today than he was 20 years ago; but a plumber still spends 20 minutes changing a washer. An increasing need for housing services in our larger cities will place a continually greater stress on the service providers. Thus, to the extent that health and safety problems are linked to a breakdown in semipublic maintenance services, there is the threat that these problems may rapidly spread. Ultimately, it may well be that housing maintenance, because of its significant public health implications, will require permanent public support.

References

DRUG ABUSE

Berg, D. Extent of Illicit Drug Use. Washington, D. C., Division of Drug Sciences, Bureau of Narcotics and Dangerous Drugs, May 1969, p. 31.

278   THE SOCIAL ENVIRONMENT

Cohen, A. Inside what's happening: sociological, psychological and spiritual perspectives on the contemporary drug scene. Amer. J. Public Health 59:2092–95, 1969.
Consumer's Union. The Medicine Show. Mount Vernon, New York, 1963.
Einstein, S. The use and misuse of drugs: a social dilemma. In Jones, H. L., ed. Basic Concepts in Health Science Series. Belmont, Calif. Wadsworth, 1970.
Glatt, M. M. Psychological and social aspects of drug dependence in adolescence. In Wilson, C. W. M., ed. The Pharmacological and Epidemiological Aspects of Adolescent Drug Dependence. New York, Pergamon Press, 1968.
Gossett, J., et al. Extent and prevalence of illicit drug use among 5600 students. J.A.M.A. 216:1464–70, 1971.
Jaffee, J. Drug addiction and drug abuse. In Goodman and Altman, eds. The Pharmacologic Basis of Therapeutics. New York, Macmillan, 1965.
Linken, A. The Pharmacological and Epidemiological Aspects of Adolescent Drug Dependence. New York, Pergamon Press, 1968.
Richards, L. C. Illicit Drug Abuse and Addiction in the United States: Scope of the Problem. Chevy Chase, Md., National Institutes of Mental Health, August, 1970.
Snyder, S. What we have forgotten about pot. The New York Times Magazine, December 13, 1970, pp. 27–8.

ALCOHOLISM

Bailey, M. P., Haberman, P. W., and Alksne, H. The epidemiology of alcoholism in an urban residential area. Quart. J. Stud. Alcohol 26:20–40, 1965.
Beeson, P. B. and McDermott, W. Cecil-Loeb Textbook of Medicine, 13th ed. Philadelphia, W. B. Saunders Co., 1971.
Berg, H. L. Effects of alcohol intoxication on self concept. Quart. J. Stud. Alcohol 32:442–453, 1971.
Block, M. A. Alcohol: man and science. N. Y. State J. Med. 2732–2740, November 1, 1970.
Campbell, P. Alcoholism held the worst addiction. The New York Times, June 29, 1971, p. 41.
Cantanzaro, R. J. The Total Treatment Approach. Springfield, Ill., Charles C Thomas, 1968.
Chafety, M. E., Blane, H. T., and Hill, M. J. Frontiers of Alcoholism. New York, Science House, 1970.
Committee on Alcoholism and Drug Dependence. Alcohol and society. J.A.M.A. 216:1011–1013, 1971.
Edwards, G. Public health implications of liquor control. Lancet, 424–425, August 21, 1971.
Falk, G. The contribution of the alcohol culture to alcoholism in America. Bost. J. Addict. 65:9–17, 1970.
Goldfarb, C. Patients nobody wants—skid row alcoholism. Dis. Nerv. Syst. 31:274–281, 1970.
Goodman, L. S. and Gilman, A. The Pharmacological Basis of Therapeutics, 4th ed. Toronto, Canada, Macmillan Co., 1970.

Guerin, J. New York City Alcoholism Study: A Program Analysis. New York City, Office of Program Analysis, Health Services Administration, January 9, 1971.

Hayman, M. Alcoholism—Mechanism and Management. Springfield, Ill., Charles C Thomas, 1966.

Iber, F. L. In alcoholism, the liver sets the pace. Nutrition Today, 2–9, Jan./Feb., 1971.

James, J. E. and Goldman, M. Behavior trends of wives of alcoholics. Quart. J. Stud. Alcohol 32:364–372, 1971.

Kammeier, M. L. Adolescents from families with and without alcohol problems. Quart. J. Stud. Alcohol 32:364–372, 1971.

Masserman, J. H. Alcoholism: disease or dis-ease? Hospital Tribune, April 19, 1971.

Medical World News. Alcoholism: America's most destructive drug problem. February 26, 1971, pp. 43–52.

Mendelson, J. H. Biologic concomitants of alcoholism. New Eng. J. Med. 283: 24–32, Part I, 1970; 283:71–81, Part II, 1970.

Mendelson, J. H. Effects of alcohol on the central nervous system. New Eng. J. Med. 284:104–105, 1971.

Roman, P. M. and Trice, H. M. The development of deviant drinking behavior. Arch. Envir. Health 20:424–435, 1970.

Rubin, E. and Lieber, C. S. Alcohol-induced hepatic injury in nonalcoholic volunteers. New Eng. J. Med. 278:869–876, 1968.

Rubin, E. and Lieber, C. S. Alcoholism, alcohol, and drugs. Science, 172: 1097–1102, 1971.

Trice, H. M. and Roman, P. M. Delabeling, relabeling, and Alcoholics Anonymous. Social Problems 17:538–540, 1970.

Ubell, E. Alcoholism: challenge to the theory that it's a disease. The New York Times, April 11, 1971, p. 7.

Vesell, E. S. Genetic factors in alcoholism. Medical Counterpoint, August 1971, pp. 37–43.

Williams, A. F., McCourt, W. F., and Schneider, L. Personality self-descriptions of alcoholics and heavy drinkers. Quart. J. Stud. Alcohol 32:310–317, 1971.

Williams, A. F., McCourt, W. F., and Schneider, L. Alcohol and Health. National Institute on Alcohol Abuse and Alcoholism. U.S. Department of Health, Education, and Welfare, December, 1971.

VENEREAL DISEASE

American Social Health Association. Today's V.D. Control Problem—1971. New York, American Social Health Association, 1971.

Brown, A. A. and Podair, S. Venereal Diseases: The Silent Menance. Public Affairs Pamphlet. New York City, Public Affairs Committee, 1970.

Brown, W. J., et al. Syphilis and Other Venereal Diseases. Cambridge, Harvard University Press, 1970.

Brown, W. J. Venereal Diseases in Preventive Medicine, Clark, D. W. and MacMahon, B., eds. Boston, Little, Brown, and Co., 1967.

Deschin, C. The Teenager and V.D. New York City, Richards Rosen Press, 1969.

Rosahn, P. D. Autopsy Studies in Syphilis. U.S.P.H.S. Pub. No. 433, Washington, D. C., U. S. Government Printing Office, 1960.
U.S. Department of Health, Education, and Welfare. Management of Chancroid, Granuloma Inguinale, Lymphogranuloma Venereum in General Practice. U.S.P.H.S. Pub. No. 255, revised 1964. Washington, D. C., U. S. Government Printing Office, 1965.

CIGARETTE SMOKING

Denson, P. A survey of respiratory disease among New York City postal and transit workers. Environmental Research, 1967.
Kahn, H. A. The Dorn study of Smoking and Mortality among U. S. Veterans: Report on Eight and One-half Years of Observation. National Cancer Institute Monograph Number 19. Washington, D. C., U. S. Government Printing Office, 1966.

ACCIDENTS

Accident Facts. Chicago, National Safety Council, 1968, 1969, 1970, 1971.
Haddon, W. The prevention of accidents. In Clark, D. and MacMahon, B., eds. Preventive Medicine. Boston, Little, Brown Co., 1967.
Hilleboe, H. and Larrimore, G. Preventive Medicine. Philadelphia, W. B. Saunders Co., 1965.
U. S. Department of Labor. State Workmen's Compensation Laws: A Comparison of Major Provisions with Recommended Standards, Bulletin No. 212. Washington, D. C., U. S. Government Printing Office, 1964.

HOUSING

Abrams, C. Man's Quest for Shelter. Boston, Mass. Inst. Tech. Press, 1965.
American Public Health Association Housing Ordinance and Maintenance Code.
De Jesus, C. Child of the Dark. New York, Signet Books, 1962.
Gremliza, F. G. A method for measuring quality of village conditions in less developed rural areas. Amer. J. Public Health 55:107–115, 1965.
Hearings before the Select Committee on Nutrition and Human Needs, 1970 of the U. S. Senate, 91st Congress. Washington, D. C., U. S. Government Printing Office, 1970.
Pan American Health Organization. Migration and urbanization: Basic housing services in shanty-town. In Pan American Health Organization Scientific Publication No. 123. Environmental Determinants of Community Well-Being.
Welner, D., et al. Housing, Environment, and Family Life. Baltimore, 1965.

CHAPTER
9
The Physical Environment

The physical environment has recently become a subject of great public interest and concern. Topics such as waste disposal and sewage treatment, which were considered trivial a few years ago, are now a cause célèbre on the women's club circuit and among college students. The words *ecology* and *pollution* have become pure magic for liberals, conservatives, Republicans, Democrats, "straights," hippies, women's liberationists, and male chauvinists alike.

Twelve miles off the New York City shoreline lies a 20-square-mile area of ocean which is quite literally a "dead sea." For four decades, industrial wastes and untreated sewage have been dumped here; and the water is discolored, malodorous, and peppered with chunks of floating feces and toilet tissue. All marine life vanished years ago.

While New York City is 12 miles removed from this vast area of dead water, the people of the city of Venice live amidst their own excrement. Once hailed as the "Queen of the Adriatic," this Italian city is now one of the pollution centers of the world. Human refuse, dead fish, drowned rats, and oil slicks from motorized barges have turned the famed canals into what is probably the world's largest open sewer. The air is filled with sulfuric acid vapor generated by a reaction of rain or sea spray with

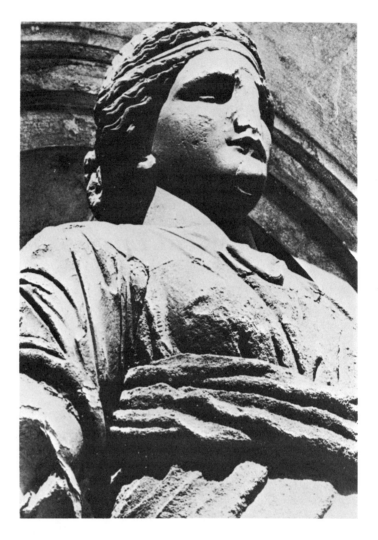

FIG. 9-1. *This statue is a victim of the sulfuric acid found in Venice's ambient air. The erosive process is colloquially known as "marble cancer." Although the Venetians suffer greatly, the prime victim of this pollution seems to be the city's fabled statuary. (Courtesy of United Press International.)*

sulfur compounds that are belched up by nearby industries. Although further research must be done to assess the definitive health effects of inhaling this acidic air, one obvious consequence is the rapid erosion of the marble statuary for which the city is noted (Fig. 9-1).

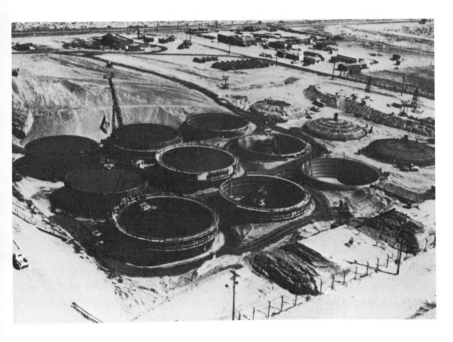

FIG. 9-2.   *Radioactive wastes stored in perpetuity at Richland, Washington. Unfortunately, some of these tanks are reported to leak. (Courtesy of Associated Press.)*

Near Richland, Washington, 140 concrete and steel tanks are buried just below the surface of the ground. These tanks contain 55 million gallons of radioactive wastes which are so toxic that a few gallons leaking into the local watershed could more or less permanently contaminate the water supply. Thousands of years must pass before this waste material is rendered harmless, and the problem is compounded by the fact that Richland is in an area subject to seismic activity (Fig. 9-2).

In Vietnam, 15 percent of the entire country has been defoliated by the years of war in that beleaguered nation. Enormous craters, 30 feet deep and equally wide, dot the barren landscape as a result of bomber attacks. It is said that some areas of South Vietnam resemble the surface of the moon more than they do a tropical country.

In light of these ecological horror stories, it is all too easy to overlook aspects of the physical environment which constituted a threat to human health long before man fouled his nest with chemicals, plastics, and non-returnable bottles. With rare exception, the prime threats to man from his physical environment are the infectious disease agents whose contacts with the human host depend on an intermediary vehicle or vector. Even in the United States, foodborne illnesses are among the most commonly reported infectious diseases, and sporadic outbreaks of mosquito-borne encephalitis recur at more or less regular intervals. In the emerging nations of the "Third World," the great threat to health is likely to be malaria or schistosomiasis rather than smog, DDT, or noise pollution.

Zoonotic and Vector-Borne Diseases

It was noted in Chapter 4 that a vector is an arthropod which transmits disease by carrying the agent from an infected host to a new, noninfected one. The infected host may be human or animal. In either case, the disease agent enters the new host as a result of a bite, through inoculation, or through the ingestion of infective materials placed on the skin.

As Table 9-1 shows, many vector-borne diseases are zoonotic. However, many zoonotic diseases do not depend on an insect vector and can reach man through direct contact, by ingestion, or from airborne or vehicular spread. Whatever their route, these diseases come to man from his surrounding environment and are therefore subject to control through primary prevention. The necessary environmental manipulations tend to be quite simple with respect to some zoonoses. Thus, trichinosis is easily avoided if one sees to it that he eats only well-cooked pork (i.e., the meat should be gray or white in color, not pink or red). This disease develops about nine days after ingestion of infected meat, with edema of the upper eyelid a common early sign. Although trichinosis is usually a mild illness, serious respiratory, neurologic, and myocardial complications are not uncommon. The essential lesion in this disease is the presence of encysted larvae in host muscle tissue. These larvae are freed when the cysts containing them are dissolved in the digestive tract of the human host. In the gut, the freed larvae mature, mate, and produce new larvae which ultimately invade human muscle and become encysted (Fig. 9-3). Since men are very rarely cannibalized, the process ends here. After experiencing an acute illness around the time of larvae penetration of his musculature, the host has no further symptoms. The prevalence of trichinosis is declining in the United States largely because of laws requiring that garbage be cooked before it is fed to hogs. One hundred fifty degrees Fahrenheit will kill trichina. The transmission cycle thus can be broken either by thoroughly cooking the garbage eaten by the pig or thoroughly cooking the pig eaten by the man. Trichinosis is widespread among rats, who often feed on raw pork in and around slaughterhouses. Once started,

TABLE 9-1. Important Zoonotic Diseases

Infection	Agent	Primary Host	Primary Mode of Transmission
Bacterial			
Anthrax	Bacillus anthracis	Hooved animals: sheep, goats, pigs, etc.	Direct contact
Brucellosis	Four variants of Brucella: B. abortus, B. suis, B. melitensis	Hooved animals	Contact, ingestion inoculation, airborne
Leptospirosis	Leptospira icterohemorrhagiae	Some hooved animals; also rodents, dogs, cats, poultry	Direct contact, vehicular (water)
Plague	Pasturella pestes	Wild rodents	Flea
Salmonellosis	Salmonella typhimurium	Rodents, fowl, swine, reptiles	Ingestion
Tetanus	Clostridium tetani	Horses	Inoculation
Tuberculosis (bovine)	M. tuberculosis	Cattle	Ingestion, airborne
Tularemia	Pasturella tularensis	Wild rodents	Contact, ingestion, various insect bites
Viral	*		
Psittacosis		Birds	Airborne
Western and eastern equine encephalitis		Birds	Mosquito
St. Louis encephalitis		Birds	Mosquito
Japanese B encephalitis		Birds	Mosquito
Rabies		Dogs, bats, skunks	Animal bites
Other			
Trichinosis	Trichinella spiralis	Hogs, rats	Ingestion
Typhus (murine)	Rickettsia mooseri	Mouse	Flea
Rocky Mountain spotted fever	Rickettsia rickettsii	Rodents ?	Tick
Rickettsialpox	Rickettsia akari	Mouse	Mite

*Viruses take the name of their disease, e.g., psittacosis is caused by psittacosis virus, etc.

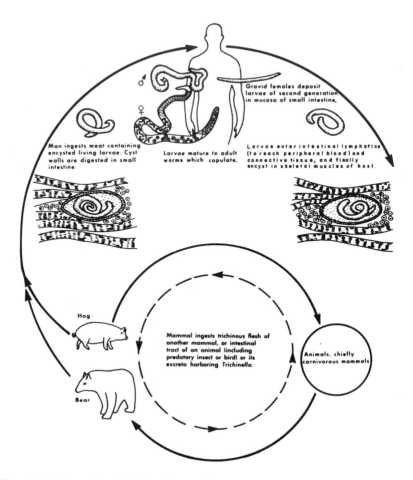

Gravid females deposit larvae of second generation in mucosa of small intestine.

Man ingests meat containing encysted living larvae. Cyst walls are digested in small intestine.

Larvae mature to adult worms which copulate.

Larvae enter intestinal lymphatics (to reach peripheral blood) and connective tissue, and finally encyst in skeletal muscles of host.

Hog

Bear

Mammal ingests trichinous flesh of another mammal, or intestinal tract of an animal (including predatory insect or bird) or its excreta harboring Trichinella.

Animals, chiefly carnivorous mammals

FIG. 9-3. *Life cycle of* Trichinella spiralis. (*From Gould,* Trichinosis in Man and Animals, *First edition, 1970. Courtesy of Charles C Thomas, Publisher and John B. Villela.*)

trichinosis is assured survival in the rat population by virtue of a tendency for these creatures to eat one another. The causative agent, *Trichinella spiralis*, is a **nematode** worm, and there is no present drug effective against it.

Tetanus is a bacterial disease commonly associated in the public mind

---

NEMATODA: a group of threadlike, roundworms, some of which are human parasites

with rusty nails, lockjaw, and childhood. The bacteria, which are **anaerobic,** live in the intestinal tract of horses and men and reach the soil in fecal matter. Once in soil, tetanus **spores** endure for long periods. Man becomes infected when spores gain entry through a puncture wound or an animal bite. Newborns develop tetanus when the unhealed umbilical stump becomes contaminated with dust and dirt. Tetanus neonatorum is an important cause of neonatal deaths in developing countries. *Clostridium tetani* produces a toxin, and it is this toxin (not the bacterial invasion *per se*) which accounts for the symptoms of the disease. Tetanus is uncommon in the United States, but it is 70 percent fatal when it occurs. Symptoms begin after an incubation period which varies from a few days to a few weeks and include pain and muscular contractions. These are especially severe in the neck muscles and those involving chewing. Death commonly results from respiratory failure. Since tetanus depends on soil contamination and, in part, on a horse population, it is not surprising that most cases are from rural areas. Urbanization has done much to control this disease and others (such as anthrax, brucellosis, and leptospirosis) which tend to thrive when men are in close proximity to animals. Although antibiotics are of little specific value in tetanus, the disease can be prevented through active immunization with tetanus toxoid. This immunization is standard for small children and should be repeated every decade or at the time of an injury.

Rabies is a viral disease spread to man by the bites of a variety of animals, especially dogs, bats, and skunks. Once it has developed, this disease inevitably produces a fatal inflammation of the brain, and death occurs within a week of onset. In cases of animal bite, every attempt should be made to identify and impound the offending animal. Because of rabies' relatively long incubation period, the victim can usually wait safely while the animal is under observation for 10 days. Should the animal die, its head is examined for characteristic signs of rabies; and if the victim's skin was broken by the bite, or if his mucous membranes were exposed to the animal's saliva, he is started on a series of vaccinations against rabies. These may be discontinued if it is established that the animal died of causes other than this disease. Some experts recommend immediate sacrifice of the animal without a period of observation. An offending wild animal usually avoids capture, and in these cases the animal is presumed rabid and the patient is vaccinated. Human vaccination against rabies is

---

ANAEROBIC: refers to a microorganism which grows in the absence of oxygen.
SPORE: an inactive bacterial form which is resistant to conditions that would be fatal to the normal bacterium

an unpleasant procedure consisting of a series of antirabies inoculations over a period of two or three weeks. This procedure carries with it a small risk that the patient will develop a postvaccinal encephalitis. For this reason, it is important that only those who are in real danger of contracting the disease be vaccinated. While little can be done to eliminate rabies in wild animals, domestic sources (dogs) can be vaccinated against the disease easily, safely, and inexpensively. Rabies immunization is secondary prevention for the dog but primary prevention for man.

The remaining zoonotic diseases are briefly described in Table 9-2.

Table 9-3 identifies the principal vector-borne diseases. Most of these tend to occur in warm climes and are neither bacterial nor viral (plague is the only bacterial disease among them). They include the great tropical diseases and a host of lesser maladies caused by bizarre organisms with highly complex life cycles. Although the housefly is believed capable of transmitting typhoid, dysentery, and other enteric bacterial infections, these illnesses are usually transmitted by the vehicular route.

TABLE 9-2. A Summary of Zoonotic Diseases Which Do Not Involve Vector Transmission

Disease	Summary
Anthrax	A bacterial disease of hooved animals. In man, primarily affects the skin but can affect GI tract, bloodstream, lungs, etc. Fatality about 20 percent. Man contracts the disease by handling hair, hides, or wool from infected animals. Responds to penicillin.
Brucellosis	Man contracts this bacterial disease by drinking infected milk or by coming into contact with infected hogs, goats, sheep, or cattle or with the products of these animals. Characterized by weakness and recurrent fever. Control is through identification and slaughter of infected animals.
Leptospirosis	Caused by a spirochete upon direct contact with an infected animal or water contaminated by the animal. Produces fever, chills, GI symptoms, and frequently jaundice and skin hemorrhage.
Salmonellosis	See text. Usually vehicular spread from man to man.
Tetanus	See text.
Tularemia	Transmitted by contact with infected wild rodents or rabbits or with their hides and carcasses. Also transmitted by ingestion of such animals. Can be transmitted by tick or fly vectors. Bacterial disease characterized by chills, fever, prostration. Rarely fatal if treated.
Bovine tuberculosis	A disease of cattle. Contracted by eating infected animal material or by airborne dissemination from cow to man. Rare in U. S. See Chapter 4.
Psittacosis	A viral disease of birds. Capable of producing fever and pneumonia. Also known as parrot fever. Spreads via airborne route.

TABLE 9–3. Principal Vector-Borne Diseases

Infection	Agent	Vector
Bacterial		
Plague	*P. pestes*	Flea
Enteric infections	Various	Housefly
Viral		
Dengue	*	Mosquito
Encephalitis		Mosquito, ticks
Hemorrhagic fever		Mosquito
Yellow fever		Mosquito
Other		
Filariasis	*Wuchereria bancrofti*	Mosquito
Leishmaniosis	*Leishmania donovani*	Sandflies
Malaria	*Plasmodium vivax, P. falciparum, P. malariae, P. ovale*	Mosquito
Onchocerciasis	*Onchocerca volvulus*	Black fly
Relapsing fever	*Borrelia recurrentis*	Lice, ticks
Schistosomiasis	*Schistosoma mansoni, S. japonica, S. hematobium*	Snail**
Typhus	*Rickettsia prowazeki*	Louse
Trypanosomiasis	*Trypanosoma gambiense, T. rhodesiense, T. cruzi*	Tsetse fly, Reduviid bugs

Viruses take the name of their disease—e.g., dengue is caused by dengue virus, yellow fever by yellow fever virus, and so on.

**Strictly speaking, not a vector.*

Yellow fever exemplifies viral diseases transmitted by vectors, in this case the mosquito *Aedes aegypti*. Yellow fever has not one but two cycles of transmission. The first is that associated with classic yellow fever. Here the reservoir is man, and disease spreads from man to man through the mosquito vector. The second is known as jungle yellow fever. This disease is indistinguishable from the classic form, except that it exists not in man but in monkeys living in the treetops of South American and African jungles. In monkeys, the vector mosquito is not *Aedes aegypti* but other Aedes mosquitoes. Man is an accidental victim of jungle yellow fever, a disease he contracts by entering the jungle environment and being bitten by one of the Aedes species which usually feeds on the monkey population. If the man in question becomes infected, he takes his newly acquired disease with him when he returns to his home. Once home, he is subject to attack by *Aedes aegypti*, which can then pass the illness on to yet another victim. The presence of a jungle fever cycle makes yellow fever zooanotic, although it is possible for the classic and jungle forms to exist quite independently of each other.

Yellow fever is an acute illness which varies in severity. In general, indigenous people from endemic areas have less severe illness than those from other locales. In the latter group, a fatality rate of 40 percent is not uncommon. Symptoms include fever, hemorrhage, **bradycardia, leucopenia,** and jaundice. The incubation period is three to six days, and the patient is capable of infecting biting mosquitoes for about three days after the onset of symptoms.

Although jungle yellow fever persists, classic yellow fever, still endemic in much of Africa, has been practically eradicated from the western hemisphere. It also does not exist in Asia, where the closely related milder disease, dengue, is endemic. In fact, many experts feel that dengue and yellow fever never coexist in the same locale.

Patients who recover from yellow fever are permanently immune to subsequent attacks. Transient passive immunity of about six months' duration is conferred on newborn infants by immune mothers. Active immunization is available, effective, and recommended for those travelling to endemic areas.

Malaria is a disease characterized by chronic intermittent fever, anemia, splenomegaly, and a wide range of potentially fatal complications. It is caused by any of four species of **protozoa** of the genus *Plasmodium.* Two of these species, *P. vivax* and *P. falciparum,* are of principal importance. Since 1955, the World Health Organization has been officially committed to worldwide eradication of malaria. This WHO project has been a modest success at best. Some nations have succeeded in eradicating the disease, but these have tended to be smaller, island countries (e.g., Taiwan). In larger areas, progress has been either slow or nonexistent. Nevertheless, the recognition of malaria as a problem of sufficient magnitude to justify a worldwide eradication effort speaks volumes about the long and close interaction of man with this stubborn and highly adaptable adversary. After almost two decades of efforts, malaria remains one of the leading causes of death and disability in the world. It is probably the world's most important disease.

BRADYCARDIA: an abnormally slow heart rate (normal is about 72 beats per minute)
LEUCOPENIA: an abnormally low number of circulating white cells in the bloodstream
PROTOZOA: a group of unicellular organisms; the lowest division of the animal kingdom

Unlike yellow fever, which runs a brief course resulting in recovery or death, malaria is a chronic condition with common relapses over a number of years. Also unlike yellow fever is malaria's susceptibility to drug therapy. Treated cases rarely end fatally, and even in untreated cases, fatality rates above 10 percent are unusual. As a leading cause of death, malaria owes its success to the large number of people affected. After all, if one million are infected, and 5 percent die each year, 50,000 victims succumb annually. It is estimated that there are over 100 million cases of malaria in the world. Malaria is not endemic in the United States.

Man is the only important reservoir of malaria, and the disease is transmitted from man to man by the bite of an Anopheles mosquito, many species of which are known to act as vectors (Fig. 9-4). The protozoan parasite has a complicated life cycle which is divided into a sexual phase (occurring in the mosquito) and an asexual phase (which takes place in man). Gametocytes, or immature male and female forms of the Plasmodium, circulate in the human bloodstream and are thus ingested by a biting mosquito. Fertilization of the female gametocyte occurs in the mosquito. The gametocyte develops into an asexual form called a sporozoite, and this is inoculated into a new host when he encounters a hungry mosquito. After a very complex process involving parasitic invasion of human red blood cells, new gametocytes are developed which ultimately find their way into another mosquito. Malaria transmission can occur without the mosquito vector when blood from a malarious patient is transfused into a nonmalarious person. At one time, malaria was a common hazard of drug addicts, who often share a common needle. It is because of malaria that heroin is usually "cut" with quinine, an antimalaria drug.

The incubation period of malaria varies somewhat with the species of Plasmodium involved, but it averages about two weeks. Patients can infect mosquitoes for as long as gametocytes remain in the bloodstream—often several years. Once infected, the mosquito remains so for life.

Malaria responds to a number of drugs, of which quinine and chloroquin are perhaps the best known. Drug therapy is appropriate for curing the individual case. However, because it has a vector, malaria can be attacked through efforts to destroy the mosquitoes necessary for transmission of the disease. Vector control is applicable in a number of diseases (e.g., filariasis) in addition to malaria (Fig. 9-5). Mosquito eradication programs are entirely responsible for the progress that has been made against yellow fever. In the absence of a vaccine against a disease—or if mass vaccination is impossible—vector control is the only practical approach to controlling the disease.

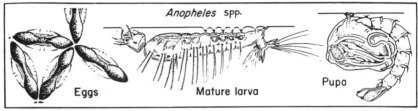

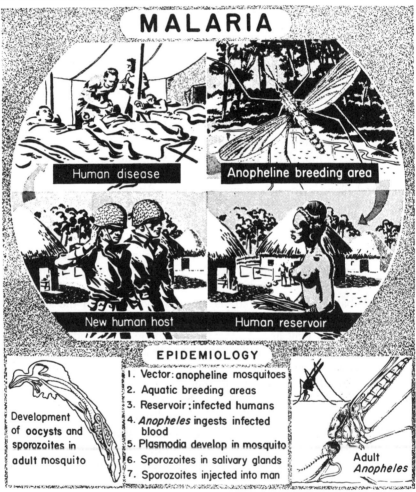

FIG. 9-4.   *(From Hunter, Frye and Swartzwelder,* A Manual of Tropical Medicine, *Fourth edition, 1966. Courtesy of W. B. Saunders Company and Martin D. Young.)*

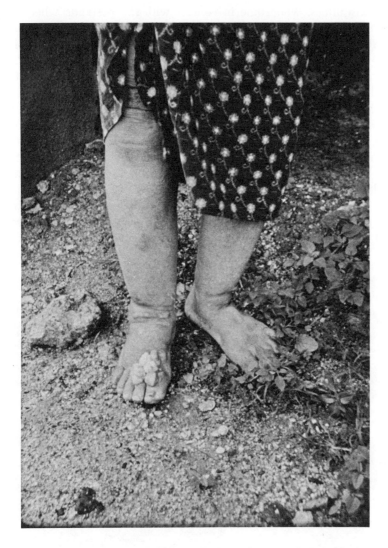

FIG. 9-5. *Elephantiasis is a condition which produces marked swelling of the legs, arms, breast, or scrotum. It is not an illness per se but rather a sign of the disease known as filariasis. Like malaria and yellow fever it is transmitted from man to man by a mosquito. Filariasis is not a great killer but limits the victim's ability to lead a happy and productive life. The agent of disease is a type of worm. The swelling results when adult worms lodge in the lymphatic system. (Courtesy of Dr. C. L. Marshall.)*

When a residual insecticide (usually DDT or one of its analogues) is sprayed on the walls of homes about every three months, it is effective against mosquitoes, who come in contact with the pesticide when they rest on the walls. Residual insecticides have long been the backbone of the WHO antimalarial campaigns; and this technique has been applied to entire countries, involving millions of individual homes in thousands of villages and towns. The tendency of mosquitoes to become resistant to DDT, the harmful effects of this chemical on some animals, and its potential but largely unknown threat to human health have brought the antimalarial people into open confrontation with those primarily concerned with the ecology. As we have seen repeatedly in this book, "there is no such thing as a free lunch"; and in the fight against malaria and other diseases the value of such insecticides as DDT must be weighed against the health hazards these chemicals represent. It is very difficult to decide whether the elimination or reduction of malaria justifies an unknown number of cases of an unknown disease in an unknown number of years.

Other methods of dealing with the mosquito population are less effec-

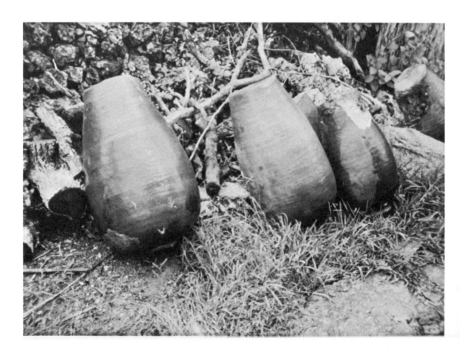

FIG. 9-6.   *Mosquito breeding depends on the presence of still water which mosquito larvae require for their development. In parts of the world without community water supplies, people store water in jars for home use. To prevent these jars from becoming breeding sites, they are left turned over. More work for the homeowner in terms of trips to the river or well, but the outcome is less malaria and filariasis. (Courtesy of Dr. C. L. Marshall.)*

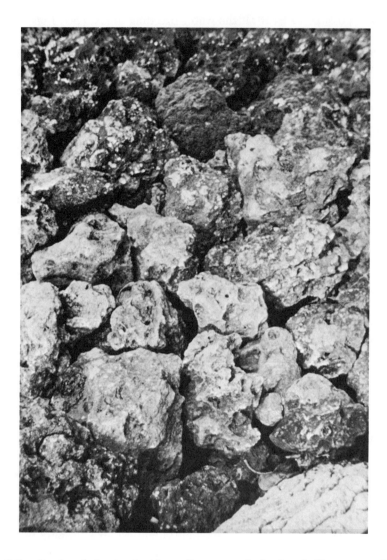

FIG. 9-7.   *Coral rock is pitted with small craters which often hold rainwater long
enough to allow the development of mosquito larvae. It is uncontrollable
breeding sites like this that make mosquito control so difficult. (Courtesy
of Dr. C. L. Marshall.)*

tive and efficient than residual insecticides. Larval forms of the mosquito
mature in stagnant water, and the treatment of water with chemicals to
kill larvae was the mainstay of malaria control before the advent of DDT
and other modern insecticides. Larviciding is inherently inefficient because

it is not possible to treat all the water breeding areas. (See Figs. 9-6 and 9-7.)

Pyrethrum sprays are useful for small quarters. These common aerosol products are used throughout the United States to kill fleas, mosquitoes, bees, and other pests. Too expensive for mass use in developing countries, these sprays also have no residual effect and must be used repeatedly— even on the same day. However, they are very useful for disinfecting aircraft departing from an endemic area and bound for a malaria-free one. Screens on windows and doors and the use of insect repellants are of value only in industrial countries, where people can afford them.

Schistosomiasis, like malaria, is a chronic infection which affects hundreds of millions of people throughout the world. The causative organism is a kind of trematode worm known as *Schistosoma*. *S. mansoni* is common in Africa, South America, and the Caribbean. *S. haematobium* is dominant in the Middle East, and *S. japonicum* is prevalent in the Orient. Adult worms lodge in the host's veins and deposit eggs in the surrounding tissues, which causes chronic inflammation and scarring. Thus, virtually any organ can be affected, although the liver and urinary bladder are particularly susceptible. Man is the most important reservoir of infection, although domestic and wild animals can act as reservoirs, especially in the case of *S. japonicum*.

Schistosome eggs are excreted by the host through urine and feces (Fig. 9-8). Frequently, this excretion occurs directly into a river, stream, lake, or fresh water source. The eggs hatch in the water and enter certain species of snail. They mature in the snail and then emerge from it in a form known as cercariae. These fork-tailed, free-swimming creatures penetrate human skin when the new host swims or bathes himself in the contaminated water source. At this point the cycle begins anew. Like malaria, schistosomiasis is theoretically vulnerable through an attack on either the disease agent itself or its snail intermediary. Unfortunately, neither is easy. Existing drug therapy for schistosomiasis is time-consuming and requires careful observation of the patient. It is therefore impractical on a mass basis. How to kill snails without killing fish or poisoning the water is a problem which has yet to be solved in a manner cheap enough to find wide application. Unfortunately, the prevalence of schistosomiasis is increasing. This disease follows the development of irrigation systems, and such projects are most important to developing countries which are trying to increase their food supplies. Again the question of a trade-off comes in. Schistosomiasis is part of the price for the development of new agricultural land through irrigation. It is a disabling disease which cannot be prevented and is difficult to treat. In some cases, agricultural output has remained static because farmers ill with schistosomiasis produce less,

TABLE 9-4. A Summary of Selected Vector-Borne Diseases

Disease	Summary
Dengue	Brief, mild, febrile disease. Transmitted by *Aedes aegypti* mosquito. Closely related to yellow fever and hemorrhagic fevers.
Encephalitis	Eastern equine, western equine, St. Louis, and Japanese B are variants of a basic mosquito-borne syndrome characterized by inflammation of the brain, spinal cord, and meninges. Japanese B and eastern equine can be highly fatal variants.
Filariasis	A tropical disease characterized by a swelling (known as elephantiasis) of the legs, arms, scrotum, and female breast. Transmitted by mosquitoes and caused by a nematode worm (see Fig. 9-5).
Hemorrhagic fevers	A group of serious hemorrhagic diseases, occurring principally in childhood and caused by a group of viruses very similar or identical to dengue viruses. Seen only in Southeast Asia, India, and the Philippines.
Leishmaniasis	A local or systemic illness due to protozoan organisms. Transmitted from human and animal reservoirs by the sandfly Phlebotomus.
Onchocerciasis	A disease transmitted by the black fly Simulium. Related to filariasis. Frequently results in blindness due to invasion of the eye by immature worms.
Plague	A zooanotic disease of rats and wild rodents. Highly fatal. Accidentally transmitted to man by fleas. Vaccine available. Responds to antibiotics.
Relapsing fever	A spirochetal infection due to *Borrelia recurrentis.* Louse- or tick-borne. In U. S., reservoir exists in wild rodents.
Trypanosomiasis	Also known as "sleeping sickness." A disabling disease occurring in an American and African form. Transmitted by cone-nosed bugs and tsetse flies, respectively. Limited to Africa and South America.

even with additional land available to them and under cultivation.

It has been said that war is too important to be left to the generals. To this, Hans Zinsser would add the argument that, until quite recently, the outcome of wars was dependent more on the occurrence of epidemic disease than on military acumen. It is as an epidemic disease and a decimator of armies that typhus is reknowned. It exists in a number of forms (see Table 9-1) but the classic form is epidemic typhus, which is transmitted from man to man by the body louse *Pediculus humanus.* Fatality rates often exceed one-third of those affected, and those who recover are subject years later to a mild recrudescence known as Brill's disease. The acute illness is characterized by fever, skin rash, and inflammatory changes in smaller blood vessels; these changes can produce

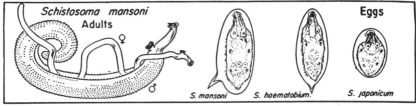

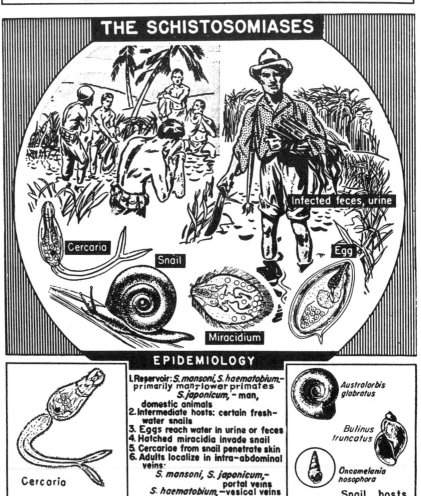

FIG. 9-8. *(From Hunter, Frye and Swartzwelder,* A Manual of Tropical Medicine, *Fourth edition, 1966. Courtesy of W. B. Saunders Company.)*

thrombosis, neurological signs, renal failure, and a host of other complications. Typhus is a disease of cold climates where groups of people live in unsanitary, louse-infested quarters. There has been no typhus in the United States for more than 50 years.

A **rickettsial** disease, typhus is caused by *Rickettsia prowazeki* and has an incubation period of one to two weeks. It is preventable through vaccination, and outbreaks can be controlled by dusting exposed persons with DDT powder. It might be noted here that this is one case in which exposure to DDT is almost surely preferable to contracting the disease. Individual cases can be treated with one of the tetracyclines or with chloramphenicol. A brief summary of other vector-borne diseases can be found in Table 9-4.

Diseases Transmitted by Inanimate Material

A vehicle is any inanimate material by means of which a disease agent is brought into contact with man. Milk, food, and water are the classic vehicles with regard to infectious disease. To this trio we will add air, the medium through which man comes into contact with the chemical agents suspended in a polluted atmosphere.

Although it has recently come under close scrutiny because of its high fat content, milk remains one of the most popular and important foods. It is a principal source of dietary calcium and a good source of protein and the vitamin riboflavin. In this country, vitamin D is added to commercially sold milk, making it a good source of this important compound. Unfortunately, milk is also especially liable to play a role in disease transmission because it serves as a good medium for bacterial growth, it comes from an animal which may be diseased and contaminate its own milk, and its processing often involves rather extensive handling by men.

As is so often the case, man himself is the most common source of contamination. Usually, this occurs as a result of direct contact between milk handler and milk, but sometimes it involves streptococcal mastitis in the cow, i.e., the streptococcal infection is traceable to man, who infects the cow's udder during the milking process. An unclean automatic milker also can act as a source of contamination, as can human and rodent feces which find their way into milk. A relationship between milk and disease

---

RICKETTSIAE: a group of very small, rodshaped microorganisms which parasitize man; they are neither bacterial nor viral

was first postulated in the mid nineteenth century in connection with outbreaks of both typhoid and scarlet fevers.

Typhoid fever is in a class with tuberculosis, malaria, and typhus as an adversary of man. A systemic bacterial infection, typhoid fever is caused by *Salmonella typhosa* and is characterized by continuous fever, spleno-megaly, a rather unique skin rash, and a tendency to produce serious complications. The bacteria, contained in the urine and feces of infected persons, gets into water, food, or milk either directly or indirectly. Some people continue to shed bacilli years after recovery from the disease. When these carriers are known, they and their families are legally pro-hibited from working as food handlers. Primary prevention is the basic typhoid control. Pasteurization of milk, purification of drinking water, treatment of sewage, and sanitary food handling in restaurants are all measures to prevent contact between man and the disease agent. Fly control is an important adjunct to these primary measures. A vaccine is available for those likely to be exposed to typhoid, and immunization is

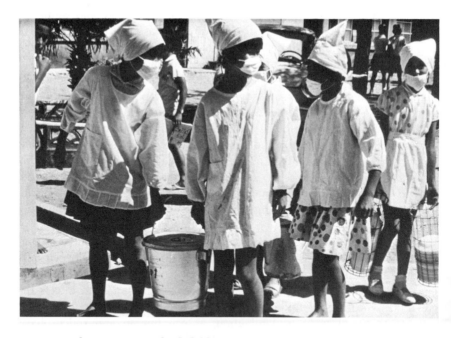

FIG. 9-9.   *These Japanese school children are specially dressed for the important job of delivering the school's lunch from kitchen to dining hall. Food that sits for a time waiting to be eaten can incubate bacteria if it has become con-taminated. Although the necessity of the costumes is debatable, the ritual of wearing it emphasizes the need to be extremely careful to avoid contami-nation of food. (Courtesy of Dr. C. L. Marshall.)*

especially recommended for travelers bound for developing countries.

In addition to typhoid and streptococcal infections, milk and milk products also transmit brucellosis, staphylococcal food poisoning, bovine tuberculosis, infections due to other Salmonella organisms, and an uncommon rickettsial disease known as Q fever. With the exception of staphylococcal food poisoning, which is caused by a toxin produced by the staphylococcus, each of these illnesses can be prevented by milk pasteurization.

Pasteurization is a procedure wherein milk is heated to a temperature high enough to destroy microorganisms. The heating process is done quickly to preserve the appearance and taste of the milk. One method raises the temperature of the milk to 140°F for 30 minutes; the so-called "flash method" employs a temperature of 161°F for 15 seconds. Prior to pasteurization, milk is tested for the presence of antibiotics, pesticides, and extraordinarily high bacterial content. (The last suggests mastitis in the supplying herd of cows.) After pasteurization, the milk is retested for bacterial content before it is distributed to retail outlets.

When they occur, outbreaks of milkborne disease are explosive in onset and infect large numbers of people simultaneously. Cream, butter, cheese, and ice cream are all derived from milk and are capable of transmitting disease. Milk products which are relatively acidic, such as buttermilk, sour cream, and cottage cheese rarely transmit disease.

FOODBORNE ILLNESS

Infections traceable to contaminated food are characterized by a brief incubation period and acute symptomatology referable to the gastrointestinal tract. The incidence of foodborne disease is increasing in the United States, partly due to increasing use of prepackaged foods such as TV dinners. The generalized community outbreak has declined in importance, and small outbreaks, often within families and traceable to a common food source, are now predominant. Like milk, most foods of animal origin readily support bacterial growth and are easily contaminated by human handling. Commercially processed foods of all kinds are subject to contamination unless scrupulous attention is paid to sanitary practices (see Fig. 9-9). Foodborne disease tends to be an especially common hazard at banquets and church suppers, where large numbers of people are served the same menu, food is prepared hours beforehand, and facilities for heating or refrigeration are makeshift or altogether lacking. Since banquets often feed hundreds of people at one time, thousands of cases can be generated by a relatively small number of outbreaks. Although outbreaks occur most frequently among families eating at home and, secondly, among persons eating in restaurants, the *number* of people affected is only 15 percent of that accounted for by banquets.

The key to the prevention of food poisoning is proper control of the temperature at which food is kept. When this is supplemented by careful personal hygiene and cleanliness of equipment, the risk of foodborne illness is virtually eliminated. Cold is bacteriostatic at temperatures below 45°F, and refrigerator temperatures should not exceed this level since some Salmonella species will grow at 50°F. Frozen foods are kept at 0°F, and these foods (especially poultry) should be thawed in the refrigerator at 45°F in preference to the common household practice of thawing these foods at room temperature. Heat is the best defense against foodborne illness. Food heated to a temperature of 162°F for two minutes will kill virtually all pathogenic microorganisms. One hundred fifty degrees for 10 minutes will achieve the same result, and temperatures of at least 150°F in cooking and no higher than 45°F in refrigeration are the two critical ones in food preparation. The main problem with TV dinners is that they are warmed in the oven before they are served, and the temperature of the food rarely reaches levels sufficient to kill bacteria which may be present. In order for them to be safe, these dinners must therefore be totally free of bacteria when frozen by the processor.

In general, all protein foods should be reheated to 150°F or more if they have been stored in a refrigerator for 24 hours or allowed to stand at room temperature for three hours or more. Foods which are pickled, corned, sugared, or salted tend to be quite safe. As a source of disease, food is far more important than either milk or water. Roughly 20,000 cases are reported each year, and estimates of unreported cases are usually placed at about one million. The causes are unknown in approximately 15 percent of reported cases, and virtually all of the others are accounted for by one of five disease agents. *Clostridium perfringens* is perhaps the most common cause of food poisoning, and produces a mild, brief illness characterized by abdominal pain and diarrhea. *C. perfringens* forms spores which resist ordinary cooking temperatures and are most commonly found in reheated cooked meat that has been contaminated with feces. The incubation period of this infection is 8 to 24 hours.

More serious, but extremely rare, is botulism, which affects the central nervous system and kills two-thirds of its victims. *Clostridium botulinum* is anaerobic in nature and is most likely to contaminate high-protein foods. Most cases arise from home-canned foods, although commercial canning companies are not immune. *Cl. botulinum* produces gas, and the bulging can is a widely recognized danger signal. This microorganism elaborates a toxin which is one of the most potent poisons known to man.

Contaminated foods containing organisms and toxin produce disease unless the food is boiled or heated to 162°F for ten minutes. Less than 1 percent of food-poisoning cases are due to botulism.

Salmonella typhimurium and other *Salmonellae* cause an extremely common form of food poisoning known as salmonellosis. The most common source of *Salmonella* are eggs, egg products, and poultry. After a brief incubation period of 8 to 24 hours, the patient is stricken with nausea, vomiting, and fever. Symptoms are usually mild but may persist for several weeks. Certain pets, such as turtles and chicks, are sources of salmonellosis which are found within individual homes.

Staphylococcal food poisoning is about as common as salmonellosis and is caused by a toxin elaborated by the staphylococcus. Unlike salmonellosis, "staph" food poisoning rarely causes fever and has a shorter incubation period of six hours or less. This disease, which usually runs a very brief course of six to eight hours, is characterized by nausea, vomiting, diarrhea, and abdominal pain. Staphylococci lodge in the nasal passages or skin lesions of food handlers and get into food from these sources. Pastries, custards, and meat products are the foods most often implicated. If left unrefrigerated, cooked food containing staphylococci will produce toxin in about five hours. Adequate cooking temperatures (above 160°F) will kill staphylococci. Adequate refrigeration of cooked food is also important.

Shigellosis is a term used to describe a group of closely related, mild syndromes caused by various species of the genus Shigella. Commonly, these entities are collectively referred to as bacillary dysentery. Shigellosis can be traced to virtually any food contaminated by infected food handlers. Flies have also been implicated as a source of contamination. Diarrhea, abdominal pain, and fever occur after an incubation period of about two days.

In the United States a large part of the problem of foodborne disease is related to the fact that laws are lax, and anyone can open a food-processing plant without adhering to a uniform set of standards. Moreover, there are 60,000 such plants, and the United States Food and Drug Administration (the agency responsible for policing facilities which process and handle food) has only 200 inspectors. Even with the relatively limited coverage that is possible under these circumstances, the agency continuously turns up food containing cockroach fragments, rodent feces, hair, and even bits of metal. Meat inspection, in contrast, is handled by the United States Department of Agriculture, which employs 8,000 inspectors who are permanently stationed in every slaughterhouse and meat processing plant in the country.

In recent years, there has been growing concern about the contamination of food by chemicals in fertilizers and pesticides and by elements such as cadmium or mercury. While few experts doubt that the presence of these inanimate contaminants is of potential harm, there is less agreement about the extent of the danger, the concentrations at which health is threatened, and what form the danger assumes. For these reasons, it has been difficult to establish standards of safety with confidence. It is known, for example, that chronic exposure to low levels of methyl mercury is a danger to health. Between 1955 and 1960, 43 persons in Japan died after eating shellfish and fish heavily contaminated with mercury. The ingestion of 0.5 grams of mercury all at once is almost always fatal; but the levels of mercury found in swordfish, tuna, and other marine life is infinitesimal by comparison. The Food and Drug Administration has established 0.5 parts of mercury per million parts of food as the upper permissible limit. This level was established not because it represents a recognized, tested, threshold value but because it is the lowest level most laboratories can detect. The Japanese have established that 10 parts per million of mercury can produce brain damage, and the FDA standard is one-twentieth that amount. At a concentration of 0.5 parts per million, one would have to consume about 4,500 pounds of food to reach the fatal dose of 0.5 grams. The presence of mercury and other chemicals in food is part of the larger problem of environmental pollution, which is discussed later in this chapter.

WATERBORNE DISEASE

Like foodborne illness, waterborne diseases classically are infections, but in recent years the health hazards of water pollution have become equal or greater in importance. Water use in the United States involves amounts difficult to imagine. Daily use approaches 300 billion gallons, or about 150 gallons per person per day. Only a third of this is used for drinking and household use; the remainder is consumed by industry to produce the goods which make such a large contribution to our high standard of living. Five hundred gallons of water are needed to produce a single yard of woolen cloth, 200 to turn out a dollar's worth of paper, and 65,000 to manufacture one automobile. Furthermore, all estimates place future use of water at still higher amounts. By the year 2000, it is expected that daily water consumption will approximate 1,000 billion gallons—an amount equal to the total available water supply. Obviously, there is a need to treat "used" water so that it can be reused over and over again.

While all water is ultimately derived from rain, man most commonly obtains water from surface sources (e.g., lakes and rivers) or from ground sources (e.g., wells or springs). Surface water is abundant and is low in mineral content, but it is also polluted with chemicals and contaminated with microorganisms. Ground water is less likely to be polluted or contaminated, but it is high in mineral content and tends to be difficult to tap in very large amounts. By the late 1960s, more than 75 percent of the American people were served by community water supplies, i.e., water which has been treated basically through chlorination and filtration. Filtration is primarily effective in rendering water colorless, odorless, and tasteless, but it also has some effect against chemicals and microorganisms. Chlorination destroys most bacterial pathogens in the water, although the addition of chlorine is not effective against viruses or the cysts of *Entamoeba histolytica*, a waterborne protozoan pathogen. Chlorination and filtration are among the most successful and important measures in man's continuing struggle against disease. The incidence rates for typhoid fever were reduced more than tenfold by these two procedures long before antibiotics came into the medical armamentarium.

Most of the infectious diseases transmitted by water are discussed elsewhere in this text. They include infectious hepatitis, tularemia, leptospirosis, schistosomiasis, amebiasis, and ascariasis, as well as the classic trio of cholera, bacillary dysentery, and typhoid fever. Amebiasis is caused by *Entamoeba histolytica* and varies from being asymptomatic to being severe causing multiple abscesses of the liver, lung, or brain. The organisms find their way into the water supply through fecal contamination and, in the form of cysts, are ultimately ingested by a new host. As we have already noted, these cysts are not destroyed by chlorination; however, they are removed from water by sand filtration. Ascariasis is a mild, usually chronic infection with the roundworm *Ascaris lumbricoides*. Although cholera has not appeared in the United States since 1911, it is still one of the world's more important diseases and is especially prevalent in India, Pakistan, and Southeast Asia. In its transmission and control, cholera closely resembles typhoid fever.

Water treatment and water pollution are intimately related. The more polluted the water, the more difficult it is to purify and the more urgent is the need to do so. Water becomes polluted from four major sources: drainage, recreational water uses, industrial wastes, and sewage. Land drainage introduces fertilizers and pesticides, while recreational use of reservoirs adds motor oil, herbicides, and trash to the water. Industrial wastes include a variety of chemicals (such as dyes, oils, mercury compounds, and so on), as well as radioactive and other materials which challenge the existing technology of treatment plants.

Sewage is a term used to describe the waste water generated by home and industry. The treatment plant and the pipes through which sewage flows to reach the plant are collectively known as sewerage. Sewage treatment consists of three parts: primary treatment, secondary treatment, and chlorination. Most American cities treat sewage, although 25 percent of municipally generated wastes are emptied untreated into nearby streams and thus create a purification problem for neighboring towns located downriver. In addition, about one-third of municipal sewage is subjected to primary treatment only. This leaves half of all sewage inadequately treated. The problem of sewage treatment is compounded by the fact that storm drainage and sewer pipes are combined in many older sewerage systems. When there are heavy rains, such systems cannot handle the runoff. This produces a situation where sewage could back up into the streets or, at the very least, contaminate the water course that normally handles runoff.

As it enters the treatment plant, sewage is 99.9 percent water, the remaining 0.1 percent consisting of solid wastes. The three-stage treatment process removes these solids, purifies the water, and thus enables its safe reuse. Primary treatment consists of a bar screen, a grit chamber, and a sedimentation tank in which solids are allowed to settle to the bottom. The bar screen and grit chamber serve to remove large objects, such as gravel, plastic items, rags, and sticks. The effectiveness of sewage treatment is measured in terms of reduced biological oxygen demand (BOD). BOD is the weight of oxygen required to oxidize the organic matter in the sewage. Primary sewage treatment reduces the BOD by 35 percent.

Secondary treatment consists of bringing the remaining sewage, or effluent, into contact with certain bacteria which digest the residual organic matter; this reduces the BOD by an additional 55 or 60 percent. Following this digestive process, the effluent flows into a second group of sedimentation tanks where any residual suspended matter settles out. Finally, the treated effluent is chlorinated and released into a local water course. In New York City, the vast amounts of sediment generated by sewage treatment is dumped into the "dead sea" area described earlier in this chapter.

In addition to domestic wastes and infectious disease agents, a variety of other pollutants threaten the water supplies. Treated sewage contains high concentrations of nitrates and phosphates. Unable to be removed, they greatly stimulate the growth of algae and other plants in the water. These plants utilize oxygen dissolved in the water and gradually cause suffocation of fish and other aquatic life. Thus, all animal life ultimately vanishes, and the water becomes "dead." The most striking example of this process is Lake Erie. Nitrates usually come from fertilizers, and phosphates from household detergents (Fig. 9-10). Heated effluent from industrial wastes or power stations raises the temperature of water and thereby re-

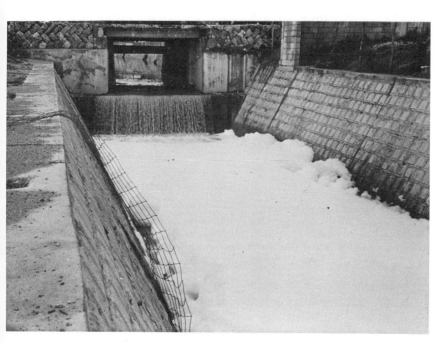

FIG. 9-10. *This phosphate-rich detergent foam in the Okinawan water supply is of a type which is not broken down into simpler compounds by naturally occurring bacteria. Consequently, it appears in drinking water where it is distasteful and may represent an undefined long-term hazard to health. (Courtesy of Dr. C. L. Marshall.)*

duces its ability to carry dissolved oxygen. This is tantamount to introducing sewage with a high BOD. Other wastes, many of which are difficult or impossible to remove, kill fish outright. Fortunately, radioactive substances in water supplies have not been a problem, although the situation in Richland, Washington, is somewhat unsettling.

As Table 9-5 illustrates, while the population of the United States increased 34 percent between 1949 and 1968, the increase in crop production, soap, and beer were modest when considered on a *per capita* basis. Although crop production per capita increased 11 percent, pesticides and fertilizer production increased 267 percent and 648 percent respectively. Fertilizer and pesticides wash into streams with the rain and introduce pollutants into the water which require expensive water-treatment facilities to remove.[1] Old fashioned soap was free of phosphates and subject to biological degradation, but soap has been increasingly displaced by detergents. The situation is similar with respect to beer bottles and the

TABLE 9-5. Pollutants in the Post-War Period

Item	Period	Percent Increase	Related Item	Percent Increase
Population	1949–68	34		
Crop production per capita	1949–68	11	Pesticides	267
			Fertilizer	648
Cleansers per capita	1946–68	0	Detergent phosphorus	1,845
Beer consumption per capita	1950–67	5	Beer bottles	595
Motor-vehicle miles per capita	1946–67	100	Tetraethyl lead	415
			Nitrogen oxides	630

Modified after Barry Commoner, The Origins of the Environmental Crisis, the keynote address before the Council of Europe, Second Symposium of Members of Parliament Specialists in Public Health, Stockholm, Sweden, July 1, 1971.

air pollutants released by motor vehicles. These statistics suggest that the pollution problem is generated not by increased population or by "affluence," but by a technology which has introduced nondegradable, non-disposable synthetic products into the environment as substitutes for previously used products which were subject to decomposition by natural elements such as bacteria.

Although solid wastes are not waterborne and do not usually produce disease, they nonetheless represent a significant aspect of the pollution problem. While we are all accustomed to "no deposit, no return" items, the act of discarding something just removes it from our presence. Aluminum cans, plastic containers, nonreturnable bottles, garbage, rubbish, and ashes are symbols of the solid-waste problem. Dumping at sea, land fills, and incineration are major ways of disposing of solid wastes. Garbage, after being boiled, is commonly fed to hogs. Land fills are rarely an adequate outlet for the volume of wastes produced, and dumping at sea adds to the already grievous problem of water pollution. Incineration is a key source of air pollution and the most expensive form of waste disposal. What to do with solid wastes is one of the great unanswered challenges to our technologically oriented society which spawned the problem in the first place.

AIR POLLUTION

We already encountered the problem of air pollution in our discussion of the etiology of bronchitis and emphysema. Although it is commonly regarded as an integral part of the ecology crisis, air pollution was identified centuries before ecologists called it to our attention. The English proclaimed it prejudicial to health as early as 1273, and its particular relationship to urban London was noted in 1661. Over the past few years, air pollution has emerged as a major public issue, and it is a rare day when some aspect of the problem fails to turn up in the press.

During the past two decades or so, temperature inversions have produced the most dramatic testimonial to the harmful effects of polluted air upon health. An inversion is said to exist when a layer of warm air traps the heavily polluted layer of air closest to the ground. This "ceiling" effect prevents dispersal of pollutants and results in an abnormally high level of them in the ambient air. Under these circumstances, it is commonly observed that the number of illnesses and deaths is greater than normally expected. One of the earliest inversions noted occurred in London in 1873 and resulted in almost 300 unexpected deaths. Since then, London has experienced serious inversions in 1952 and 1956. In 1948, an acute episode in the small coaltown of Donora, Pennsylvania, resulted in over 7,000 illnesses. As might be expected, New York City has had its share of serious inversions; these occurred in 1953, 1956, and 1966.

Needless to say, air pollution affects most of the American population to a greater or lesser degree. Urban areas are most heavily affected, and it is estimated that 90 percent of persons living in cities are exposed to polluted air. The irony of air pollution is the extent to which it represents the dark side of affluence. The industries which feed our prosperity pollute our atmosphere. Electric power generators, paper factories, oil refineries, steel mills, incinerators, and home coal and oil burners all represent important pollution sources. However, none is in a league with the automobile when it comes to the generation of air pollutants. Industry and power generators tend to produce primarily oxides of sulfur; but the auto produces not only sulfur oxides but carbon monoxide, nitrogen oxides, various hydrocarbons, and a range of particulate matter. The last includes soot, ash, and smaller particles which provide a nucleus for the formation of water droplets. In the aggregate, these droplets make up an aerosol. Small-particle aerosols account for the blue haze in polluted urban areas, while large particles are partly responsible for the brilliant sunsets so sought after by photographers. Aerosol particles often coalesce with each other or combine with gasses such as sulfur dioxide, nitrogen oxides, or carbon monoxide. These combinations produce chemical compounds whose health effects may be quite different from that of a single, uncombined pollutant.

Air pollution is basically of two types. The first is the photochemical haze widely known as smog. Smog results from the oxidation of hydrocarbons and nitrogen oxides. Compounds are produced which irritate the

For Doctors

Advice for Patients During Air Pollution Episodes

1. The population risk consists mainly of patients with chronic heart and lung diseases especially in the older group. During an alert it may be desirable for susceptibles to stay indoors and reduce their activities. Routine household chores such as sweeping, cleaning, shopping, etc., should be avoided if necessary. Rest in a chair or a bed is helpful.

2. Since the pollutant content of ambient air in an apartment is usually lower than outside, windows should be kept closed so far as practicable. It is advisable to use air conditioning which recirculates room air. This is better than letting in outside air. Filters, preferably those with activated charcoal, are helpful. Diurnal measurements of air pollutants such as sulfur dioxide and particulates indicate that they are usually at their lowest levels in the early afternoon and late at night. Therefore, during nonsummer months, ventilation of rooms for brief intervals is best done at these times. During summer months, however, when oxidant levels tend to peak during bright sunshine hours, ventilation of rooms is best done after dark or early in the morning.

3. The effects of air pollution are exacerbated by smoking which in itself is a primary bronchial irritant and markedly raises the carbon monoxide content of the blood. All smokers should be urged to discontinue smoking during an alert.

4. Bronchospasm with wheezing and asthma in susceptible patients should be treated *early*. Ephedrine and related compounds, aminophyllin by various routes, corticosteroids, and compressed air are among the measures known to be useful.

5. Prophylactic tetracycline or other suitable antimicrobials may be indicated for some patients with chronic bronchitis especially when there is a past history of exacerbations or pneumonitis.

FIG. 9-11.

eyes, nose, and throat but which are not thought to present a serious threat to health. More dangerous are the particulate matter, sulfur dioxide, and other materials generated by the burning of fossil fuels such as coal, oil, or gasoline. Most inversion episodes are associated with abnormal concentrations of sulfur dioxide.

There can be little doubt about the harmful effects of acute pollution episodes such as the Donora disaster; in addition, heart and respiratory disease have long been associated with chronic exposure to lower levels of pollutants. Just how these effects come about, which pollutants are to blame, and which levels of these pollutants should be considered dangerous is presently unclear. Nevertheless, long experience with air pollution in our great urban centers has led to the identification of those segments of the population at greatest risk and to the advocacy of measures and precautions most likely to minimize risk. Figure 9-11 reproduces an advisory notice which was mailed to all physicians by the Health Commissioner of New York City.

This brief and circumscribed review of factors related to water and air pollution reflects only a very small part of the total and urgent ecologic and environmental pollution problems which face our world. The discussion which follows presents a broader look at these problems and considers some further specific issues of concern in these areas.

Ecology and Environmental Pollution

"We are not interested in pollution control projects which would cost us money and impede our industrial progress." This remark comes not from an American industrial tycoon but from an official in the government of an industrializing African country. In a nutshell, it sums up the central issue to be grappled with in all problems relating to environmental pollution.

Environmental pollution can be defined as the cumulative addition of harmful substances to the biosphere, i.e., the earth's thin film of living matter. Human beings must now begin to question the consequences implicit in two very important facts: (1) man now uses increasing portions of the energy that runs the biosphere and (2) man is increasingly filling the biosphere with toxic substances that reduce the energy available to him. The health worker, in particular, must pay special attention to the ways in which environmental pollution can specifically damage human health. Energy cycles, food chains, ecosystems, seabed contaminants, soil abuse, eutrophication and the health hazards of air pollution are complex issues and frequently provoke acrimonious controversies. This is not surprising in view of the vastness of the overall problem and its countless economic, social, and political implications.

POLLUTION AND ECOLOGY

Ecology is the study of the interrelationships between biological communities and their environments, both of which comprise the biosphere. The effects of pollution on the biosphere's many complex cycles for the transfer of food, energy, air, water, nitrogen, carbon, and other vital substances form the basis of the widely publicized ecologic and environmental crisis. In the past 20 years, ecology has received recognition as a science with its own methods, hypotheses, and data. Energy use, population pressure, the effects of technological change on environmental

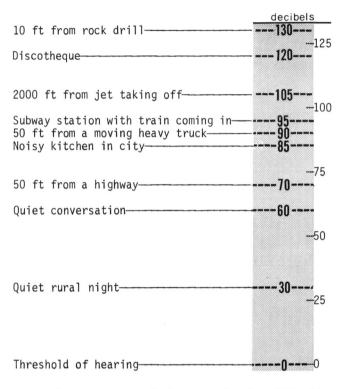

FIG. 9-12. *Sustained exposure to noise levels greater than about 75 decibels can lead to permanent hearing loss. Deafness is thus an occupational hazard for subway workers, airport employees and construction workers. Those who spend much time listening to loud music are similarly endangered. (Courtesy of Office of Noise Abatement and Control, U.S. Environmental Protection Agency.)*

quality and human health are all matters for the ecologist's concern. For this reason, ecology has become a field which is attracting many students who wish to combine an interest in science with service to mankind.

In somewhat less grandiose terms, an ecologic approach can be applied to any environment which is seen as interacting with a community. We can observe and study how any specific community is affected by a change or set of changes in the environment. In the slums of New York City, for example, a tenement apartment with poisonous lead paint peeling from the walls serves as the environment for a community of young children. Here, environmental "pollution" has little to do with changes within naturally occurring energy cycles, but it has a great deal to do with the health of a specific human sub-community and, for that matter, public policy and morality.

Along the same lines, it is becoming increasingly clear that exposure to high levels of noise can have a detrimental effect on hearing. This phenomenon is commonly referred to as noise "pollution" and is summarized in Figure 9-12.

ENVIRONMENTAL POLLUTION AND HUMAN HEALTH: ASBESTOS AS AN EXAMPLE

There are many situations in which a change in the environment has very specific and damaging effects on human health, though the effect on the biosphere-at-large may be insignificant. These situations require special steps for prevention and control and are of particular interest to health workers. As a case study of the medical, economic, and political issues entangled with the problem of environmental pollution, let us consider the problems associated with the contamination of air by asbestos.

Asbestos is a mineral that can be woven into cloth. Many of the largest quarry-like areas from which asbestos is mined are in North America. As a naturally occurring mineral element, it sits quietly and harmlessly in the ground. According to geologists, asbestos originated millions of years ago when upheavals in the earth's surface created rock fractures which were penetrated by hot water from the earth's interior. These waters dissolved some of the rock surface and thus allowed crystals of asbestos to grow within the fractures. Asbestos is of immense industrial interest because it can withstand intense heat, it is resistant to erosion and decay, and it is light but as strong as piano wire. For these reasons, it is often called "the magic mineral." Roof shingles, insulation board, casings for electric motors, fireproof curtains, conveyor belts, ironing board covers, airplane fittings, brake linings, automobile mufflers and hoods, floor tiling, and pipes to carry water, gas, and sewage all contain asbestos because of its marvelous properties. It has doubtless saved the lives of many people by insulating girders against the heat of a fire. The uses and industrial value of asbestos are attested to by the rise in production, from 500,000 tons in 1930 to four million tons in 1970.

Unfortunately, when sprayed onto a surface, asbestos releases fibers into the air which are lethal environmental pollutants. Doctors have discovered that construction and shipyard workers occupationally exposed to asbestos tend to develop a crippling lung disease called asbestosis; they are also at great risk of developing cancers of the chest and abdominal wall. If they smoke, they are 92 times more likely to contract lung cancer than the average man. Those of us who are not construction workers, but who live in cities, are exposed to smaller concentrations of asbestos, as is evidenced by the presence of asbestos fibers in the lungs of autopsied city dwellers. In the 1970s, the air in Manhattan contained six times as much asbestos as that of the New Jersey suburbs.

What are the effects of this contamination of the air on the health of children, adults, or the aged who breathe it daily? No one can really say. What happens to people in air-conditioned buildings with asbestos-lined ducts and channels? It has been shown that these ducts offer up asbestos fibers which, once circulated, are inhaled. No one knows what will happen when, 75 to 100 years from now, wreckers demolish the asbestos-lined buildings constructed in the last few years and thus fill the air with asbestos dust.

These questions and the need to analyze and study them illustrate the kinds of problems associated with many contemporary environmental pollution issues. The pollutant, harmless in its natural state, is commercially widespread because of its usefulness. To remove or eliminate it by law, penalty, or the discovery of something equally useful but less dangerous initially means that someone or everyone would have to surrender certain benefits or conveniences. The cost resulting from the spraying of asbestos cannot be eliminated. At present, it is being paid by workers occupationally exposed to the pollutant and possibly by those communities of people who are inhaling smaller, nonoccupational doses. The cost can be redistributed only through the use of less dangerous but possibly more expensive insulating material (such as masonry) or by the time-consuming application of asbestos as a wet paste. Both alternatives involve more expense. Someone must be willing or required to pay the extra cost associated with reduced disease. *In every environmental pollution issue, the problems of control and prevention are basically questions of cost, of who will pay, and of how they will pay—with money or with disease.* Again, we are confronted with the fact that no benefit exists without a cost, even if that cost is poorly recognized for years.

Asbestos, of course, is merely one of the many examples of an environmental contaminant whose adverse effect on human health is the penalty of indiscriminate and improper use. Another, more publicized example is lead, which is a widespread air pollutant because it is so useful as an anti-knock agent in automotive fuels. Although there is disagreement as to the effects of urban ambient concentrations of lead, available evidence suggests that these concentrations are much higher than in former years and are therefore a cause for concern. However,

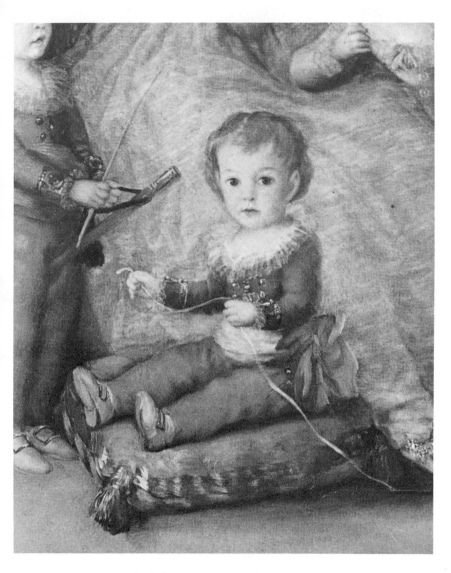

FIG. 9-13A.   *A new medical theory conjectures that Goya's drastic change of artistic style was due to the effects of lead poisoning produced by his daily exposure to large quantities of white lead-based paint. Others have attributed the change to either syphilis, schizophrenia, thrombosis, or the natural artistic progress of a genius. A. Detail from* The Duke of Asuna and his Family, *1789. B.* Saturn Devouring his Son, *1820, by Francisco Goya (Courtesy of Museo del Prado, Madrid.)*

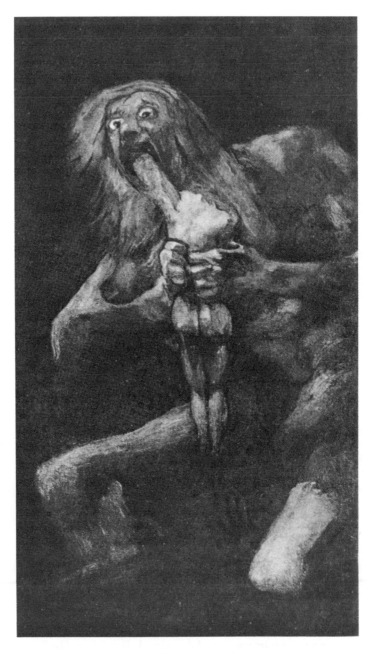

FIG. 9-13B.

when consumers are given a choice between leaded and unleaded gasoline, they are presently unwilling to buy the latter because it costs more, has a lower octane rating, and provides lower performance.

Because of their utility, asbestos and lead are substances which are difficult to "eliminate." They are prototypes of a vast number of substances which have either been extracted from the ground or synthesized in the test tube for industrial or commercial use (see Fig. 9-13A, B). It is only in the last few years that we have begun to ask whether man can introduce countless new substances, technologies, and processes into his environment without risking disastrous consequences for human health and natural ecosystems.

As was suggested by the African official, the poorer, newly industrializing countries of Africa, Asia, and Latin America appear to be less enthusiastic than the industrialized nations of Europe and North America about efforts to control environmental pollution. For these poorer countries, such efforts are perceived as adding to the economic costs of industrialization and thus as reducing the competitiveness of their products in world markets. As was the case in Europe and the United States, the costs of industrialization will be paid in terms of damaged health and shortened lives, especially among hazardously exposed workers, as well as through despoliation of the natural environment. At present, and much to the regret of health workers, econometric models of national growth and development do not take such effects into consideration.

ENVIRONMENTAL POLLUTANTS AND LONG-TERM EFFECTS

When the smokestack of a factory spits out dirty smoke, everyone notices. The smoke may or may not be harmful, but it is a nuisance—ugly, embarrassing to the community, and temporarily irritating if it gets in one's eyes. This is the kind of problem that is relatively easy to act on because many people are *immediately* bothered. However, today's major environmental pollution problems often produce subtle consequences which do not manifest themselves until many years have passed. For this reason, there are many pollutants which are not readily associated with adverse effects. Asbestos and lead again serve as excellent examples. Breathing asbestos is not discomforting, but the effects 20 years later can be fatal. It is suspected that it may be damaging to health to inhale the lead in the air of our cities. However, many possible adverse effects from this may not be apparent until years after the onset of exposure. Indeed, we are just beginning to realize that, with few exceptions, next to nothing is known about the long-term effects on human health of exposure to varying kinds of environmental pollutants in our air, water, ground, and food, and in the products we use. For this reason, standards and regulations promulgating "safe" air, water, or food must be recognized as tentative and subject to future revision in the light of facts yet unknown. It goes without saying that investigation of the long-term effects of environmental pollutants on human health is a major future horizon in medical research. In any case, it is frequently very difficult to generate public support for control of pollutants whose adverse effects occur years or generations later, or which, in many cases, are not even known. All of us tend to be influenced far more strongly by an insignificant but discomforting event occurring today than by the possibility of a truly dangerous one 20 years from today. This behavioral principle, coupled with man's tremendous and perhaps excessive capacity to adapt to the unpleasant, is a major barrier to the implementation of measures against environmental pollution.

ENVIRONMENTAL POLLUTION AND PLANET EARTH

"We human beings exist and enjoy life only by virtue of conditions created and maintained at the surface of the earth by the microbes, plants, and animals that have converted its inanimate matter into a highly integrated living structure. Any proposed disturbance in the ecological equilibrium is a threat to the maintenance of human life as we know it now." (Rene Dubos)

Eutrophication of freshwater lakes exemplifies the accuracy of this statement. As we have already seen, eutrophication, meaning enrichment, usually refers to the addition of nitrogen and phosphorus to such lakes from their surrounding fertilizer-enriched shores. When certain aquatic organisms, such as algae and other plants, are provided with this extra supply of nitrogen and phosphorus, they are enabled to increase their body mass and to grow. This is known as "algae bloom." When these algae and other aquatic plants decay and die, their mass gravitationally sinks to the bottom of the lake. The decaying mass becomes organic debris that serves as food for oxygen-consuming organisms, and the total availability of oxygen in the waters is thereby reduced. This, in turn, means that there will ultimately be lessened amounts of oxygen available for animal life in the lake, and the former will diminish. If industrial waste is also added to the waters, the amount of life which can be supported by the lake is reduced even faster. In time, if preventive measures are not taken, the lake's bottom will be encrusted with the debris from dead algae, and the water will be unable to support any life at all.

This encrustration can become progressive and eventually result in the disappearance of the lake itself. In short, eutrophication resulting from nitrogen and phosphorus "run-off" can produce a dead or dying lake.

There are many complex issues involved in eutrophication. Nitrogen and phosphorus fertilizers enrich the soil and comprise the basis for modern agriculture in western and "westernized" countries. The industrial plants pouring their chemical wastes into the lake are all producing products which people want to purchase, and, moreover, these plants provide jobs for many workers. No one's physical health seems to be immediately affected. Yet a serious problem not only exists but, according to ecologists, could initiate a cycle which would result in the inability of surrounding shoreline environments to support natural life. Again, the problem of saving the lake becomes one of cost, of defining the nature of the cost, and of ascertaining who will pay the price. Should the farmers reduce their use of fertilizers containing nitrogen and phosphorus? Should they be compensated for doing so? Should they be penalized for not doing so? Should industries reduce their effluent wastes and pass on to the consumer the costs of implementing this reduction? Should industries be subject to fines so high that they act as true deterrents? Should government subsidize a clean-up program and the construction of sewage-treatment plants with tax monies from everyone? Eutrophication is an example of environmental pollution which has no widespread or immediately obvious health effects. And yet, these questions and many others will have to be answered not only in the interests of saving the lakes but, in the words of Dubos, "human life as we know it."

ENVIRONMENTAL POLLUTION AND POPULATION

For the first two million years of man's existence, he lived as a hunter, an herbivore, and a scavenger. Under these circumstances, the maximum population the earth could support was about 10 million people. Ten thousand years ago, man domesticated plants and animals and began to use the biosphere for his own purposes. As man exploited the earth's capacity for food production, human population increased. As pointed out in Chapter 2, it took two million years for the world's population to reach one billion; but between 1960 and 1975, it will rise by another one billion and reach four billion. There is the strong temptation, therefore, to point to the enormous increase in population as the major reason for environmental pollution. However, this is a conjecture which requires careful examination. There is evidence that pollution is not most directly related to the sheer increase in population or, for that matter, to national affluence but rather to the fact that in the last 25 years, innumerable technological processes have been introduced without consideration of their environmental consequences.

It is useful to review the evidence which suggests this conclusion. From 1946 to 1968, the population of the United States increased 48 percent. Affluence, which is most simply measured by the Gross National Product, increased about 50 percent. However, various types of pollution (such as smog, algae in Lake Erie, and bacteria in harbors) increased by 200 to 1,000 percent At the same time, the production of plastics (which results in many adverse environmental effects because of that product's high degree of inertness, or nondegradability) increased by 1,024 percent; the production of nitrogen fertilizer increased by 574 percent, detergents by 300 percent, and electric power (a big source of air pollution) by approximately 76 percent. Thus, as ecologists have pointed out, the critical factor in this country's environmental degradation appears to be neither population nor affluence but rather the impact of technological changes associated with the increasing production of certain commodities.

These observations do not mean that continued expansion of the global population poses no threat to our environment. Indeed, in terms of the rampant introduction of new technologies, every baby born into the world adds a further threat to its pollution, and the more industrialized the country of his birth, the greater is the threat. In other words, the addition of an extra American baby to the world's population is accompanied by far more serious environmental consequences than is the addition of an extra baby from India, China, Indonesia, or Brazil. Once the American baby grows up, he will require 180 **BTU**s of energy per year (based on 1961 figures) to run his car, refrigerator, air conditioner, and other devices. He will purchase a myriad of products whose production and use can exacerbate environmental pollution. And he will be fed by an agricultural system which many authorities think is already dangerously overdependent on fertilizers. In adulthood, the baby from a less-developed country will require between 2 and 5 BTUs per year (36 to 90 times less than estimated for the American infant) at current levels. He will own few, if any, appliances, and he will be fed by an agricultural system that is not dependent on fertilizers containing nitrogen and phosphorus. Thus, population increases in countries with new polluting technologies and high per capita rates of energy consumption will result in much more environmental pollution than similar increases in countries which are both poorer and less apt to use these technologies. This situation is ironic

---

BTU: British thermal unit; a measure of heat energy

in view of the intense efforts of both the United States government and wealthy American foundations to encourage and finance "family planning" efforts in underdeveloped countries. In terms of environmental impact, one American indirectly produces perhaps 50 times the pollution generated by a Nigerian or a Burmese.

ENVIRONMENTAL POLLUTION AND ENERGY CONSUMPTION

Only recently has attention been focused on the world's increasing per capita consumption of energy as it relates to environmental pollution. Figure 9-14, which correlates Gross National Product with per capita energy consumption, can also be a fairly useful guide as to which countries have air pollution problems associated with the burning of oil, gas, and coal.

It is frequently stated that not only will the amount of energy consumed rise simply as a result of population increase, but each person will himself require more energy than has hitherto been the case. If this produc-

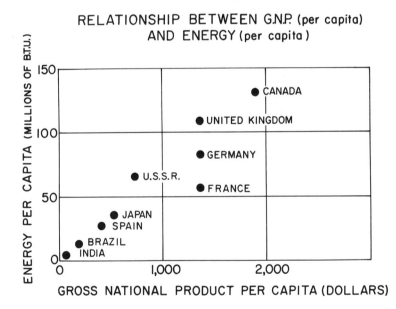

FIG. 9-14. *A high gross national product per capita is associated with high energy consumption per capita which, in turn, requires the use of large amounts of fuels. (From Singer, Human energy production as a process in biosphere. Scientific American, 223, Sept. 1970. Courtesy of W. H. Freeman and Company.)*

tion is borne out, slogans aimed at "eliminating the source of air pollution" are naive. For this very reason, it is now being questioned whether per capita increases of energy consumption should be *allowed* to occur. Even after the world exhausts its fossil fuel supplies, new problems will be created by the use of electric power and nuclear-energy power sources. In the meantime, the tasks facing government, industry, and communities to protect community health and the natural environment from fossil fuel pollution will be formidable.

ENERGY PRODUCTION, AIR POLLUTION, AND SOCIAL PLANNING

By the twenty-third century, man probably will have used up the fossil fuel supplies which he uses to run his automobile and all other machines powered by internal combustion engines. Until then, he will have to live with (or perhaps suffer from) the health and esthetic consequences of air pollution. In the United States, 90 percent of all energy consumed annually comes from fossil fuels. In addition to the solid particulates, the major air pollutants resulting from the burning of fossil fuels are carbon monoxide, the sulphur oxides, hydrocarbons, the nitrogen oxides, and photochemical oxidants such as ozone. Each of these pollutants is now suspected of adversely affecting the health of excessively exposed populations. The effects vary, depending on complex interactions of the pollutant with such factors as climate, preexisting health, and intensity of exposure. Excess mortality, aggravation of preexisting illness, interference with the mechanics of breathing, irritation of the eyes, nose, and throat, and general impairment of well-being have been some of the consequences noted to occur in populations living in polluted areas, especially during peak periods of air pollution. Carbon monoxide, in concentrations produced by heavy urban traffic, can subtly impair mental judgment; sulphur dioxide can irritate the membranes of the respiratory tree, and the oxidants can produce irritation of the eyes, nose, throat, and lungs. In addition, air pollution affects the quality of life in cities and adjacent areas; it results in dirty clothes and window sills, damaged crops, and blackened stone buildings.

The major sources of air pollution are automobiles, industry, electric power plants, space heating, and refuse disposal. From Figure 9-15 it is apparent that control of air pollution will have to depend much more heavily on public measures regulating the uses of power and much less on campaigns aimed at changing the behavior of individual citizens. Air pollution will not be eliminated by radio and television announcements

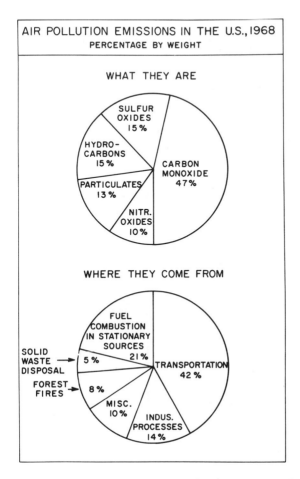

AIR POLLUTION EMISSIONS IN THE U.S., 1968
PERCENTAGE BY WEIGHT

WHAT THEY ARE

SULFUR OXIDES 15%
HYDRO-CARBONS 15%
CARBON MONOXIDE 47%
PARTICULATES 13%
NITR. OXIDES 10%

WHERE THEY COME FROM

FUEL COMBUSTION IN STATIONARY SOURCES 21%
SOLID WASTE DISPOSAL → 5%
TRANSPORTATION 42%
FOREST FIRES → 8%
MISC. 10%
INDUS. PROCESSES 14%

FIG. 9-15. *(Courtesy of National Pollution Control Administration, Department of Health, Education and Welfare.)*

exhorting drivers to idle their automobiles in neutral drive. A more potent approach would be based on measures requiring the installation of pollution control devices in all sources of power, on improved mass transit (which transports the largest number of people per unit of fuel expenditure), and on technological changes and controls in those industries which are the biggest polluters (Fig. 9-16). As has been the case with the previous examples we have discussed, all of these steps involve complex issues of costs and benefits; and doing something about air pollution in any community or region involves ascertaining its major sources of air

COMPOSITION OF STATE POLLUTION BOARDS

Note: This table is not a classification of states' air and water pollution conditions

● Means state pollution board with regulatory authority contains members associated with basic pollution sources (industry, agriculture, county and city governments).
O Means state board is free of such representation.

"No Boards" means air and water pollution regulation statewide is handled by a full-time state agency.

	Air Board	Water Board	Combination Air-Water Board		Air Board	Water Board	Combination Air-Water Board
Alabama	O	O		Montana			O
Alaska		No Boards		Nebraska			●
Arizona		No Boards		Nevada			●
Arkansas			●	New Hampshire	●	●	
(1)California	O	●		New Jersey		No Boards	
Colorado	●	●		New Mexico			O
Connecticut		No Boards		(2)New York		No Boards	
Delaware			●	North Carolina	●	●	
Florida			O	North Dakota	●	●	
Georgia	●	●		Ohio	●	●	
Hawaii			O	Oklahoma			●
Idaho	●	O		Oregon			●
Illinois		No Boards		Pennsylvania			●
Indiana	●	●		Rhode Island		No Boards	
Iowa	●	●		South Carolina			●
Kansas			O	South Dakota	●	●	
Kentucky	●	●		Tennessee	●	●	
Louisiana	●	●		Texas	●	●	
Maine			●	Utah	●	●	
Maryland		No Boards		Vermont	O	O	
Massachusetts	O	O		Virginia	O	O	
Michigan	●	●		Washington		No Boards	
Minnesota			●	(3)West Virginia	●		
Mississippi			●	Wisconsin			●
Missouri	●	●		(4)Wyoming	●		

(1) Pollution sources represented in regional branches of State Water Board. (2) State Environmental Board is advisory.
(3) Water pollution under State Division of Water Resources.
(4) Water pollution under State Department of Health and Social Services.

FIG. 9-16. *Pollution control policy is often determined by the polluters themselves. This is like asking the tobacco industry to condemn cigarettes. (Courtesy of* The New York Times.)

pollution, the benefits associated with these sources, the costs, and ways of redistributing these costs and benefits.

OCCUPATIONAL HEALTH: THE TIP OF THE ICEBERG

As our case study of asbestos and asbestosis has already shown, many of the health-related community-wide problems in environmental pollution concurrently are problems in occupational health. In polluted work environments, industrial workers are exposed to an array of health-damaging agents in the course of their work. Regrettably, the United States and, for that matter, most other countries, have not come anywhere near reaching the goal of a safe and healthy work environment for all working people.

For many of the pollution-related health problems of concern to the general population, "the tip of the iceberg" can frequently be found in the excessive and, at times, disabling or fatal exposures to dusts, fumes, mists, smokes, solvents, vapors, aerosols, chemical hazards, pesticides, plastics and synthetic resins, physical hazards such as ultraviolet, infra-red, microwave, and ionizing radiation and noise experienced by occu-pationally exposed persons for many years of their lives. The National Occupational Health and Safety Act of 1970 represented belated recogni-tion of this situation and may help to spur efforts both in occupational health and safety and community-wide environmental pollution resulting from industrial processes.

In occupational health, the strategies for eliminating adverse exposures for definable work populations are fairly well-defined. These strategies can frequently serve as prototypes for problem-solving in health-related community-wide pollution problems. For example, it is an axiom in occu-pational health that prevention should be external to individual human behavior and attitudes and should not have to rely on the behavior of individuals.

This axiom from occupational health happens to be a more traditional way of saying what we have already said about community-wide environ-mental pollution: Public policy rather than individual behavior must be the primary locus of intervention in any community effort to "control" or "eliminate" specific kinds of environmental pollution.

CONCLUSION

By now, it is no longer enough for governments and com-munities to describe and measure environmental pollution where and when it occurs. The real challenge increasingly appears to be one of antici-pating possible future sources of environmental pollution *in advance*. Power plants yet unplanned, nuclear explosions still unscheduled, paper mills still on the drawing boards, and super highways not yet funded must all be scrutinized for their potential effects on environmental quality. Should there be an oil pipeline through the perma-frost of Alaska? Should more oil exploration be carried out along the continental shelf? Should a super highway, rather than a mass transit system, be built in yet another city? Should asbestos be sprayed on the steel girders of another skyscraper? These are all questions which are part of what has been called the "politics of ecology."

This brief discussion could not hope to review all the varieties of environmental pollution. Furthermore, no one can expect to be an expert on its every aspect; but those who do become knowledgeable about any one specific issue will always be challenged to defend their statements with data on costs and benefits—economic, social, medical, and so on. Unless the environmentalist can ask the questions which force people to provide such data, he will have difficulty contributing to the control of any given environmental pollution problem. Health workers especially must be vigilant. On the one hand, they must become alert to ways in which environmental pollution may affect health. On the other hand, they must be wary of the "double negative" fallacy: If no ill effects on health have yet been ascribed to a specific pollutant, the reason for this may be that these effects have not been sought, especially if they occur only after a long period of time. Again, it must be emphasized that the kinds of questions which have to be asked about any environmental pollution problem are as important as the answers.

Radiation

The planet Earth may be regarded as a spaceship hurtling through the universe on its way to a fate as unknown as the void from whence it came millions of years ago. Of all the animate creatures which inhabit the Earth, only man is aware of his past, conscious of his present, and capable of influencing his future. While it is a fact of life that man is subject to certain hazards from outer space, it appears quite likely that long before humanity succumbs to these uncontrollable forces, man will have destroyed himself precisely because of his ability to influence conditions in his immediate earthly environment. Our discussion of environmental pollution has already pointed out some ways in which this destruction could occur. In somewhat more detail, let us explore what is perhaps one of the best examples of this: the relationship between man and electromagnetic radiation.

THE ELECTROMAGNETIC SPECTRUM

Electromagnetic radiation refers to a spectrum of energy sources which travel at the speed of light (186,000 miles per second) in a wavelike configuration. The shorter the **wavelength,** the greater the number of waves which can occur in a given time interval. The term "cycles" is often used instead of wave; and the number of waves, or cycles, occurring in a second is known as frequency. The energy delivered by the source of radiation is directly proportional to the frequency and, therefore, inversely proportional to the wavelength. Regardless of the type of radiation involved, the frequency times the wavelength equals the speed of light. The waves involved in the transmission of radio broadcasts are very long, often many miles. In contrast, the wavelength of x-rays is less than one-millionth of a millimeter.

The most readily obvious forms of electromagnetic radiation are heat and light. Both have profound effects on man. For example, heat is largely responsible for the differing life styles of Eskimos in Antartica and tribesmen living in the sweltering jungles of New Guinea. Temperature also exerts a major effect on the diseases to which men are exposed. In particular, infectious diseases transmitted by vectors are influenced by the latter's ability to survive at a range of temperatures. There is no malaria in cold climes, largely because the mosquito vector cannot survive lower temperatures. Sunlight, of course, is ultimately related to temperature, but some of its effects are independent of heat. Cancer of the skin is most common in farmers and others whose skin is continuously exposed to sunlight. The role of light, particularly ultraviolet light, in producing the widespread malady known as "sunburn" is well recognized. Less obviously, the recurring cycle of day and night constitutes a kind of "biologic clock" by which many basic bodily functions seem to be regulated. When this **circadian rhythm** is disrupted by rapid jet travel across several time zones, a "jet-travel syndrome" occurs which is characterized by fatigue, lassitude, confusion, and often by impaired judgment. This syndrome disappears when one's biologic rhythm has become acclimated to the new time zone. Although heat and light are the most readily apparent radiation sources, ionizing radiation is, without doubt, the most widely publicized and the most widely feared.

IONIZING RADIATION

Radiation is a term used to describe the emission of discrete particles, or rays, from a substance. Sources of radiation are said to be

---

WAVELENGTH: the distance between the crests of two or more waves
CIRCADIAN RHYTHM: refers to that which recurs on a daily basis

radioactive. Ionizing radiation is that which is capable of splitting atoms in the process of traversing through a medium, such as a human body. The atoms within the body which are split as a result of exposure to a radioactive source are said to be ionized, meaning that they are divided to positively and negatively charged particles.

Radioactivity has been known to science since the late nineteenth century, but most people first learned of it in August of 1945, when atomic bombs obliterated the Japanese cities of Hiroshima and Nagasaki. About 150,000 persons died outright in these holocausts. An equal number survived the explosions, only to succumb, in the days and weeks that followed, to burns, injuries, or a disease new to man—radiation sickness.

The types of radiation of concern to health workers are alpha and beta particles, and gamma and x-rays. The former rarely present hazards to health because neither alpha nor beta particles penetrate the body to any great extent. On the other hand, gamma and x-rays do penetrate the body and cause a wide variety of physical effects. The effects of radiation depend on the dose absorbed and on the duration of exposure. The unit of exposure is known as the Roentgen, and it approximates the Rad, or unit of absorbed dose. The Rem (Roentgen-equivalent-man) is defined as the quantity of radiation which produces the same effects on man as those resulting from the absorption of one Roentgen of gamma or x-radiation. Dose and duration relate to each other, such that the effects of a small dose over a long period of time differ from those of a large dose all at once.

Man is continuously and unavoidably exposed to radiation. Some foods are naturally radioactive, and man is bombarded daily with cosmic rays and with the residual of past atomic and hydrogen bomb tests. The importance of this so-called background radioactivity lies in the effects of cumulative exposure over a lifetime. Twentieth-century man is exposed to more radiation than were any of his ancestors. Part of this additional exposure is the result of weapons testing, but most of it comes from medical sources, particularly **radioisotopes** and x-rays. Both of these sources are vital to the diagnosis and treatment of disease, and it is therefore necessary to balance the benefits of radiation against its harmful effects.

The effects of prolonged and continuous exposure to small doses of radiation are both genetic and physical. The genetic effect is the stimu-

---

RADIOISOTOPE: a variation of a chemical element which is radioactive and which can be traced in the human body; used in medicine as a diagnostic tool

lation of **mutations.** Once they appear, mutations are a permanent part of the organism unless they are incompatible with life, in which case the mutation dies with its phenotypic manifestation. Physical effects depend on the size of the chronic dose and sensitivity of the particular tissue involved. Leukemia, cancer of the skin, and bone cancer are related to prolonged exposure. About one-quarter of all pregnant women are x-rayed during pregnancy; and radiation can effect unborn children as well as adults. Fetal exposure to radiation during the first trimester of intrauterine life is associated with various cancers during childhood. As might be expected, leukemia has long been recognized as an occupational hazard of health personnel, such as radiologists and dentists, who work continuously around sources of radiation.

Exposure to large doses of radiation over a brief period of time produces radiation sickness. The severity of this syndrome depends on the dose absorbed. Doses below 100 R (Roentgen) produce no symptoms, while doses above 1,000 R are usually fatal. Between these extremes lie a wide variety of disease manifestations. Chances for recovery are greater at the lower end of the dosage spectrum. Fever, nausea, abdominal pain and discomfort, skin ulceration, **purpura,** leukopenia, hemorrhage, **epilation,** and a host of neurologic symptoms may all be present in severe cases; while mild cases may consist of nothing more than fever, nausea, and perhaps diarrhea. Radiation sickness begins as a **prodromal** period of vague malaise which lasts from a few hours to a couple of days. This is followed by an asymptomatic latent period of two to three weeks, after which the illness becomes overt. If the victim does not die, a long convalescence (up to five or six months) is commonplace. Diarrhea occurring during the prodromal period indicates moderately severe exposure, while convulsions and other signs of disturbances in the central nervous system usually precede a fatal outcome. There is no specific treatment for radiation sickness. The most valuable assistance medicine has to offer is antibiotic therapy to control the infections which accompany leukopenia and a general decline in the body's ability to resist bacterial invaders.

The collective experience of Japanese who survived the destruction of Hiroshima and Nagasaki has demonstrated that the dangers of large doses

---

MUTATION: a spontaneous change in a gene, which produces an alteration in future generations of the organism.
PURPURA: a condition characterized by the presence of purple-colored patches on the skin and mucous membranes due to small discrete hemorrhages under both
EPILATION: the process of hair falling out at the root
PRODROME: a group of premonitory symptoms; premonition

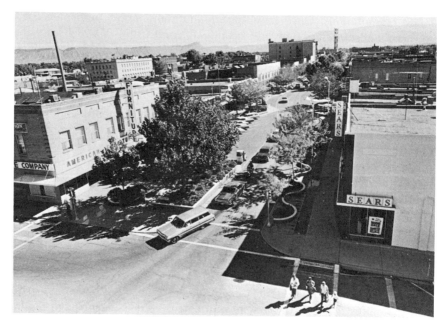

FIG. 9-17.   *Grand Junction, Colorado, may turn out to be as real a victim of the atomic age as Hiroshima or Nagasaki, although on a far smaller scale. Since the end of World War Two, most victims of America's nuclear might have been the Americans themselves. (Courtesy of Gary Settle, The New York Times.)*

of radiation do not end once the victim survives an acute episode of radiation sickness. Pregnant women delivered babies whose heads were abnormally small and who developed into mentally retarded children. Leukemia and cancers affecting the breast, lung, and thyroid have all been especially common in bomb victims, particularly those who were within a mile of the blast center.

Since life in close proximity to radioactive sources seems to be a continuing reality, it becomes a matter of great importance that the public be protected against unnecessary exposure. The Atomic Energy Commission controls the safe distribution, use, and disposal of radioactive sources from nuclear reactors, and the United States Public Health Service is responsible for monitoring and interpreting radiation levels in water, air, and milk and other foods. State health departments promulgate regulations covering the sources of radiation and controlling the transport and storage of these sources. Regardless of the regulatory agency involved, the aims are to prevent unnecessary exposure and to minimize necessary exposure.

Recently, a study of birth and death records from the town of Grand Junction, Colorado, has produced much public skepticism about the effectiveness of all the governmental regulations. In Grand Junction, extensive use was made of radioactive sand in building homes and other structures. This sand is a by-product of uranium processing and is known as "tailings" (Fig. 9-17). Tailings contain the element radium, an element which undergoes radioactive decay and which, during this process, is converted to a radioactive gas known as radon; and radon, being a gas, can be inhaled. It appears that exposure to these radioactive sources in Grand Junction has resulted in a lower birth rate and more genetic problems and cancer than would normally be expected in a population the size of Grand Junction's. In addition, and as yet unknown, are the potential effects on millions of Americans of exposure to radioactive fallout from atmospheric atomic testing. This compounds the skepticism about the degree to which the public has in fact been protected against the hazards of radiation.

During the second week of August, 1945, just after the bombing of Hiroshima and just before the Nagasaki disaster, American planes dropped leaflets over Japan. They bore the following message:

TO THE JAPANESE PEOPLE

America asks that you take immediate heed to what we say on this leaflet.

We are in possession of the most destructive explosive ever devised by man. A single one of our newly developed atomic bombs is equivalent in explosive power to what 2,000 of our giant B-29s can carry on a single mission. This awful fact is one for you to ponder and we solemnly assure you that it is grimly accurate.

We have just begun to use this weapon against your homeland. If you still have any doubt, make inquiry as to what happened to Hiroshima when just one atomic bomb fell on that city.

Before using this bomb to destroy every resource of the military by which they are prolonging this useless war, we ask that you now petition the Emperor to end the war. Our President has outlined for you the thirteen consequences of an honorable surrender. We urge that you accept these consequences and begin work of building a new, better, and peace-loving Japan.

You should take steps now to cease military resistance. Otherwise, we shall resolutely employ this bomb and all our other superior weapons to promptly and forcefully end the war.

Evacuate your cities now!

(From J. Toland's The Rising Sun, *New York, Random House, 1970, p. 799)*

Twenty-six years later, the Colorado State Department of Health was busy drawing up a letter to be sent to 5,000 homeowners in Grand Junction. A draft of this communication read as follows:

SUGGESTED LETTER TO OWNERS OF PROPERTIES
WHERE RADIATION LEVELS EXCEED THE SURGEON
GENERAL'S GUIDELINES

Dear _____,

An official report on our survey of your property for the presence of uranium mill tailings is enclosed.

You will note that our study has confirmed the presence of uranium tailings on your property and that the radiation exposure rate is higher than the level at which the U. S. Surgeon General feels corrective action is suggested.

We wish to point out to you, in all honesty, that there is little precise scientific information about the long-term health effect of low-level radiation, such as exists in your home. We strongly recommend, however, that you make every effort to lower the radiation exposure level in your home by removing the uranium tailings from your property.

(*From P. Metzger's article* Dear Sir: Your House is Built on Radioactive Uranium Waste, *New York Times Magazine,*
October 31, 1971)

After the expenditure of billions of dollars since the end of World War II to develop the nuclear weapons needed to "deter aggressors," it is perhaps a supreme irony that the only people victimized by this hazard to date are the Americans themselves.

Pests

In this final section we will consider a group of man's natural enemies who add danger, discomfort, and displeasure to his life on this planet.

The bites of scorpions, black widow and brown recluse spiders, and the stings of bees and wasps constitute a form of environmental hazards which potentially threaten human life. Scorpion bites and those of the two spiders inject a poison which commonly requires specific treatment with an antidote. Bee and wasp stings too frequently produce a rapidly fatal anaphylactic shock in those persons who have been sensitized by previous stings.

In addition to these insects, a large number of other arthropods are implicated in a variety of bites and stings which itch, burn, hurt, swell, or otherwise annoy the victim. Ticks, chiggers, and mites are well known pests, as are bedbugs, gnats, sand flies, houseflies, and the ubiquitous cockroach. This last pest does not bite, and efforts to establish a relationship between roaches and human disease have been inconclusive. However, their presence in a home is often one of the most distressing situations in the human experience. Although roaches are ignorant of social class and totally oblivious to economic status, infestations are most common and most severe in urban slum areas. Tenements are literally alive with roaches. When the lady of the house sets the table for dinner, she takes the utensils from a drawer full of roaches. The casserole in the oven comes out covered with dead roaches who failed to leave their home in the oven soon enough to avoid being cooked along with the dinner. Sleep frequently brings with it the unpleasant experience of having a curious roach crawl into the nose or ear.

In addition to its role in the transmission of typhus, the louse is another pest in its own right. Different types of lice affect different parts of the anatomy. Some live in the hair on one's head, others prefer the body; and one type, the crab louse, inhabits the pubic hair, where it is responsible for a condition usually transmitted by the venereal route and popularly known as "crabs."

In spite of the ingenuity, flexibility, and universality of insects, the nonpareil among pests is unquestionably the rat. There are two important varieties of domestic rats. The Norway rat (*Rattus norwegicus*) is the larger and more populous variety. It thrives in urban areas, where it lives under buildings or in piles of trash. Female rats begin breeding at three or four months of age, and each one can be expected to produce up to 80 offspring a year. The average lifespan for rats is about one year. The smaller roof rat (*Rattus rattus*) prefers roof dwelling-places and is found primarily in rural areas and coastal cities.

Rats are an important health problem for a number of reasons. For one thing, more than 60,000 rat bites are reported annually in the United States, and children are probably the most common victims. In addition to being painful, rat bites transmit an infectious disease known as rat-bite fever. This condition is caused by either of two bacteria. In the United States, the offending agent tends to be *Streptobacillus moniliformis*, while *Spirillum minus* predominates in Asia. The Streptobacillus infection is also known as Haverhill fever. In untreated cases, fatality rates may be as high as 10 percent.

Leptospirosis is a disease caused by several types of Leptospira bacteria. Severe cases are relatively uncommon, but when they occur, they lead to severe dysfunction of the liver and kidneys and are fatal in about 20 percent of cases. Leptospirosis is a zoonosis whose reservoirs include a variety of wild and domestic animals, among which is the rat. Humans usually contract the disease by drinking water contaminated with rat

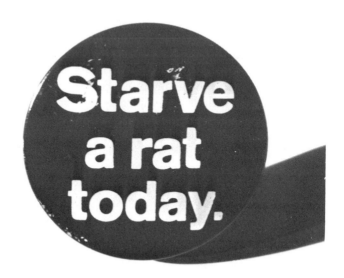

FIG. 9-18.   *Although this button is now remembered principally as a cliché of the late 1960's, it nevertheless sums up a basic principle of rat control. (Courtesy of Dr. C. L. Marshall.)*

excreta. Fortunately, leptospirosis is an uncommon disease in the United States. Only 67 cases were reported in 1967. Food contaminated by rat excreta transmits a rare type of tapeworm infection as well as the extremely common Salmonella food poisoning.

Rats themselves are often the victims of disease which may, under certain circumstances, infect man. Rats dying of trichinosis are sometimes eaten by pigs which, in turn, are consumed by man. Rats infected with murine typhus and bubonic plague carry fleas which transmit these diseases from rat to man if the latter is bitten by the rat.

Rats are ravenous eaters whose economic cost is enormous. Not only do they eat food earmarked for human consumption but they often also contaminate what food they leave behind. Their habit of constantly gnawing is believed responsible for fires, which can occur after rats have gnawed through the insulating material surrounding electric wiring. Indeed, some officials believe that as many as 25 percent of fires of unknown causes are in fact related to rats. It is estimated that the American rat population is about 100 million and the cost of supporting this population is as high as a billion dollars each year (Fig. 9-18).

It is often assumed that the key to rat control is the use of poisons. However, this animal is so prolific that the best that can be hoped for from poison campaigns is a temporary reduction in the size of the population. While the appearance of dead rats in baited areas gives the pest-control official reason for optimism, the true key to rat eradication is to eliminate the food and harborage on which they depend. This is best accomplished by placing garbage (a prime food source) in water-tight, rust-resistant, well sealed containers. Efforts to rat-proof buildings involve measures to prevent rats from entering through drainpipes, doors, basement windows, skylights, chimneys, and even electric wires running from the street.

This chapter has attempted to highlight those aspects of the physical environment and man's relationship to it which are of primary concern, especially to the health worker. The references for this chapter provide many sources for further exploration of the specific areas that have been reviewed.

Footnote

1   It should be noted that contamination of potable water sources by nitrates which have washed off from the soil is known to produce a condition called methemoglobinemia. This condition afflicts babies and is a form of anemia in which the synthesis of hemoglobin is impaired. As in other anemias, there are deficiencies in oxygen transport; and this can result in the infant's death. Methemoglobinemia is seen in babies whose bottled milk has been diluted with water from nitrogen-contaminated sources.

References

GENERAL

Benenson, A., ed. Control of Communicable Diseases in Man, 11th ed. New York, American Public Health Assn., 1970.

Cipolla, C. The Economic History of World Population. Baltimore, Pelican Books, 1962.

Colbourne, M. Malaria in Africa. London, Oxford University Press, 1966.

Hunter, G., Frye, W., and Swartzwelder, J. C. A Manual of Tropical Medicine, 4th ed. Philadelphia, W. B. Saunders, 1966.

Kilbourne, E. D. and Smillie, W. S. Human Ecology and Public Health, 4th ed. Toronto, Macmillan Co., 1969.
The New York Times, September 26, 1971.
Wintrobe, M. *et al.* Harrison's Principles of Internal Medicine, 6th ed. New York, McGraw-Hill, 1970.

FOODBORNE DISEASE

Fleck, A. C., Colorn, C., and Salvato, J. Milk-borne illness. *In* Hilleboe, H. and Larimore, G., eds. Preventive Medicine, 2nd ed. Philadelphia, W. B. Saunders, 1965.
Ingraham, H., Colorn, C., and Salvato, J. Food-borne illness. *In* Hilleboe, H. and Larimore, G., eds. Preventive Medicine, 2nd ed. Philadelphia, W. B. Saunders, 1965.
Johnson, P. E. Food additives. Public Health Reports 81:244, 1965.
The New York Times, December 16, 1970.
The New York Times, December 20, 1971.

WATERBORNE DISEASE

American Public Health Association. Standard Methods for Examination of Water and Waste Matter, 12th ed. New York, American Public Health Assn., 1965.
Burton, L. and Smith, H. Public Health and Community Medicine. Baltimore, Williams and Wilkins, 1970.
National Academy of Sciences. Waste Management and Control, Publication 1400. Washington, D. C., U. S. Government Printing Office, 1966.
The New York Times, October 24, 1971.

AIR POLLUTION

Commissioner of Health, City of New York. Advisory Bulletin for Physicians Regarding Air Pollution. New York, Office of the Commissioner of Health, 1971.
Commoner, B. The Origins of the Environmental Crisis. Stockholm, Sweden, Keynote address before the Council of Europe, Second Symposium of Members of Parliament Specialists in Public Health, July 1, 1971.
Commoner, B. The Closing Circle. New York, Alfred Knopf, 1971.
Iglauer, E. The ambient air. New Yorker Magazine, April 13, 1968.
McCarroll, J. Influence of the physical environment on health and disease. *In* Kilbourne, E. and Smillie, W., eds. Human Ecology and Public Health, 4th ed. Toronto, Macmillan, 1969.
The New York Times, January 31, 1972.
Public Health Service Publication No. 1556. The Effects of Air Pollution. Washington, D. C., U. S. Government Printing Office, 1967.

Public Health Services Publication No. 1548. The Sources of Air Pollution. Washington, D. C., U. S. Government Printing Office, 1966.

ECOLOGY AND ENVIRONMENTAL POLLUTION

Commoner, B. The Closing Circle. New York, Alfred Knopf, 1971.
Dubos, R. Elements of Adaptibility, The Environmental Handbook.
Edelson, E. The Battle for Clean Air. Public Affairs Pamphlet Nos. 403 and 381.
Gafater, W., Ed. Occupational Diseases: A Guide to Their Recognition. Washington, D. C., U. S. Department of Health, Education, and Welfare, Public Health Service Publication No. 1097, Washington, D. C., U. S. Government Printing Office.
Health Resources Statistics, List of Health Occupations. Washington, D. C., U. S. Department of Health, Education, and Welfare, February 1971.
Scientific American. The Biosphere. September, 1970. Special Issue.
Scientific American. Energy and Power. September, 1971. Special Issue.
The New York Times, July 18, 1971.

RADIATION

Baetjer, A. Radiation. In Sartwell, P., ed. Maxcy-Rosenau Preventive Medicine and Public Health, 9th ed. New York, Appleton-Century-Crofts, 1965.
Hilleboe, H. and Larimore, G. Preventive Medicine. Philadelphia, W. B. Saunders Co., 1965.
Johnson, K. Ionizing radiation. In Kilbourne, E. and Smillie, W., eds. Human Ecology and Public Health, 4th ed. Toronto, Macmillan, 1969.
Metzger, P. Dear Sir: Your House is Built on Radioactive Uranium Waste. The New York Times Magazine, October 31, 1971.
Toland, J. The Rising Sun. New York, Random House, 1970.
Whittenberger, J. The physical and chemical environment. In Clark, D. and MacMahon, B., eds. Preventive Medicine. Boston, Little, Brown, 1967.

PESTS

Barnako, D. Rats, J.A.M.A. **218**:5, 1971.
Davis, D. E. Control of rats and other rodents. In Sartwell, P. E., ed. Maxcy-Rosenau Preventive Medicine and Public Health, 9th ed. New York, Appleton-Century-Crofts, 1965.
Sawitz, W. G. Medical Parasitology. New York, McGraw-Hill, 1956.
Zinsser, H. Rats, Lice, and History. New York, Bantam Books, 1967.

10

Trends Affecting Health Care

The preceding chapters have included a general consideration of health and disease as well as an introduction to certain disease entities and the methods used in their study and control. In addition, we have explored various factors related to the promotion of health, the causation and prevention of illness and disability, and the diagnosis and treatment of a number of specific diseases.

In the remainder of this book we will examine in some detail the relationships and arrangements through which medical and related health services have been, are, and might be made available to individuals, families, and to the population at large. Attention will be given to those factors which affect the nature, the structure, and the organization of these services, to their costs, and to the methods by which costs are met. Finally, we will discuss some of the variables which affect the ways and the extent to which medical care services are utilized.

HISTORICAL BACKGROUND

In today's world most industrialized nations recognize health care as a basic necessity which, along with food, clothing, and shelter, should be available to the entire population. This idea and many others which characterize contemporary health care systems have their roots in the past, and it is thus of interest to sketch briefly an historical framework within which we can visualize where we were and where we are, before we consider where we seem to be going.

Evidence of social concern for the health of people in early societies is plentiful. In primitive cultures the physician was also a priest and sorcerer. He was called a shaman (medicine man), and shamanism consisted of consulting the oracles to determine the nature of a person's illness and the proper technique to cure it. The Babylonians developed surgical codes for their physician-priests: The Code of Hammurabi (2250 B.C.) specified certain conditions of medical practice and stipulated what fees physicians might charge. In early Hebrew history we can find the roots of some of our present concern with sanitation and dietetics. In fact, Hebrew biblical prohibitions constitute what amounts to the first historical concern with preventing epidemics and promoting community health.

Medicine in ancient Greece was an itinerant vocation, and the Hippocratic physician wandered from town to town practicing his craft. Medical care in small towns was available only in this manner. Physicians would arrive, open small shops (iaterons), and finally move on when business became slow. In larger Greek cities, physicians were employed by the municipal government and given a salary raised from a specific tax. By the end of the fifth century B.C., this pattern of providing care was generally followed in all Greek cities and wherever Greek culture existed.

In the early days of the Roman Republic, health care was delivered first by priests, later by slaves, and then by freedmen. Around 3 B.C., Greek physicians began to migrate to Rome and became well known for their abilities. For the most part, only the wealthy classes benefited from the practice of medicine during the Republican period and the early years of the Roman Empire. By the second century, however, the Greek model became predominant, and municipal physicians (archiatri populares) were appointed in Roman towns and cities to provide services to all the residents, but especially to the poor.

Other forms of medical practice are also found in Roman history. Most physicians were in private practice similar to the prevailing pattern in the United States today. There were also groups of salaried doctors attached to the military, the imperial court, gladiatorial schools, and the baths. Other physicians were employed by prominent families who paid them an annual fee to provide whatever services were needed during the year.

During the Middle Ages, the practice of medicine again became closely associated with religion. All of medieval society was dominated by the Church, and health care was no exception. Physicians were usually clerics, financially supported by the Church, so that medicine could be practiced in a charitable manner. By the eleventh century, however, laymen began to enter the medical profession and, as had been a pattern in ancient Greece and Rome, accepted salaried posts as municipal doctors or became associated with prominent families. The great intellectual expansion which characterized the Renaissance led to an increasing emphasis on science, and during this period (roughly from the middle of the fourteenth century to the middle of the seventeenth century) physicians began to receive training in universities. They also began practicing in guilds, an arrangement which was something of a forerunner of modern group practice.

During the eighteenth century the Industrial Revolution began to transform the Western world from an essentially rural culture to an industrial society. The problem of the urban laboring-poor commanded significant attention from those concerned with shaping social policy; and this policy was addressed primarily to the question of poverty. It was through this concern that social philosophers began to consider the problems of sickness and health care. In the United States our present health care programs for **indigent** and **medically indigent** persons have their ideological roots in this period. In addition, the idea of collective protection—one of the basic tenets of contemporary health insurance—emerged in France in the late 1700s as a direct result of conditions produced by the Industrial Revolution. Many social organizations in Europe began to apply the principles of **collective protection** to meet exigencies which threatened employed persons, e.g., funeral expenses, unemployment, sickness, forced retirement, and the need for survivor benefits.

INDIGENT: needy; destitute; unable to provide food, clothing, shelter, and health care for oneself

MEDICALLY INDIGENT: financially unable to provide health care for oneself, although able to afford other basic necessities, such as food, clothing, and shelter

COLLECTIVE PROTECTION: sharing the economic risks of illness and disability by spreading the hazards over a large population group

During the nineteenth century in Europe, health care increasingly became an area of national concern. In 1865 a program of public medicine (zemstov) was introduced in Czarist Russia. In 1883 Bismarck, the leader of a conservative government in Germany, responded to social demand and instituted a national program for compulsory sickness insurance for workers (Krankenkasse). As the turn of the century approached, other European countries developed programs which reflected a growing recognition that health care was a national responsibility and that health services for the majority of people could not be provided on a private basis. In 1911 the British Prime Minister Lloyd George established a system of national health insurance which was the precursor of England's present National Health Service.

While these changes, triggered principally by the Industrial Revolution, were going on in Europe, major developments in health care were also occurring in the United States. Although they were primarily concerned with survival in a new and often hostile land, the early settlers of our nation did direct some private and public resources to the sick and the poor. During the colonial period, public funds were allocated to build several almshouses in more populated areas, and health care was provided through municipal physicians and midwives. Private resources, elicited through voluntary subscriptions, were responsible for the development of this country's first hospital (Pennsylvania Hospital) in 1786. Later in that century, the College of Philadelphia established a professorship in the theoretical and practical aspects of medicine. This move marked the beginning of the first American medical school, and this school soon became affiliated with Pennsylvania Hospital.

Towards the end of the eighteenth century, the first local health department was formed in Baltimore, Maryland; and in 1798 an act of Congress established the Marine Hospital Service, which provided temporary relief and maintenance for sick and disabled merchant seamen. Financed through compulsory taxes and federally administered, this was the country's first organized and nationally significant effort to protect groups of people against the risks of ill health. The Marine Hospital Service later evolved into our present national Public Health Service. During the middle and late 1800s, both the American Medical Association (1847) and the American Dental Association (1889) were formed. In addition, it will be remembered from Chapter 7 that this was a period of relative enlightenment in the treatment of mental illness; and the crusading efforts of such prominent citizens as Dorothy Dix helped spur the building of state hospitals for the care of the mentally ill.

From the middle of the nineteenth century to the early twentieth century the pressures of industrialization and urbanization were felt in this country, and the health problems of urban wage-earners received increasing attention. Many private groups with varying special interests in health were organized, and public support was solicited for many different programs in health-related areas. These private groups included the American Public Health Association, the American Red Cross, the National Health Council, and so on. During this period, the Flexner report, which documented the state of medical education in Canada and the United States, was published. This report significantly influenced the development of quality standards for medical school graduates and had the effect of reducing considerably the number of medical schools which had proliferated in the United States. In the public sector, the Children's Bureau was established and became a powerful force in promoting measures to safeguard the health of mothers and children. There was also the passage of the Federal Food and Drug Act and workmen's compensation laws. In fact, during the early 1900s vigorous national debate was centered on workmen's compensation, a program which had already been widely accepted by other industrial countries since its introduction by Bismarck. The concern which this question mobilized led to an increased interest in establishing a broad-based national health insurance program. Today, almost 50 years later, compulsory national health insurance is still a prominent and controversial issue. It is interesting to note that during the early years of the American labor movement, the American Medical Association favored national action for health care, whereas organized labor was opposed to such action; today the reverse is true.

While the question of compulsory national health insurance remains unsettled, there has been a growth of various prepaid health insurance plans during the last 30 years. In addition, there have been several amendments to the Social Security Act which have authorized federal matching funds to states for direct payment of medical care services to patients who receive public assistance or who are medically indigent. Most famous of these amendments was the one (passed in 1965) establishing Titles XVIII and XIX—Medicare and Medicaid, respectively. Medicare provided a federally administered program of health insurance for the aged. This included hospital insurance financed through social security taxes and a voluntary program of supplementary benefits, financed by matching contributions. Title XIX, known locally as Medicaid, provided for an expanded and unified program of grants to states for medical assistance and was intended eventually to replace existing medical care provisions under all public assistance programs. The growth of social concern with health care in the United States, the existing national programs, and potential programs are discussed in greater depth in Chapter 12.

We have briefly summarized some of the significant historical developments to which, in part, the origins of modern health care systems and, especially, the current American system can be traced. Actually, the pattern of health care in every era of history up to the present reflects an interaction between available technology and the existing social structure. Changes in scientific, technologic, social, demographic, and economic factors change the shape and nature of these patterns in a society. In the remainder of this chapter we will identify significant trends in these areas and examine general trends in health and medical care which themselves have an impact on and create problems within the health care system.

TRENDS IN SCIENCE AND TECHNOLOGY

Technological and scientific advancements related to health have been both dramatic and significant. The discovery and development of penicillin and other antibiotics have, of course, been milestones in medical progress. While organ transplants are among the most spectacular medical achievements in recent years, it is perhaps of greater importance that our newly discovered ability to synthesize active DNA has paved the way for increased knowledge of the gene, of virus infections, and of life itself. Often, the medical advances of just a few years produce major changes which alter practice standards and, of equal importance, the expectations of patients.

Complicated diagnostic and laboratory equipment, long available only in hospitals, is now being developed for use in patients' homes. A vast array of equipment already aids the physician and other health personnel in the prevention, diagnosis, and treatment of disease and illness and in the rehabilitation of patients. The computer, a major example of such equipment, now appears to be a necessary part of medical technology. Within the laboratory, the computer's usefulness ranges from keeping track of samples to producing final reports. With its ability to monitor care and provide vital information continuously, the computer is becoming an essential part of intensive care units. In addition, computers are now engaged in determining the availability of hospital beds, in dispensing drugs, in scheduling hospital services, and in calculating, storing, and retrieving data of all kinds.

Progress in science and technology has dramatically expanded medicine's overall capacity to help the patient. With this expanded capacity for effectiveness, medical science has also become increasingly more complex; as a result, more and more attention must be given to the organization and delivery of health care. As medicine has changed from an individualized profession to a labyrinthine and interdependent industry, not only have diagnostic and therapeutic procedures become more complex, but the relationships between different types of health care personnel have been altered significantly. It is no longer possible for a single physician to provide the complete gamut of medical care as he did in years past. The sheer mass of knowledge and skills, ever increasing, cannot be effectively absorbed by any single physician or health worker. For this reason, health manpower has become increasingly specialized. For example, diagnostic services often require the particular skills of the x-ray technician, medical technologist, laboratory assistant, cytotechnologist, histologic technician, and a host of others. The same is true for therapeutic services, where skills are provided by specialists in inhalation therapy, social work, speech pathology, physical therapy, and so on. Specialization among physicians themselves has been increasing for a number of years, with a corresponding decrease in the number of general practitioners. As shown in Figure 10-1, general practitioners represented about four-fifths of the active practicing physicians in 1931, while full-time specialists made up about one-fifth. At present, the trend has changed, with the specialists comprising more than half of all physicians actively practicing their profession.

Related both to scientific and technologic advances and to the associated increase in specialization is an overall decline in the private, fee-for-service practice of medicine. The number of physicians with full-time salaried positions in hospitals and medical schools, in administrative, laboratory, and preventive medicine, and in research is steadily increasing. Excluding physicians in the federal government, doctors in private practice represented about two-thirds of all active physicians in 1960; today they account for less than 60 percent.

Although the proliferation of knowledge and skills has obvious benefits, it is not entirely without disadvantages and problems. For example, one consequence of specialization is fragmentation. The continued decline in the number of general practitioners in active practice is partly responsible for the overcrowded hospital emergency rooms and outpatient departments which are so familiar today. In such settings, care tends to be episodic, depersonalized, and uncoordinated. On the one hand, medical science becomes more and more effective as scientific and technologic progress is implemented; on the other hand, progress in medical science has produced serious inefficiencies in the delivery of medical care services.

Scientific and technologic advances also contribute to another problem area, namely, rising costs. Newly developed diagnostic and therapeutic equipment is purchased by hospitals and other health care institutions

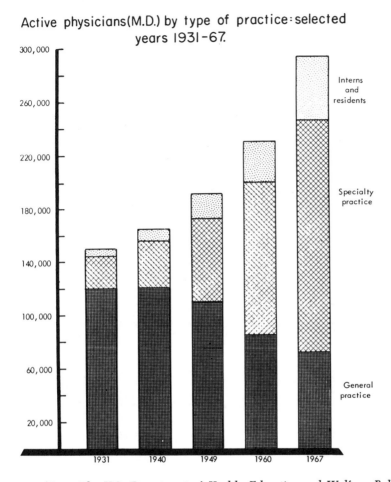

Active physicians(M.D.) by type of practice=selected years 1931-67.

FIG. 10-1. *(From The U.S. Department of Health, Education and Welfare, Public Health Service, Health Manpower Source Book. PHS. no. 263, Section 20, Washington, D.C., U.S. Government Printing Office, 1969.)*

which, in turn, must employ the needed additional personnel. The costs incurred are reflected in increased fees and charges to patients or **third-party payers.** Over the past 15 years, **private-consumer expenditures** for

---

THIRD-PARTY PAYERS: groups or sources, such as private health insurance, federal, state, and local governments, employers, and others who purchase or provide health services on behalf of individuals or groups of people

health care have increased by about $20 billion annually. Of this increase, over 37 percent represents scientific and technologic advances and a correspondingly greater demand and utilization of services. In addition, although the **consumer price index** (CPI) for all types of goods and services shows a continuing and steady rise, the index for health care is rising even faster. During the ten-year period between 1960 and 1970, for example, the CPI for all items increased by about 28 percent compared to a 42-percent increase for medical care (Fig. 10-2).

If just the CPI hospital and physician components are considered, a sharper rise can be seen in daily hospital service charges than in physicians' fees. In 1945 it cost **community hospitals** an average of $9.39 per day to treat one patient; at present, this figure exceeds $70 per day. Of course, the amount the hospital charges the patient is higher than the cost of providing the services. The current average charge in a community hospital is close to $100 per day, and it is even higher in many large medical centers and teaching hospitals.

Given the further development and implementation of scientific and technologic knowledge, and some degree of inflation, health care prices are bound to show an unrelenting increase. It therefore seems most likely that the public and third-party payers will find it even more difficult to meet the costs of future health services unless consumers and health professionals alike seek ways to insure economy in the delivery of these services.

SOCIOECONOMIC AND DEMOGRAPHIC TRENDS

A number of socioeconomic and demographic factors are related to health care; in fact, such factors constitute the major deter-

---

PRIVATE-CONSUMER EXPENDITURES (for health care): all direct payments for health care made by individuals themselves or on their behalf; includes private health insurance but excludes government expenditures

CONSUMER PRICE INDEX: a technique to measure changes, over a period of time, in the average price of goods and services, including health care

COMMUNITY HOSPITAL: according to the American Public Health Association, "a facility having an organized staff providing services especially for inpatient care of individuals who require definitive diagnosis and treatment for illness, injury, or other disability, and which also regularly make available at least clinical laboratory services, diagnostic x-ray services, and other equipment and services for definite clinical treatment." The term is frequently used to describe a hospital which is not associated with a medical school.

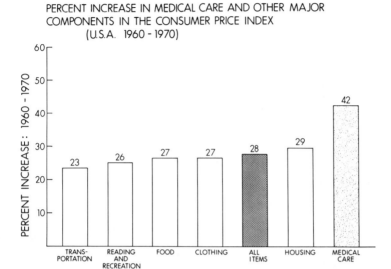

PERCENT INCREASE IN MEDICAL CARE AND OTHER MAJOR
COMPONENTS IN THE CONSUMER PRICE INDEX
(U.S.A. 1960 - 1970)

FIG. 10-2. (*Adapted from* Medical Chart Book, *University of Michigan, School of Public Health, Third Edition, Revised 1968.*)

minants of health care utilization (see Chapter 12).

Population increase is one of the most important demographic trends, since an absolute increase in total population results in increased demand for health services. In 1970 the population of the United States approximated 205 million. The Bureau of the Census projects an increase to over 361 million by the year 2000.

Of at least equal importance is a pronounced shift in the proportion of various age groups in the total population. Persons under 20 continue to make up an increasing proportion of the population; between 1960 and 1999 the number of such young persons will increase from 38 percent of the total population to over 42 percent. Aged persons also show a percentage gain, and projections indicate that by 1990 over half of the population will be under 20 or over 65 years of age. Since persons between these ages constitute the major portion of the labor force, about half of the nation's population will be working to support the other half by the end of this century.

A further factor to be considered is the high mobility of this country's population, about 20 percent of which moves each year. Much of this moving reflects a decided trend toward urbanization. The farm population, as a percent of total population, has decreased markedly over the past 50 years, from 30 percent in 1920 to about 5 percent at present. In addi-

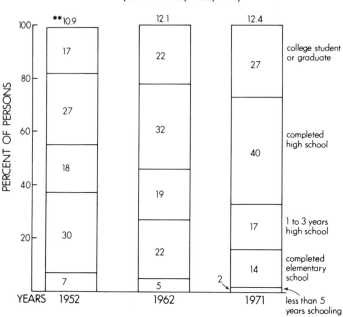

FIG. 10-3. (*Adapted from statistics in* Statistical Abstract of the United States, *U.S. Department of Commerce, 1971.*)

tion, information from the Bureau of the Census indicates that between 1950 and 1970 urban population increased from 64 percent of the total population to about 74 percent, whereas rural population decreased from 36 to 27 percent. Population in urban fringe areas increased from about 14 to over 27 percent, while the population of central cities remained relatively stable at about 32 percent of all types of urban areas.

Education and income provide some measure of national achievement, and there is a definite relationship between these social factors and the use of health services. That the nation is becoming better educated is reflected in the steady decline in the percentage of the population which is illiterate. Educational attainment is also measured by the number of high school and college graduates, the number of earned degrees, and the median school years completed—all of which continue to increase (Fig. 10-3). Of particular importance is the increased percentage of 17-

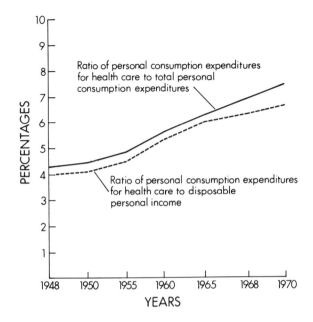

FIG. 10-4.   *Ratio of personal consumption expenditures for health care to total personal consumption expenditures and to disposable personal income, selected years 1948–1970, U.S.A. (From* Source Book of Health Insurance Data, *Health Insurance Institute, 1971–1972.)*

year-olds who complete high school. At the turn of the century only 6 percent were graduates; the number had increased to over 50 percent just prior to World War II, to over 65 percent by 1960, and to over 78 percent by 1967. Moreover, the **median** number of school years completed rose from 10.9 in 1952 to 12.4 in 1971; during this period, there was a considerable increase in the number of earned degrees conferred by institutions of higher learning.

In addition to education, it is important for the purposes of health care planning to have a measure of national economic well-being. One such measure is the Gross National Product (GNP). Growth in the GNP has been persistent, and indicates that this nation is the most affluent in the world. In 1940 the GNP was calculated at about $100 billion; it had increased to about $504 billion by 1960, and quite recently it approximated $750 billion. However, more important than the aggregate GNP

MEDIAN: a numerical value which divides a series so that one-half or more of the items are equal to or greater than the value

figures are the continuing increases in **per capita income, disposable personal income, and personal consumption expenditures.** Greater consumption expenditures reflect augmented spending ability, given the rise in per capita and disposable income. Between 1950 and 1968 per capita income increased by $865, disposable personal income increased by $686, and personal consumption expenditures rose over $600. The service component of the last increased most rapidly, and, according to the Public Health Service, personal consumption expenditures for health care have increased steadily, and represent the greatest percentage increase.

Figure 10-4 shows the relationship between all personal consumption expenditures and those for health care. The amount spent privately for health care more than quadrupled between 1948 and 1970. The ratio between expenditures rose from 4 percent to almost 8 percent. A similar increase (4 percent to almost 7 percent) is shown for the ratio of personal expenditures for health care to total disposable income.

Although the United States is an affluent country, about one-fourth of all families still had incomes of less than $5,000 in 1967, and over 12 percent had incomes of under $3,000. (In 1950 about 60 percent of all families had incomes of under $5,000; by 1960 the percentage had decreased to about 36 percent.) Middle-income ($5,000 to $9,999) families made up over one-third of the population in 1950, 44 percent in 1960, and 40 percent in 1967. Families with incomes of $10,000 or more comprised 8 percent of the population in 1950, 20 percent in 1960, and 25 percent in 1967. Between 1950 and 1967, median family income increased over $3,360, from $4,611 to $7,974.

HEALTH AND HEALTH CARE TRENDS

Scientific, technologic, socioeconomic, and demographic changes have influences which, in turn, generate trends in health and health care; and these trends ultimately affect the nature and organization of the health care system. For example, mortality and morbidity patterns reflect the changing population structure. Mortality rates have shown a steady downward trend since 1900, with a corresponding increase in life expectancy. Longevity gains have resulted largely from the conquest of acute, infectious diseases; and a larger proportion of the

---

PER CAPITA INCOME: national income divided by the population
DISPOSABLE PERSONAL INCOME: income after taxes
PERSONAL CONSUMPTION EXPENDITURES: purchases of goods and services by individuals or families

Private and Public Expenditures for Health and Medical Care
(U.S.A.,Selected Years,1928-1929—1968-1969).

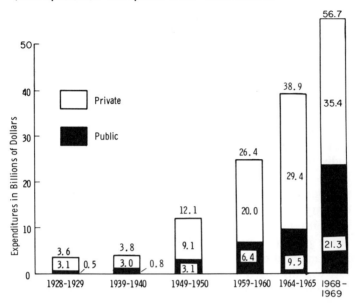

FIG. 10-5. *(After* Medical Chart Book, *University of Michigan, School of Public
Health, Third Edition, Revised 1968.)*

population now reaches middle and old age, where chronic, long-term illnesses predominate. The reader will recall that Table 4-7, which contrasts
the 10 leading causes of death in 1900 with those in the late 1960s, indicated the changing patterns from acute to chronic disease.

As a review of Chapter 5 will confirm, morbidity patterns reflect the
decline in infectious illness and a corresponding increase in chronic disease. Data from the U.S. National Health Survey reveals that over 40
percent of the population reported one or more chronic diseases or impairments during a recent year, with an average of two conditions per
person. Heart disease, arthritis, and rheumatism were the leading causes
of activity limitation. As age increases, so does the proportion of persons
with chronic conditions; 80 percent of persons aged 65 or over had at
least one chronic illness, while this was true in only 20 percent of those
aged 17 or younger.

The various trends reviewed in this chapter have a telling impact on
health economics and medical care organization. That medicine is big
business is clearly shown in the amount spent nationally for health and

medical care: $56.7 billion in the fiscal year 1968 to 1969, an increase of over $17 billion from the fiscal year 1964 to 1965. The increasing economic importance of health is underscored further if national expenditures are viewed since 1928 to 1929, at which time total health expenditures were $3.6 billion, or 3.6 percent of the GNP. In the fiscal year 1949 to 1950 this figure increased to over $12 billion and 4.6 percent of the GNP; and the 1968-to-1969 total health expenditures of $56.7 billion represents 6.6 percent of the GNP (Fig. 10-5). During these years there has been a simultaneous trend toward greater public expenditures for health and medical care. From 1928 to 1929 public sources contributed only 13 percent of the total cost. This figure increased to about 25 percent from 1964 to 1965, and presently exceeds 37 percent.

Appendix 9 provides a detailed analysis of health and medical care expenditures.

Developments related to medical care personnel, facilities, and services are as dramatic as those in health economics. The changing mortality and morbidity patterns, coupled with the demographic shifts already mentioned, have produced urgent problems in terms of the supply and distribution of medical care resources. The trend toward specialized health manpower was discussed earlier in this chapter. Trends in overall supply of health manpower show that during the period 1955 to 1965 population increased by 17 percent, but the number of active practicing physicians rose only 22 percent and that of active nonfederal dentists increased only 13 percent. The greatest growth was in the supply of supportive health manpower and professional nurses. The percentage increase in the number of physicians is higher than the percent of population increase, and this may imply some improvement in the ratio of physicians to population. However, because of an increased demand for and utilization of physicians' services, this slightly better ratio is still far from adequate, and there remains a shortage of physicians in this country. Moreover, the National Advisory Commission on Health Manpower has pointed that in spite of an expected increase in the number of medical school graduates, this shortage will become even more acute as the demand for care grows. Maldistribution of health manpower is also a problem, and plans have emerged to redistribute personnel in order to meet the needs of a population which has shifted increasingly to metropolitan areas.

With regard to facilities, the number of community hospitals increased about 8 percent since 1960, and there are now over 5,850 such hospitals in the nation (if all federal, psychiatric, and other nonfederal long-term hospitals are included, the total number is over 7,100). During this same period, however, the number of community hospital *beds* increased over 29 percent, mushrooming from 639,000 to 826,000. **Skilled nursing care** homes and beds have also increased, particularly since the introduction of Medicare in 1965. Such facilities grew from 7,000 in 1954 to 11,600 in 1967, with a corresponding rise in the number of skilled nursing care beds from 180,000 to 546,000.

In just the last few years, the number of community hospitals has remained relatively stable, although the population continues to increase. In addition, many of these facilities are in need of modernization or replacement. Most were built to accommodate only persons with short-term, acute conditions, and physically cannot provide the comprehensive array of hospital and related services required by the increasing number of chronically ill persons. Little rational *organization* of facilities exists at present. Although there are voluntary controls on the distribution and number of community hospital beds, many areas of the country can build at will, with minimum attention to actual need. Cooperation among hospitals and between hospitals and other health care institutions is not strong enough to be viewed as a definite pattern. Cooperation may exist in such administrative areas as joint purchasing and standardization of records, but there is no specific national mandate for patient care coordination among facilities.

Extended care facilities, including skilled nursing care institutions, are now increasing at a slow rate, with the number of beds growing somewhat faster. Whether such facilities are in the mainstream of medical care is doubtful. Although forced by federal regulations to develop relationships with community hospitals, nursing homes remain on the periphery of institutional health care.

Along with the trends in the supply of medical care resources are those in medical care services; of particular note are hospital-based **home care** and **family health maintenance** programs. Home care services were initiated in 1947 at Montefiore Hospital in New York City, and there are

---

SKILLED NURSING CARE HOME: a facility which makes available services primarily for inpatient care of persons who require significant nursing care and related medical services but who do not require hospital care

EXTENDED CARE FACILITIES: a term developed by the federal government to describe those facilities which participate in the Medicare program and provide more types of medical and nursing services than one would expect to find in the usual nursing home

HOME CARE: services provided in the patient's home by nurses, physical therapists, and other health workers and under the aegis of an organized agency

FAMILY HEALTH MAINTENANCE: a number of interrelated preventive, educational, social, and rehabilitative services, coordinated for application to the family as a group rather than on behalf of an individual patient or family member

now about 100 home care programs throughout the country. They are located primarily in urban settings and provide a variety of services, ranging from housekeeping assistance to a complex array of nursing, medical, and social services needed by the homebound patient. Within recent years, health maintenance programs which focus on families rather than individuals have been established in large medical centers and in some prepaid medical groups.

Another organized service (initiated after World War II) is multiphasic screening. At present, there are approximately 15 such screening programs, many of them funded by grants or contracts from the Public Health Service. Basically preventive in nature, these programs focus on the mass detection of diseases by using sophisticated, frequently automated tests and techniques. Multiphasic screening programs are based mostly in large medical centers and municipal or state health departments, although some are found within prepaid medical groups or in association with industrial medical care programs. (Some of the problems related to screening programs have been reviewed in Chapter 3.)

Home care, multiphasic screening, group medical practice, and family health maintenance programs appear to have developed because of gaps in the existing medical care process. There is, in addition, concern with the need to provide **comprehensive services.** Every segment of the medical care process receives organizational attention, and service programs such as home care or neighborhood health centers are usually viewed and evaluated as independent units within a whole system. This, by itself, is not enough; they must additionally function and be assessed as integrated components of the macrocosm—the totality of medical care services.

This chapter has summarized the evolution of health care, the forces and motivations which influenced that evolution, and the nature of certain major trends in science and society which have an impact on health care system in the United States. The last two chapters will examine some aspects of that system in more detail, namely, its resources, its organization, and the delivery of health services.

COMPREHENSIVE SERVICES: those varied health services directed at maintaining health, preventing disease, diagnosing and treating conditions and diseases, and rehabilitating the patient who has suffered illness or injury; it is important that the gamut of needed services be readily available and effectively coordinated

References

American Medical Association. Distribution of Physicians, Hospitals and Hospital Beds in the United States by Census Region, State, County and Metropolitan Area. Chicago, American Medical Association, 1966.

Health Insurance Institute. 1971–1972 Source Book of Health Insurance Data. New York, Health Insurance Institute, 1971.

National Advisory Commission on Health Manpower. Report of the National Advisory Committee on Health Manpower, Washington, D. C., U. S. Government Printing Office, Vol. 1, 1962.

Peterson, P. Q., and Pennell, M. Medical Specialists, Health Manpower Source Book, PHS Pub. No. 263, Sec. 14, Washington, D. C., U. S. Government Printing Office, 1962.

Rice, D. P., and Cooper, B. S. National health expenditures, 1929–70. Social Security Bull., 34:3–18, 1971.

Rosen, George. A History of Public Health, New York, MD Publications, Inc., 1958.

Sigerist, H. E. On the History of Medicine, Mart-Ibañez, F., ed. New York, MD Publications, Inc., 1960.

Somers, A. R. Health Care in Transition: Directions for the Future, Chicago, Hospital Research and Educational Trust, 1971.

U.S. Department of Health, Education, and Welfare. National Center for Health Statistics. Vital and Health Statistics: Data from the National Health Survey, PHS Pub. No. 1000, Ser. 10, Washington, D. C., U. S. Government Printing Office, 1970.

U.S. Department of Health, Education, and Welfare, Public Health Service. Health Manpower Source Book, PHS Pub. No. 263, Secs. 18, 20, 21, Washington, D. C., U. S. Government Printing Office, 1969, 1970.

CHAPTER

11

Resources for Health Care

Facilities

In the United States there are numerous types of facilities in which persons receive health services: hospitals, nursing homes, extended care facilities plus a myriad of others which are primarily custodial or educational in function but which do undertake health-related activities, e.g., facilities for the deaf, blind, physically handicapped, and mentally retarded, as well as those for unwed mothers, dependent children, and alcoholics. Of primary concern to us are those facilities, such as nursing homes and hospitals, which provide inpatient services for individuals undergoing active medical treatment.

NURSING HOMES AND RELATED FACILITIES

A nursing home is a facility in which 50 percent or more of

the residents receive one or more **nursing services;** the facility must have at least one registered nurse (RN) or licensed practical nurse (LPN) employed 35 or more hours per week. As such, the nursing home should not be confused with those accommodations, often referred to as nursing homes, which are essentially boarding facilities and do not provide nursing services in the medical sense. Additional terms are used to describe such facilities: (1) **personal care home with nursing,** (2) **personal care home,** and (3) **domiciliary care home.**

Prior to the mid 1930s, indigent aged persons were often wards of local or state governments, and numerous localities had a "public almshouse." This was sometimes referred to as the state or county farm, or, more commonly, the "poor farm." When the Social Security Act was passed in 1935, many indigent aged began to receive **social insurance** rather than public assistance. Partly as a result of the increased purchasing power thus afforded the aged population, public almshouses gave way

---

NURSING SERVICES: refer to services which include nasal feeding, catheterization, irrigation, hypodermic injection, intravenous injection, oxygen therapy, full bed-bath, enema, temperature-pulse-respiration, blood pressure, application of dressing or bandage, and bowel and bladder retraining

PERSONAL CARE HOME WITH NURSING: a home in which either (1) some, but less than 5 percent of the residents, receive nursing care from RNs or LPNs or (2) more than 50 percent of the residents receive nursing care, but no RNs or LPNs are employed full-time on the staff

PERSONAL CARE HOME: a facility that routinely provides three or more personal services but no nursing services (personal services include rub or massage, assistance with bathing, dressing, correspondence or shopping, walking or getting about, or eating)

DOMICILIARY CARE HOME: a facility that routinely provides less than three of the personal services and no nursing services; this type of facility provides a sheltered environment primarily to persons unable to care for themselves

SOCIAL INSURANCE: in the United States, refers to such programs as Social Security, as opposed to private insurance or welfare; four major elements which characterize social insurance: (1) protection exists as a matter of right and not as a benevolence of a government, institution, or employer; (2) all citizens are eligible for coverage regardless of class, income level, race, and so on; (3) the individual, within the limits of his earnings, contributes to the program; (4) financial contributions are also made by the employer; existing social insurance programs include Old Age Insurance, Survivor Insurance, Disability Insurance, and Medical Insurance for the Aged; this combination is referred to as OASDMI, or the Social Security Program

to **proprietary** nursing homes and boarding facilities.

Two additional factors have contributed significantly to the growth of nursing homes in this country. First, the number of aged persons in the population is growing; and this growth, along with the shift in disease patterns from acute to chronic, has resulted in an increased demand for health care services which do not require hospitalization. Secondly, amendments to the Social Security Act now allow payment under Medicare and Medicaid for care in certain types of nursing homes. The Medicare program covers a certain amount of extended care in a facility certified to provide the skilled nursing services described above. Under the Medicaid program (limited to persons eligible for financial assistance in those states that instituted programs), an additional level of nursing care—intermediate care—is being developed in some states. Intermediate care is rather broadly explained as being less than the skilled nursing care provided in extended care facilities but more than domiciliary care usually associated with boarding homes. At present, many aged persons who are recipients of state assistance are located in skilled nursing homes even though they do not medically require such placement. The intermediate-care facility provides long-term institutional care with limited nursing services.

Tables 11-1, 11-2, and 11-3 present recent information about the various kinds of nursing homes in the United States. In 1939 there were only 1,200 such homes and about 25,000 beds. By the late 1960s they numbered 19,150, with a total of over 836,550 beds. Of all the nation's homes, 56 percent are nursing homes (as defined earlier in this chapter), 23 percent are personal care homes without nursing services, 20 percent are personal care homes with nursing services, and 1 percent are domiciliary care homes.

The greatest number of these facilities are in California (2,973), followed by Ohio (1,126), New York (1,081), Massachusetts (952), and Illinois (914). States with the least number are Alaska (4), Nevada (22), Wyoming (30), Delaware (33), and Idaho (56). As to the number of beds, figures indicate that there are 44.5 total beds per 1,000 people aged 65 and over. However, considerable variation exists when this rate is viewed by state. Iowa is the state with the highest ratio of beds to population (81.4) and West Virginia the one with the lowest ratio (11.5).

Table 11-2 presents information about the size of these homes in terms of the number of beds. Of the total number of homes, about 45 percent have under 25 beds, and one-fourth have less than 50 beds; only 9.2 percent

---

PROPRIETARY: privately owned, as opposed to public and nonprofit corporate-owned facilities

TABLE 11-1. Beds in Nursing Care and Related Homes:
United States, 1967

Beds	Total Beds	Nursing Homes	Personal Care Homes With Nursing	Without Nursing	Domiciliary Care Homes
Number	836,554	584,052	181,096	66,787	4,619
Number per 1,000 population aged 65 and over	44.5	31.0	9.6	3.6	0.2

Source: Adapted from U. S. Department of Health, Education, and Welfare. Health Resource Statistics, PHS Pub. No. 1509, Washington, D. C., U. S. Government Printing Office, 1969, pp. 260–261.

of all homes have 100 or more beds. Table 11-3 indicates the ownership of these health-care facilities. Over three-fourths of all types of long-term care facilities are proprietary and operated for profit; 15 percent are nonprofit, and just a little over 7½ percent are in the government sector. Of those classified as nursing homes (10,636), over 83 percent are proprietary, 11½ percent nonprofit, and 5 percent owned and operated by state and local governments.

It has been said that nursing home facilities must be brought into the mainstream of modern health care. This statement reflects concern with the low level of health care that exists in many facilities of this type. There is also a shortage of nursing home beds, as is revealed by an analy-

TABLE 11-2. Percent Distribution of Nursing Care and
Related Homes by Bed Size: United States, 1967

Bed Size	Total Homes	Nursing Homes	Personal Care Homes With Nursing	Without Nursing	Domiciliary Care Homes
			Percent Distribution		
Under 25 beds	44.6	25.1	48.6	85.3	85.4
25–49	25.4	32.8	22.7	10.8	9.8
50–74	14.1	20.2	11.4	2.5	2.0
75–99	6.7	10.0	5.2	0.5	0.8
100–199	7.5	10.1	8.7	0.8	0.4
200–299	1.1	1.2	2.1	0.1	0.4
300–499	0.5	0.5	1.0	...	1.2
500–999	0.1	0.1	0.2	...	...
1,000 beds or more	0.0	0.0	0.1	...	...

Source: Adapted from U. S. Department of Health, Education, and Welfare. Health Resource Statistics, PHS Pub. No. 1509, Washington, D. C., U. S. Government Printing Office, 1969, p. 262.

TABLE 11-3. Ownership of Nursing Care and Related Homes:
United States, 1967

| Ownership | Total Homes | Nursing Homes | Personal Care Homes | | Domiciliary Care Homes |
			With Nursing	Without Nursing	
Total	19,141	10,636	3,853	4,396	256
			Percent Distribution		
Government	7.6	5.0	8.0	13.2	14.0
Federal	0.1	<1	0.1	0.3	...
State-local	7.5	5.0	7.9	12.9	14.0
Proprietary	77.5	83.5	62.5	76.3	73.4
Nonprofit	14.9	11.5	29.4	10.4	12.5
Church	5.2	3.9	11.7	2.9	3.5
Other	9.7	7.6	11.7	7.5	9.0

Source: Adapted from U. S. Department of Health, Education, and Welfare, Health Resource Statistics, PHS Pub. No. 1509, Washington, D. C., U. S. Government Printing Office, 1969, p. 262.

sis of the ratio of beds to population aged 65 and over. In addition, many nursing homes are unacceptable under the standards of the Hill-Burton Act in that their nursing personnel are not only in short supply but often are inadequately trained, and there is frequently little provision for medical care. A large number of nursing homes and related facilities lack the resources necessary to provide rehabilitative or restorative services. All too frequently patients are left in bed for an excessive period of time and receive only minimal custodial care.

New federal standards under the Medicare program and new requirements (federal and state) under the Medicaid program are helping to resolve some of these problems. It is also important that there be closer and more formal affiliations of nursing homes with community hospitals and with the teaching programs of medical centers. Classification of nursing homes and patients is needed so that there is a more appropriate matching of the patient's need to the resources of a particular nursing home.

A recent study of nursing homes and their patients was conducted in New Haven, Connecticut. One of the major sets of recommendations resulting from this study focused on the need to expand the public health codes governing nursing homes. The researchers found that the medical records revealed serious gaps in such areas as the transfer of information from hospitals to nursing homes and in the charting techniques used by nursing home personnel. Expansion of public health codes to correct deficiencies is a necessity, but the mere expansion of regulations or the promulgation of new standards becomes an academic exercise unless they are applied.

HOSPITALS

Hospitals have played a major role both in providing health services and in shaping the present system of health care. Table 11-4 highlights some selected information about hospitals in this country during the 1960s.

According to the American Hospital Association, there were over 7,100 hospitals of all types in 1969. Between 1960 and 1969 the total number of hospitals increased by about 4 percent, while the number of hospital beds actually decreased slightly. As shown in Table 11-4, the reduction in beds occurred in noncommunity or long-term facilities. Although the total number of hospitals increased about 4 percent during the decade, the number of admissions rose by almost 23 percent, and the number of **outpatient** visits increased sharply, by about 64 percent. As if to keep up with the increased patient load, the number of hospital personnel rose by almost 52 percent. Of special concern to consumers of health services is the dramatic increase in the total hospital expense, which rose by almost 163 percent between 1960 and 1969.

The term *community hospital* was defined earlier in this chapter. However, additional explanation is needed. Community hospitals are those facilities in which most people receive hospital care. Because community hospitals predominate, they will receive particular attention in this discussion. In the aggregate, community hospitals are the major providers of health services and, in the words of the American Hospital Association, "tend to reflect the pattern of advancement in medical service." During the period 1960 to 1969 the number of these hospitals increased by over 8 percent, their beds by over 29 percent, and the number of admissions by 23 percent. A further look at Table 11-4 reveals that the percentage change in all categories of items increased more for community hospitals than for

---

HOSPITAL: a facility which has an organized medical staff providing services primarily for inpatient care of individuals who require definite diagnosis and treatment for illness, injury, or other disability, and which regularly makes available at least clinical laboratory services, diagnostic x-ray services, and other equipment and services for definitive clinical treatment

OUTPATIENT: a patient who is not lodged in a hospital at the time he receives its medical, dental, or allied services

TABLE 11-4. Selected Hospital Information: United States, 1960-69

Item	United States—Total			Community Hospitals[a]			Noncommunity Hospitals[b]		
	1960	1969	Percent Change	1960	1969	Percent Change	1960	1969	Percent Change
Number of hospitals	6,876	7,144	+3.9	5,407	5,853	+8.2	1,469	1,291	-12.1
Number of beds (000s)	1,658	1,650	-0.5	639	826	+29.3	1,019	824	-19.1
Number of admissions	25,027	30,729	+22.8	22,970	28,254	+23.0	2,057	2,475	+20.3
Average daily census[d] (000s)	1,402	1,346	-4.0	477	651	+36.5	925	695	-24.9
Number of outpatient visits (000s)	99,382[c]	163,248	+64.3	70,727[c]	120,831	+70.8	28,655[a]	42,417	+48.0
Total expense (000,000s)	$8,421	$22,103	+162.5	$5,617	$16,613	+195.8	$2,804	$5,490	+95.8
Payroll expense (000,000s)	$5,588	$13,803	+147.0	$3,499	$9,813	+180.5	$2,089	$3,990	+91.0
Personnel (000s)	1,598	2,426	+51.8	1,080	1,824	+68.9	518	602	+16.2

[a]Community hospitals is the term used to describe all short-term, nonfederal institutions providing general and selected special hospital services.
[b]Noncommunity hospitals include all federal hospital institutions, all psychiatric institutions, and all other long-term nonfederal hospitals.
[c]Data are for 1962; data are not available for 1960 or 1961.
[d]Average daily census is the average number of inpatients per day for each year.

Source: American Hospital Association. Hospitals (Guide Issue) 44:(15) 463 (1970).

Short-term hospital: hospital in which 50 percent of all patients admitted have a length of stay of less than 30 days
Long-term hospital: hospital in which 50 percent of all patients admitted have a length of stay of 30 days or more
Psychiatric hospital: includes hospitals in the following categories: psychiatric, epilepsy, mental retardation and alcoholism and/or addictive diseases

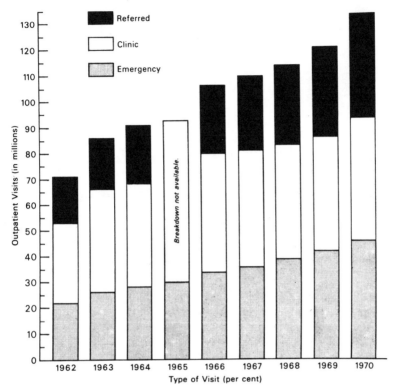

NUMBER AND TYPE OF OUTPATIENT VISITS TO COMMUNITY
HOSPITALS, 1962-1970

Fig. 11-1.   *Since 1962, the proportion of clinic visits has decreased while the percentage of referred visits has increased. Perhaps this indicates the emphasis in community hospitals on replacing the diagnostic and therapeutic
services previously offered in physicians' offices.* (From Hospitals, American Hospital Association, Guide Issue, Volume 45, August 1, 1971.)

all types of hospitals and also more than the single category *noncommunity hospitals.* Studies have shown that the dramatic increase in outpatient visits to community hospitals reflects the fact that patients have
turned to the hospital emergency room and clinics for their nonemergent
care (Fig. 11-1). In other words, many persons use these **ambulatory care**

AMBULATORY CARE: refers to all types of services which may be provided on an outpatient basis, in contrast to services provided in the home or to
persons who are inpatients; while many inpatients may be ambulatory, the term *ambulatory care* usually implies that the
patient has come to a location to receive services and has de-
parted the same day after receiving those services

TABLE 11-5. Hospitals by Ownership and Type of Service: United States, 1969

	Hospitals		Beds		Admission		Average Daily Census	Occupancy	Average Stay (Days)
	Number	Percent[a]	Number	Percent[a]	Number	Percent[a]			
All hospitals	7,144	100.0	1,650,000	100.0	30,729,000	100.0	1,346	81.6	18.0
Nonfederal (total)	6,729	94.2	1,480,000	89.7	29,000,000	94.3	1,206	81.5	15.8
Short-term general and other special	5,853	81.9	826,000	50.1	28,254,000	91.9	651	78.8	8.3
voluntary	3,428	48.0	579,000	35.1	20,338,000	66.2	468	80.8	8.2
proprietary	759	10.6	48,000	2.9	1,893,000	6.2	36	74.6	6.8
state and local gov't.	1,666	23.3	198,000	12.0	6,023,000	19.6	146	78.9	8.8
Psychiatric	509	7.1	570,000	34.5	565,000	1.8	490	85.9	402.6
Tuberculosis	107	1.5	20,000	1.2	36,000	0.1	13	64.7	140.7
Long-term general and other special	260	3.6	63,000	3.8	105,000	0.3	52	82.5	183.7
Federal (total)	415	5.8	170,000	10.3	1,769,000	5.7	140	82.7	38.8
General	333	4.7	87,000	5.3	1,461,000	4.8	71	81.4	19.9
Psychiatric	35	0.5	47,000	2.8	69,000	0.2	40	84.5	336.2
Tuberculosis	2	...	200	...	600	...	127	58.5	409.0
Other special	45	...	35,000	2.1	238,000	0.7	30,000	76.5	60.4

[a]Percentages may not total due to rounding.
Source: Adapted from American Hospital Association. Hospitals (Guide Issue) 44:(15) 472–480, Tables 1–4 (1970).

facilities of the hospital as others use private doctors.

Table 11-5 presents a rather complex listing of types of hospitals. Basically, hospitals are divided into two categories: nonfederal and federal. Within each major category, there are a number of subcategories. The nonfederal hospitals are divided into four subgroups: (1) short-term general and other special hospitals, (2) psychiatric, (3) tuberculosis, and (4) long-term general and other special hospitals. The subcategory of short-term general and other special hospitals is further divided by type of ownership; that is, whether the hospitals are owned by voluntary or proprietary bodies or by state and local governments. Federal hospitals, the second of the major categories, are also divided, but here the distinction is by type of care rendered in the facility, i.e., general hospital care, psychiatric care, and care for tuberculosis, drug addiction, leprosy, and so on.

Table 11-5 further indicates that the overwhelming number of hospitals (94 percent) are nonfederal and that the majority of these are mainly short-term facilities (which are listed as "community hospitals" in Table 11-4). Although these facilities are predominantly voluntary institutions, there are a significant number of government hospitals: 1,666 community hospitals, or not quite one-fourth of all the hospitals in the United States, are short-term institutions owned and operated by state and local government agencies.

Note that the number of beds in community hospitals has increased, while beds in psychiatric facilities have decreased. In 1968 community hospital beds represented 41 percent of the total number of hospital beds in this country; by 1969, this figure had increased to slightly over 50 percent. Psychiatric beds represented 46 percent of the total in 1963, and this figure had decreased to 34 percent in 1969. However, this is still rather dramatic in that over one-third of all kinds of hospitals beds in the United States are devoted to the care of the mentally ill. It is of interest that the 617,000 psychiatric beds are located in only 544 hospitals; the 826,000 community hospital beds are in over 5,853 hospitals.

Table 11-5 also lists percent of occupancy and average stay. The average length of stay in a community hospital is 8.3 days, but notice how long the average stay is in psychiatric, tuberculosis, and long-term hospitals; in some cases it exceeds a year. Similarly, the **occupancy rate** is generally higher in long-term facilities than in short-term hospitals.

Hospitals in the United States are descended directly from those in

---

OCCUPANCY RATE: the ratio of the number of inpatients to the number of beds

eighteenth-century England. Our early hospitals adopted the form of the English voluntary (nongovernment) nonprofit charitable institution as well as its primary mission, the care of the poor. Many English hospitals additionally functioned as old age homes, foundling homes, or orphanages. Early hospitals in the United States offered little more than custodial care for the sick poor or a facility where the ill could be isolated from the rest of society.

The advent of **asepsis** and anesthesia produced significant changes, and hospitals began to develop into more sophisticated medical institutions, caring for both rich and poor. Other types of institutions (chronic disease hospitals, nursing homes, and tuberculosis sanatoria) began to assume the custodial and isolation functions. At one point in time, the threat existed that the hospital itself might be fractionated into a series of specialty facilities—eye infirmaries, **lying-in hospitals,** or hospitals for bone and joint diseases. Though this "specialty-hospital era" did not last long, the growth of institutions caring for those with long-term illness has continued to the present. In fact, the number of nursing home beds in the United States almost matches that of the acute beds available in community hospitals.

The current problem facing the American hospital must be viewed principally as those of the central institution within a total health care system. There is a widespread tendency for hospitals to function as insular and circumscribed components of this system, and coordination is the exception rather than the rule. A major problem is to determine how the hospital can best relate to other health care facilities with similar roles, as well as to those whose roles are different. A basic question is whether differentiated roles are as important as once thought, or whether the total needs of the patients and a corollary emphasis on continuity of care are of sufficient priority to reduce the importance of ownership or specific function.

THE HOSPITAL AND SOCIETY

The community hospital is a social institution and, as such, is subject to pressures from several identifiable sources within the society it serves. The providers of health care constitute one such source of pres-

---

ASEPSIS: freedom from infection; the aseptic technique is one in which not only surgical instruments and the hands of the surgeon are sterile but the entire operating room and the air within it are completely free of living germs

LYING-IN HOSPITAL: an inpatient facility limited to obstetric care

sure. Primarily physicians in the community, they comprise the medical staff of the hospital but, with few exceptions, do not carry any responsibility for its management. The hospital's clients represent another source of pressure; that is, patients are beginning to make strong and direct demands on the hospital for improved services. Ethnic minority groups and the poor, though essentially part of the hospital's clientele, add special dimensions in their demands for new and improved services. Among other things, they have a particular investment in pressuring the hospital to increase its training and educational opportunities and to open them to specific groups within the community. Other social organizations and government legislation represent further sources of pressure.

It is important to note that the pressure from these various sources may be felt with equal intensity by the hospital and yet be in direct conflict with each other. For example, clients of a hospital may be interested in expanded medical services while its governing body is more concerned about the escalation of hospital costs. In responding to the various pressures, this body (or Board of Trustees in a voluntary nonprofit hospital) must allocate the institution's limited resources under the constraint of preserving its fiscal viability. In addition, various kinds of hospitals may be subject to different mixtures of these pressures. Teaching hospitals, for example, are particularly sensitive to the demands of medical school faculty and consequently may be less responsive to community needs unless they coincide with those of the medical staff.

The provider groups, who have dominated hospital planning and program development, can be considered as two subgroups: the physicians, or medical staff, and the hospital employees. Physicians are primarily concerned with the "scientific excellence" of the hospital. They are quite likely to want the most sophisticated equipment and services to be available to their patients regardless of cost or the probability of use over a period of time. Such services are epitomized in the "special care units" which have resulted in remarkable decreases in the mortality of selected diseases, particularly heart disease and diseases of early infancy. It is a serious question whether it is logical for each hospital to have every newest machine or scientific advancement. Frequently, duplication results in such minimal utilization of specialized patient-care resources that they are economically wasteful, especially since they are usually very expensive to acquire, maintain, and staff. Of particular concern is that the additional costs, though borne to some extent by the hospital, are frequently passed on to the consumer through increased room charges. Hospital employees, both professional and technical, are demanding higher wages to correspond with the level of those employed in industry and comparable service organizations outside the health care system.

Since hospitals are "labor-laden," i.e., about 75 percent of hospital expenses are labor costs, these pressures also contribute to higher costs for hospital care.

In many communities, patients are coming to the hospital's emergency room in ever-increasing numbers—a previously mentioned trend which is transforming this former accident service into a first-line general medical care facility. Other than in the emergency room and clinics, it is rather difficult for a patient to make use of a hospital's services without a physician's intervention. Therefore, in the name of the patient, the medical staff often "translates" client pressures to the hospital. It is not yet clear how much this will be intensified or affected by the Medicare and Medicaid programs with their specific provisions for payment of care from private physicians.

Through the formal channels of government regulations, recent federal and state legislation has reshaped the hospital's role and broadened its social responsiveness. Medicare and Medicaid have done more than merely develop a fiscal relationship between hospitals and federal and state governments. Measurements of the quality of patient care are required under Medicare's **utilization-review** concept, and existing federal legislation extends the application of this concept to other programs. Under the required **transfer agreements** between hospitals and extended-care facilities, the former have been placed on notice that closer formal relationships between the various components of the system can be expected shortly. Further, the Comprehensive Health Planning Act, enacted in the late 1960s, is more than a statement of each citizen's right to high-quality medical care; it is an attempt to bring the consumer's concerns into the health planning area. Regional Medical Programs is another national program enacted at about the same time. Its scope, originally limited to education and logistic support for heart disease, cancer, and stroke, has been extended to include the development of new approaches to the

---

UTILIZATION REVIEW: a systematic approach directed at determining whether facilities such as hospitals and nursing homes are being used effectively; the approach usually taken is to review admissions to the facility, duration of stays for various patients, and professional services furnished; frequently, there is a review of those cases which are considered to be of extended duration

TRANSFER AGREEMENT: a formal agreement, usually between a hospital and an extended-care facility, which facilitates continuity of care and expedites appropriate care for the patient; to that end, the agreement provides reasonable assurance that transfer of patients will be effected between the two facilities whenever the attending physician determines that such transfer is medically indicated

delivery of medical care. An additional example of social action is that several new state laws require that hospitals receiving public funds be accountable for the cost and quality of the care they deliver.

Hospitals and other health care institutions are under the threat of further government legislation. As a result, many are actively pursuing voluntary planning, monitoring, and quality control by cooperating with planning agencies in various states and regions. These agencies have undertaken the role of coordinating interhospital planning and program development; in a few areas they have provided the impetus for shared services between hospitals (e.g., laundry, purchasing, bill collecting, and so on). Some prepayment agencies, such as Blue Cross, have begun to put financial teeth into the recommendations of voluntary planning groups by creating different rates for those hospitals which spontaneously participate in regional planning programs.

Disadvantaged and minority groups in the community are making increasing demands on hospitals. In the larger cities, the demand for a patient **ombudsman** in hospital outpatient departments has become fairly common. The composition of Boards of Trustees is being questioned and minority representation requested. Some black organizations are attempting to achieve policy control of the hospitals within their communities or are agitating for some way of negotiating community demands outside the federal administrative channels.

Historically, hospitals have provided educational opportunities leading to social and economic upward mobility. Formal education programs, such as those for nurses and laboratory technicians, and various in-service training programs for health manpower groups (e.g., medical stenographers and nurses' aides) have offered opportunities for minority groups to move into various technical, semiprofessional, and professional positions. These educational efforts are expensive, particularly if they are more than just apprentice programs. It is a significant social question whether the patient should be charged for these costs or whether the community should assume financial responsibility as it has for other programs within the formal school and college systems.

The hospital, as the primary provider-oriented facility, finds it difficult

---

OMBUDSMAN: a person, usually employed in the role of patient advocate, who intercedes on the behalf of patients in their relationships with medical and health institutions, facilities, and personnel; the role of the advocate is twofold: (1) to receive the concerns and grievances of patients and to investigate situations and make recommendations for appropriate change, and (2) to appraise various programs in order to determine whether they are serving people effectively to deal with demands such as those described above. Hospitals have yet to discover how to give their constituents a voice in management. There is also an uncomfortable feeling that to do so may result in severe constraints on the administration of the institution. Those in hospital administration are particularly concerned about two crucial areas: (1) the increased costs associated with new programs in a labor-laden industry, and (2) the type and size of institution that can be most responsive to the needs of patients and specific population groups within the community.

HOSPITAL COSTS

Operating expenses for all types of hospitals rose from about $2 billion in 1946 to over $22 billion in 1969. These figures, although dramatic because of the $20-billion increase, have an even greater impact when one views changes in operating expenses on a per-patient-day basis (Table 11-6). From 1946 to 1969 operating expenses for nonfederal short-term hospitals increased from just $9 dollars per patient-day to over $70. These figures do not represent patient charges, i.e., the amount the patient is billed for a day of care in the hospital, but what the hospital spends to provide the services. Patient charges may be higher because the patient's bill may include additional items, such as bed-debt allowances, losses for outpatient-department expenses, and so on.

The outlook is for still higher costs per patient day because the costs of operating a hospital are bound to increase in an inflationary economy; the hospital itself must pay more for supplies if they go up in price, and justifiable salary demands require higher operating costs. In addition, hospital operating expenses will increase due to the costs of already-expanding outpatient services.

Expenses involved in an average hospital stay can be determined by

TABLE 11-6. Nonfederal Hospital Operating Expense per Patient Day: United States, Selected Years 1946–1969

Type of Hospital	Year				
	1946	1950	1960	1965	1969
Short-term general and other special	$9.39	$15.62	$32.23	$44.48	$70.03
Psychiatric	1.39	2.43	4.91	7.50	13.61
Tuberculosis	4.57	7.22	10.13	17.39	29.47
Long-term general and other special	2.97	5.39	8.06	19.79	29.77

Source: American Hospital Association. Hospitals (Guide Issue) 44:(15) 472–473 (1970).

Table 11-7. Expenses Involved in an Average Hospital Stay in
Community Hospitals[a]: United States, Selected Years 1946–1970

Expenses and Related Items	Year				
	1946	1950	1963	1968	1970
Total expense per patient day (in dollars)	9.4	15.6	38.9	61.38	81.01
Average stay (in days)	9.1	8.1	7.7	8.4	8.2
Total cost per stay (in dollars)	85.5	126.5	299.7	581.3	664.3

[a]*All nonfederal, short-term general, and other special hospitals.*

multiplying the total expense per patient day by the average length of
patient stay (Table 11-7). The average length of a hospital stay was
slightly over nine days 1946, was about eight days in 1950, decreased
during the early part of the 1960s, rose during the latter part of that
decade (probably due to Medicare and Medicaid), and now appears
to be approaching the 1950 level again. Although the pattern of hospital
use varied during this quarter of a century, total expense continued its
steady upward trend. This produced an unremitting increase in the average expense per hospital stay from $85 in 1946 to a sizeable $664 in 1970.
Despite the reductions in average stay, the cost per stay has doubled
since 1963.

Some indication of the factors behind rising costs is provided by analyz-
ing the rise in health care expenditures in general. A recent study by
Herbert E. Klarman and others showed that over the past four decades
(1929 to 1969), prices contributed to one-half the increase and population growth was responsible for about one-third. Rice and Cooper (from
the Social Security Administration, U.S. Department of Health, Education,
and Welfare) show that from 1966 to 1970, expenditures for hospital
care increased by $11.5 billion. Price increases represented over three-
fourths of this rise, whereas population represented 7 percent, and all
other factors (such as greater utilization, improvements, and so on) represented about 17 percent.

Whatever the causes, rising costs in hospitals may be contained in two
ways: the first is to lower the cost of each day of service, and the second
is to decrease the number of hospital days used per unit of population
per year. Both routes must be explored if the community and individuals
are to be able to afford and pay for hospital care.

Hospital mergers and interhospital cooperation are recent trends which
might offer both economic and quality advantages. These actions ap-

proach the cost problem by attempting to provide a better basis for the organization of hospital services. There are some indications that **economies of scale** can be achieved if hospitals share services, equipment, manpower, and other resources. New technologic and scientific advances have helped to promote this trend. For example, the rapid processing and communication of information such as laboratory results makes it less critical that a given laboratory be located in each hospital. In terms of quality of care, there may be real differences between hospitals of varying sizes; and the larger hospitals seem to have the edge, possibly due to more stringent professional standards or the greater availability of sophisticated support services. However, though there may be some economies in large-scale institutions, their atmosphere and the patient care they provide almost inevitably tends to be impersonal. Hospitals are vulnerable to the dangers of depersonalization because their services require decisions by various groups—professionals, administrators, service personnel, and consumers.

Mergers, cooperative and formal affiliations between hospitals, and questions of optimum facility size present classic organization problems involving centralization and decentralization. Currently, there is no mandate for an organizational scheme that relates hospitals to each other and to other facilities. Voluntary cooperation and coordination began during the mid 1940s. Although there are significant examples of worthwhile cooperative endeavors, the national pattern is one in which each hospital works in isolation. What is needed is an effectively planned format for delivering well-balanced community health services. The economic and organizational questions which face today's hospital, its inability to appraise the quality of institution care satisfactorily, and the need to plan the type, size, and location of medical care institutions which most effectively meet patient and community needs are particularly urgent problems. They cannot be met by the hospital alone; they must be resolved by a comprehensive approach involving all components of the health care system. (This aspect of the organization of health care services is discussed in Chap. 12.)

Personnel

We have thus far discussed some of the major facilities which house and deliver health care services in this country, and we are now

---

ECONOMIES OF SCALE: the relationship between the resources brought to bear to achieve organizational goals and objectives and the cost of achieving them

ready to consider the personnel who provide these services. This section will first focus briefly on the physician—the principal autonomous health professional—and then examine the developing field of allied health personnel.

THE PHYSICIAN

The demand for health care is usually expressed when a person perceives a medical need, and most often he seeks the advice and assistance of a physician. In the early part of this century this process almost always resulted in a home visit by the doctor. This situation was reversed through the years, and the physician's office increasingly has become the central point for providing medical care. Although there was an added efficiency to office visits versus home visits, the demands of a growing population were frequently found to be overwhelming. Some relief was provided as advances in scientific technology resulted in equipment which was not only labor-saving but which frequently improved diagnostic accuracy. However, this sophisticated instrumentation proved too costly for the average physician in private practice, particularly when he had the added office expense of paying for the services of a registered nurse.

In response to the increasing demands of their practices, a growing number of physicians have entered **group-practice** arrangements. The combined resources of several physicians, plus their aggregate patient demand, permits the purchase and utilization of equipment usually not found in the solo practitioner's office. Personnel can also be more efficiently and economically used, and, in addition, studies have suggested that the quality of care often improves when physicians practice under these circumstances. In 1969 the Public Health Service reported that in the United States there existed over 6,000 group-practice arrangements and about one-half were limited to a particular speciality (e.g., pediatrics, internal medicine, obstetrics-gynecology, and so on) (Fig. 11-2). It should be reemphasized here that the number of general practitioners, once the mainstays of American medicine, has been steadily declining since 1950 (Fig. 10-1), and the attraction to specialty practice, as opposed to general practice, is likely to continue.

There are significant differences not only in types of practice but in where physicians choose to practice (Fig. 11-3). In 1967, the Middle Atlantic region of the country had 171 active physicans (nonfederal

---

GROUP PRACTICE: an organization arrangement of three or more physicians working together in one location and sharing the income of their efforts

Per Cent Distribution Of Group Practices And Group Practice Physicians By Type Of Group, 1969

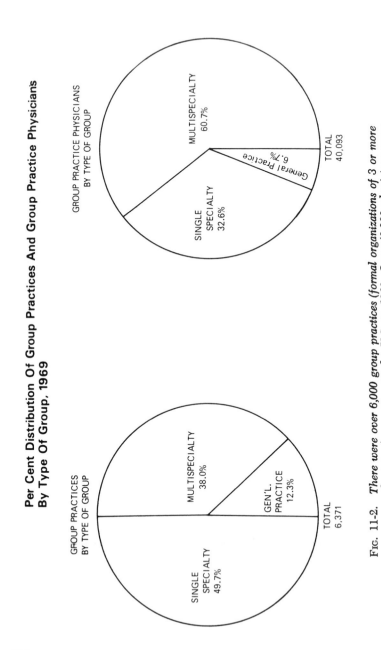

GROUP PRACTICES
BY TYPE OF GROUP

SINGLE
SPECIALTY
49.7%

MULTISPECIALTY
38.0%

GEN'L.
PRACTICE
12.3%

TOTAL
6,371

GROUP PRACTICE PHYSICIANS
BY TYPE OF GROUP

MULTISPECIALTY
60.7%

SINGLE
SPECIALTY
32.6%

General Practice
6.7%

TOTAL
40,093

Fig. 11-2. *There were over 6,000 group practices (formal organizations of 3 or more physicians) operating in the U.S. in 1969. Over 40,000 physicians were practicing in these group settings. (From Reference Data on Socioeconomic Issues of Health, 1971 revised edition, American Medical Association.)*

374

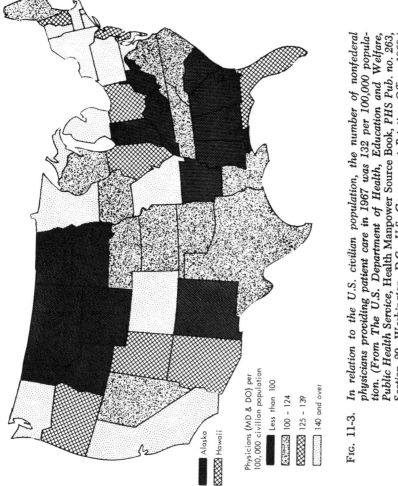

Physicians (MD & DO) per
100,000 civilian population

Alaska

Hawaii

Less than 100

100 – 124

125 – 139

140 and over

Fig. 11-3. In relation to the U.S. civilian population, the number of nonfederal physicians providing patient care in 1967 was 132 per 100,000 population. (From The U.S. Department of Health, Education and Welfare, Public Health Service, Health Manpower Source Book, PHS Pub. no. 263, Section 20, Washington, D.C., U.S. Government Printing Office, 1969.)

M.D.s and Doctors of Osteopathy) per 100,000 population, while the south central region had only 94 per 100,000. A glance at four states during the same year highlights even greater variation. The highest physician-to-population ratios were found in New York and Massachusetts, with about 190 physicians per 100,000. Mississippi and Alaska had the lowest ratios of approximately 69 physicians per 100,000. On a smaller scale, Figure 11-4 shows urban and rural distribution of physicians involved in general practice and specialty practice. Larger metropolitan areas average approximately 118 physicians per 100,000 population, while less urbanized areas (isolated rural) have about 42 physicians per 100,000. The ratio of general practitioners to all population areas is approximately the same.

The trend toward urbanization and specialization among physicians has significant implications for the country's health industry. Many of the

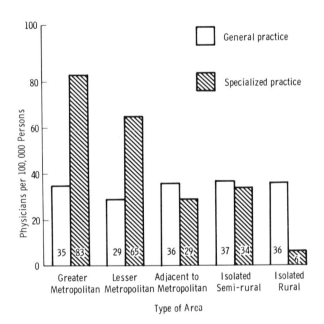

* Includes only physicians in active practice and not employed by the Federal Government.

FIG. 11-4.   (From Medical Chart Book, University of Michigan, School of Public Health, Third Edition, Revised 1968.)

traditional functions of the general practitioner are being absorbed by medical specialists, nurses, social workers, and other personnel. In areas where there are shortages of physicians, other types of specially trained personnel must try to fill the void. The growing number of specialists intensifies the demand on medical centers to provide the intellectual climate, the equipment, and the staff that will allow maximum use of the specialist's skills and talents.

THE HEALTH INDUSTRY

In 1970 the nation's health industry (medical goods and services) represented 7 percent of the Gross National Product, or $67.2 billion. The government absorbed 37 percent of this cost, which left 63 percent to be borne by the private sector of the economy. Eighty-three percent of the $37.6 billion spent by the private sector purchased services (e.g., physician's services, dental treatment, and physical therapy treatments). The remaining 17 percent purchased medical goods such as drugs, eyeglasses, and wheelchairs. The disproportionate demand for services versus goods reflects the labor-laden character of the health care industry.

In 1969 the country's demand for medical services resulted in 840 million visits to physicians, 293 million dental appointments, and over 28 million admissions or discharges from general hospitals. In terms of the average consumer, this indicates that in 1969 each person in the United States visited a physician 4.3 times and a dentist 1.5 times (see Fig. 5-6). For every 1,000 people, about 144 were admitted to a hospital. In this same year, hospital outpatient departments had 120 million visits (see Fig. 11-1). The magnitude of this demand for medical services is responsible for the employment of approximately four million people, which means that about one out of every 20 workers has a job in the health industry.

Table 11-8 shows that in 1967 physicians who actively practiced medicine or **osteopathy** numbered about 305,000. This represented an increase of 250 percent over their total number in 1900. However, as Fig. 11-5 points out, the supply of physicians declined over that same time period, from 35 percent to 9 percent of the total health manpower. The percentage of

---

OSTEOPATHY: the official definition of osteopathy is provided by the American Osteopathic Association as follows: "that system of the healing art which places the chief emphasis on the structural integrity of the body mechanism as being the most important single factor to maintain the well-being of the organism in health and disease"

TABLE 11-8. Estimated Employment in Health Occupations: 1900 and 1967

Health Occupation	Number of Workers	
	1900	1967
All health occupations	350,000	3,515,000
Physicians (M.D. and D.O.)	123,000	305,500
Medical related	60,000	651,300
Dentists	30,000	98,700
Dental related	5,000	137,000
Registered nurses	12,000	659,000
Other nursing	109,000	1,095,000
Environmental health engineers, scientists, and technologists		54,500
Environmental health technicians, assistants, and aides	11,000	163,500
All other		350,500

Source: Public Health Service estimates.

persons employed in other health occupations (excluding nursing) has increased about 25 percent since the turn of the century. The table also

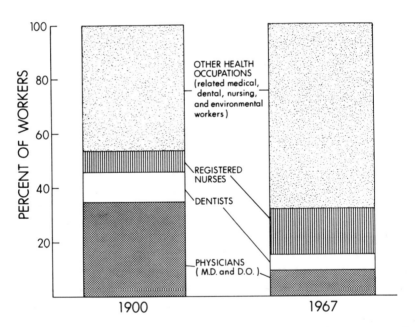

FIG. 11-5. *Percent distribution of health workers (U.S.A. 1900 and 1967). (From The U.S. Department of Health, Education and Welfare, Public Health Service, Health Manpower Source Book, PHS Pub. no. 263, Section 21, Washington, D.C., U.S. Government Printing Office, 1970.)*

reveals that in 1900 there were three health workers for every one physician, and that by 1967 this ratio was 10:1. Who are these health care workers? What do they represent in terms of educational backgrounds? How great is the need for their services?

In his recent book, *Allied Health Manpower: Trends and Prospects,* Harry I. Greenfield divides allied health personnel into three separate components: allied health professionals, allied technicians, and allied health assistants. The basis for each division is the level of education attained. For example, allied health professionals have attained at least a baccalaureate degree. For the most part, the allied health technicians have received training on the community-college level. The allied health assistants include the remainder of the people employed, and have generally had no more than a high school education. Physicians, dentists, and other doctoral-level professionals are in the separate and distinct classification of "autonomous health personnel."

The listing of personnel in Table 11-9 is grouped by this system of classification. The first group, as the title implies, are independent personnel and bear ultimate responsibility for the patient. The personnel in group 2 work closely with the physician and under his general direction. Persons in groups 3 and 4 work under the direction of the other two groups and usually have explicitly defined areas of responsibility.

In 1965 there were an estimated 2,838,800 people employed in the health field. As is shown in Table 11-10, physicians comprise 10.7 percent of all health manpower; dentistry and its allied services represent 8.1 percent; and the field of nursing and related services accounts for about one-half of the total and represents the largest block of people employed in health. The remaining 31.6 percent includes 32 specific health fields, and the rest of our discussion of allied health manpower will be directed primarily to the personnel in these 32 fields.

SPECIAL CHARACTERISTICS OF ALLIED HEALTH MANPOWER

Over two-thirds of all allied health personnel are employed in hospital settings. The remaining third are found in physicians' offices, clinics, nursing homes, and the like. The distribution of allied health personnel is therefore similar to that of the over 7,000 hospitals scattered throughout the country. Hospitals, except for those in large urban areas, are generally situated considerably distant from each other, and each hospital requires a multiplicity of skills represented by small groups of personnel.

With the possible exception of some members of the nursing and

TABLE 11-9. Classification of Allied Health Personnel

1. *Autonomous Health Professionals*
   Physicians
   Osteopaths
   Dentists
   Podiatrists
   Optometrists
2. *Allied Health Professionals*
   Professional nurses
   Clinical psychologists
   Cytotechnologists
   Dental hygienists
   Dieticians
   Food technologists
   Hospital administrators
   Immunochematologists
   Medical illustrators
   Medical record librarians
   Medical technologists
   Biostatisticians
   Computer programmers
   Health economists
   Manual arts therapists
   Recreation therapists
   Psychometlists
   Mycologists

Allied Personnel in Health Manpower

   Nuclear medical technologists
   Nutritionists
   Occupational therapists
   Physical therapists
   Rehabilitation counselors
   Speech pathologists and audiologists
   Virologists
   X-ray technologists
   Pharmacists
   Bioengineers
   Health administrators
   Health educators
   Music therapists
   Medical social workers
3. *Allied Health Technicians*
   X-ray technicians
   Registered nurses (Associate degree or diploma)
   Medical records technicians
   Occupational therapy assistants
   Medical technicians
   Medical and dental assistants
4. *Allied Health Assistants*
   Licensed practical nurses
   Nurse's aides
   Psychiatric aides

TABLE 11-10. Estimated Employment in Health Field
by Occupation, 1965

Health Field	Estimated Employment	Percent of Total
All Fields	2,838,800	100.0
1. Nursing and related services	1,409,000	49.6
2. Medicine and osteopathy	305,000	10.7
3. Dentistry and allied services	230,900	8.1
4. Secretarial and office services	200,000	7.1
5. Pharmacy	118,000	4.2
6. Clerical laboratory services	90,000	3.2
7. Radiologic technology	70,000	2.5
8. Basic sciences in health field	44,200	1.6
9. Visual services and eye care	40,400	1.4
10. Medical records	37,000	1.3
11. Administration of health services	34,250	1.2
12. Environmental health	33,750	1.2
13. Dietetic and nutritional service	30,000	1.2
14. Chiropractic and naturopathy	25,000	0.90
15. Veterinary medicine	23,700	0.80
16. Social work	17,500	0.62
17. Health education	16,700	0.59
18. Food and drug protective services	16,500	0.58
19. Speech pathology, audiology	14,000	0.49
20. Physical therapy	12,000	0.42
21. Psychology	9,000	0.32
22. Library services in health	8,000	0.28
23. Podiatry	7,600	0.27
24. Biomedical engineering	7,500	0.26
25. Misc. hospital services	6,200	0.22
26. Occupational therapy	6,000	0.21
27. Specialized rehabilitation services	5,600	0.20
28. Midwifery	5,000	0.18
29. Health information and communication	5,000	0.18
30. Vocational rehabilitation and counseling	4,200	0.15
31. Orthopedic and prosthetic appliances	3,300	0.12
32. Health and vital statistics	1,900	0.07
33. Anthropology and sociology	700	0.02
34. Economic research in health	500	0.02
35. Automatic data processing	300	0.01

Source: Health Resource Statistics, Public Health Service Publication No. 1509 (Washington, D. C., 1965).

medical staffs, the personnel complement of a hospital is usually drawn from its own community. The allied health personnel generally are trained in the hospital or at some nearby vocational center. In view of the diversity of health manpower required to operate a hospital, this can be a costly proposition. At any given time a hospital may have several training programs underway for very small groups of people.

In contrast to all other industries in the United States, most people entering the health field are women. During the 1960s about 70 percent of the employees in industry (excluding health services) were male, while 30 percent were female. The reverse was true in the health services industry, where 70 percent of the employees were female and 30 percent were male. With the exception of physicians, men traditionally have remained on the periphery of the health field because of its low salaries and poor opportunities for advancement.

Until recently there has been little possibility of changing the level of salaries in the health services industry. Before 1966 hospitals were excluded from the Fair Labor Standards Act, since most of their services are rendered on an intrastate basis. An amendment to this act became effective in February, 1971, and provided, for the first time, a minimum wage for hospital and nursing home workers. In many states the nonprofit nature of hospitals also has excluded their employees from minimum wage laws and unemployment benefits. In addition, hospital employees have been a captive working group, since many of their particular medical skills are not transferable to other settings in the community. In selected geographic areas, however, there has been marked improvement in the salaries of health personnel. In 1960 the Bureau of Labor Statistics indicated that the average weekly salary in the manufacturing industries of New York City was $84.36, and in accredited general hospitals it was $69.20. In 1965, the average salary in both industries was approximately $100 a week; and by late 1966 hospital workers were averaging $104.87—$2.92 more than those in the manufacturing industries.

ALLIED HEALTH EDUCATION AND TRAINING

Allied health workers acquire the skills necessary for their roles through a variety of education and training programs. Education programs focus on general knowledge, with some emphasis on a vocational area. Training programs, on the other hand, are specific in nature and provide the person with the skills essential for a definite job. Historically, allied health workers received on-the-job training in hospitals, clinics, and physicians' offices. This training method was patterned after the traditional apprenticeships of nurses and doctors. As medical science expanded and the demand for more and better services grew, responsibilities were delegated to personnel other than the physician and nurse. Apprenticeship programs could not meet the need for trained people. The magnitude of the demand can be appreciated when it is realized that 75 percent of all employees in today's hospital are required to meet educational criteria and to possess a definite set of skills.

The majority of health positions require basic knowledge in the biologic sciences, others entail familiarity with the social sciences, and still other positions depend on the acquisition of a specific technical skill. Basic education in the biologic and social sciences can usually be provided most effectively in a university setting. Technical skills can best be developed in a clinical situation, and a hospital, by virtue of the volume of its services, is the ideal clinical location for this type of training. Some positions, of course, require the benefits of both university and hospital.

Hospitals are responsible for most of the health service training, and their training programs emphasize clinical experience. Such programs cost the student little or nothing, and some of the expense to the hospital is offset by the student's free labor. Yet, as medical training of every type becomes more involved, many hospitals are reconsidering the financial arrangements and reviewing the ethics of distributing teaching costs to the patients. In addition, attempts are being made to incorporate health education programs as much as possible in established institutions of higher learning. This would distribute education costs more evenly and also provide the student with a certificate or degree readily recognized in any community.

There are a number of allied health occupations whose members presently receive their credentials after four years of college, e.g., pharmacy, physical therapy, and dental hygiene. There is also a wide selection of courses available below the college level. Junior colleges (which provides two years of education after high school) have programs in over 40 health occupations that are essential to the community. Programs are offered in nursing, inhalation therapy, and surgical technology, to mention a few. Technical or vocational schools prepare people in one year or less for positions as practical nurses, x-ray technicians, occupational therapists, and so on. Figure 11-6 gives some indication of the extent to which institutions of higher learning share with hospitals the task of developing the manpower needed for today's health care industry.

Although adequate data are not yet available for objective evaluation of the allied health training programs, some observations can be made. The length of the programs thus far established varies from institution to institution and from course to course. One nurse's aide program may continue for only 3 weeks, while another may extend beyond 40 weeks. These differences depend in part on the educational background of the enrollees or the urgency of the hospital's employment needs. In addition to length of the programs, training standards vary. The American Medical Association has provided in its *Essentials of an Accredited Curriculum*

Calendar of health careers

The calendar on the following pages gives you a quick check on how many years of education, after high school, you should count on for the representative health occupations listed here. The lines and symbols show what is customary—some people take only minimum required training; many take more.

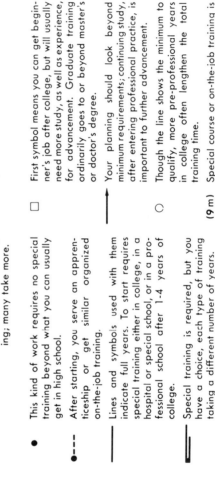

●   This kind of work requires no special training beyond what you can usually get in high school.

●---   After starting, you serve an apprenticeship or get similar organized on-the-job training.

│   Lines and symbols used with them indicate full years. To start requires special training either in college, in a hospital or special school, or in a professional school after 1-4 years of college.

▮   Special training is required, but you have a choice, each type of training taking a different number of years.

□   First symbol means you can get beginner's job after college, but will usually need more study, as well as experience, for advancement. Graduate training ordinarily goes to or beyond master's or doctor's degree.

↑   Your planning should look beyond minimum requirements; continuing study, after entering professional practice, is important to further advancement.

○   Though the line shows the minimum to qualify, more pre-professional years in college often lengthen the total training time.

(9 m)   Special course or on-the-job training is shown in number of months.

Fig. 11-6A. (*From Health Careers Guidebook, U.S. Department of Labor, 1960, Washington, D.C., U.S. Government Printing Office.*)

384

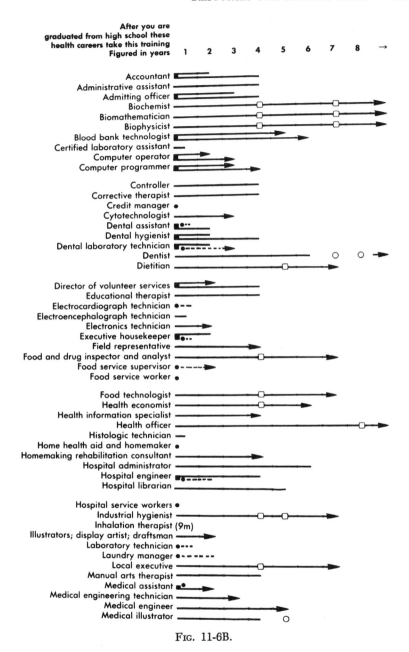

After you are graduated from high school these health careers take this training
Figured in years — 1 2 3 4 5 6 7 8 →

Accountant
Administrative assistant
Admitting officer
Biochemist
Biomathematician
Biophysicist
Blood bank technologist
Certified laboratory assistant
Computer operator
Computer programmer

Controller
Corrective therapist
Credit manager
Cytotechnologist
Dental assistant
Dental hygienist
Dental laboratory technician
Dentist
Dietitian

Director of volunteer services
Educational therapist
Electrocardiograph technician
Electroencephalograph technician
Electronics technician
Executive housekeeper
Field representative
Food and drug inspector and analyst
Food service supervisor
Food service worker

Food technologist
Health economist
Health information specialist
Health officer
Histologic technician
Home health aid and homemaker
Homemaking rehabilitation consultant
Hospital administrator
Hospital engineer
Hospital librarian

Hospital service workers
Industrial hygienist
Inhalation therapist (9m)
Illustrators; display artist; draftsman
Laboratory technician
Laundry manager
Local executive
Manual arts therapist
Medical assistant
Medical engineering technician
Medical engineer
Medical illustrator

FIG. 11-6B.

the criteria necessary for each of the programs the Association endorses. However, these criteria are not yet universally applied. Frequently, each

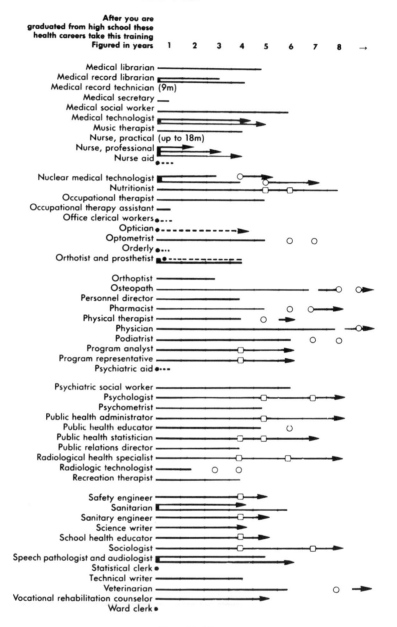

FIG. 11-6C.

state determines the qualifications required for teaching positions. When shortages of teachers exist, many programs must be taught by people who have not fulfilled normal degree or certification requirements. Also, training for a particular occupation may vary from one hospital to another simply because of the difference in job definition from institution to institution.

Appendix 10 lists professional health organizations which can provide health career information on request.

ALLIED HEALTH MANPOWER NEEDS

Recent national estimates of health manpower requirements indicate that the projected demand far exceeds the present supply of allied health personnel. It should be emphasized that the projections are merely estimates and should be interpreted accordingly. There are several techniques for estimating requirements: budgeted vacancies, ratios to total population, perceived needs, ratios to patient populations, requirements per unit of service, and staffing patterns. Table 11-11 presents estimates of health manpower requirements by the year 1975. Based on information from assembled professional judgments, census computations, projections by the Bureau of Labor Statistics, and manpower needs as reported in a 1966 survey of hospitals, it can be seen that a sharp increase in demand is forecasted. Professional judgments project an increase of

TABLE 11-11. Health Manpower Requirements: 1966 and 1975 Estimates

Occupation	Number of Workers in 1966	Percent Increase Required by 1975 on the basis of:		
		Professional Judgments	Highest Region	BLS[a] Projection
All health occupations	2,786,200	34	36	43
Selected medical allied occupations Baccalaureate level (total)	114,000	165	35	76
Clinical laboratory technologist	40,000	75	31	88
Dietitian and nutritionist	30,000	...	...	27
Medical record librarian	12,000	33	1	50
Occupational therapist	6,500	731	92	200
Physical therapist	12,500	332	42	116
Speech pathologist and audiologist	13,000	123	42	...
Sub-baccalaureate level (total)	122,000	...	...	64
Clinical lab technician and aide	50,000	...	...	100
Radiologic technician	72,000	39	28	39

[a]*Bureau of Labor Statistics.*
Source: Department of Health, Education, and Welfare. Health Manpower Source Book, Sec. 21. Public Health Service Publication, No. 263 (Washington, D. C., 1970).

TABLE 11-12. Hospital Manpower Requirements: 1966 Estimates

Occupation	Number of Workers in 1966	Percent Increase Required in 1966 on the Basis of Hospital Judgment National Average
Hospital Manpower Only		
All professional and technical	1,332,100	19
Selected medical allied occupations Baccalaureate level (total)	73,100	26
Clinical laboratory technologist	36,500	17
Dietitian and nutritionist	12,700	28
Medical record librarian	6,300	29
Occupational therapist	4,100	56
Physical therapist	8,500	34
Recreation therapist	3,800	42
Speech pathologist and audiologist	1,200	47
Sub-baccalaureate level (total)	125,700	19
Clinical lab technician and aide	36,500	17
Food service manager	5,400	16
Medical record technician	10,100	18
Occupational therapy assistant	3,800	31
Pharmacy aide	5,600	17
Physical therapy assistant	5,200	21
Radiologic technician and aide	30,000	16
Physician's aide (surgical)	17,600	22
Electrocardiograph technician	5,900	14
Inhalation therapist and aide	5,600	40

34 percent in the need for people in all health occupations, and the Bureau of Labor Statistics predicts a 43-percent increase. A 36-percent increase is predicted if each of the four census regions were to need and be provided with the manpower now available in the region with the highest rate of utilization. In selected medical allied occupations on the baccalaureate level, a total increase of 165 percent was projected by professional judgments, a 35-percent increase by highest region (and a 76-percent increase by the Bureau of Labor Statistics). In the sub-baccalaureate level, the Bureau of Labor Statistics projected, by selected medical occupations, an increase of 64 percent over the needs as reported in 1966.

The current shortage of manpower indicated for hospitals, the major employers of health workers, is shown in Table 11-12. Based on the perceived needs of the hospital, a 19-percent increase in their professional and technical personnel was required. The hospitals further indicated a 26-percent shortage in selected medical occupations on the baccalaureate level and a 19-percent shortage for selected occupations on the sub-baccalaureate level.

The expanding technology of medicine, the need for better coordination of complex medical resources as well as for their more rational organization, and the potential from improved standards of professional work, all underscore the importance of developing cooperating teams of health personnel. In addition, the shortages of health manpower will continue to create a demand for more efficient ways of using personnel. Of particular importance is the increasing need to train allied health workers to perform some of the more routine tasks which prevent the professional staff members from using their time and skills most effectively.

References

American Public Health Association. A Guide to Medical Care Administration, Vol. I: Concepts and Principles. New York, American Public Health Association, 1965.

Brown, H. J. Delivery of personal health services and medical services for the poor. The Milbank Memorial Fund Quarterly (Part 2) **XLVI**:203–224 (1968).

The New York Academy of Medicine. The 1971 Health Conference of the Academy. Bull. N.Y. Acad. Med. **48**:(1) (1972).

Schaefer, Morris. Current issues in health organization. Amer. J. Pub. Health **58**:1192–1199 (1968).

Stevens, R., and Stevens, R. Medicaid: anatomy of a dilemma. Law & Contemp. Prob. 35:348–425 (1970).

Somers, H. M. and Somers, A. R. Medicare and the Hospitals: Issues and Prospects. Washington, The Brookings Institution, 1967.

White, Kerr L. Organization and delivery of personal health services. The Milbank Memorial Fund Quarterly (Part 2) **XLVI**:225–258 (1968).

CHAPTER

12

The Provision of Medical Care Services: Organization, Financing, and Utilization

We have seen how medical care has evolved from a rather simple and primitive art to an extremely complex technology, we have examined the network of interacting factors which affect and are affected by this technology, and we have discussed the principal health resources which house and deliver medical care services. We can now turn our attention to some of the problems involved in organizing the resources so that they are optimally effective in delivering the services and in organizing the services so that they are responsive to the needs of the people who use them. In addition, we will explore the major ways in which delivery and receipt of medical care is financed by provider and consumer, respectively. The final section of this chapter will discuss the utilization of medical care services.

Before we deal with these areas, there are several aspects of the very services to *be* organized, financed, and utilized which are important to consider. What, for example, constitutes adequate medical care? Actually, there is no precise definition of this. Among the patient population, perceptions of this concept vary considerably from individual to individual and from time to time. How a person defines adequate medical care in a period of stress or when faced with a serious illness may be quite different from his view at other times or from the view of the professional community. Indeed, health professionals themselves are not in complete agreement about what is meant by adequate medical care. Nevertheless, there are some essential and generally accepted observations which can be made.

The concept of adequacy can be viewed both qualitatively and quantitatively. The former implies the formulation of certain standards or criteria, many of which have been postulated as critical to good medical care. The five which are generally considered most basic and inclusive were advanced by the late Dr. George James who proposed that good medical care programs must be (1) comprehensive, (2) continuous, (3) family centered, (4) preventive in emphasis, and (5) of the highest quality.

For the community, comprehensive medical care means the availability of the total gamut of medical care services, including all specialty and auxiliary medical skills needed to deal with problems of disease in the population. For the individual, comprehensive medical care makes available to each patient all the techniques and services he requires— including health professionals, health care facilities, and health care supplies.

Continuity of care means that each patient should be cared for by the same health professional or health team through the course of any given episode of illness. If such an arrangement is not possible, then at the very least the same clinical record of the illness should be available to all the health professionals responsible for care of the patient. It should be noted that the increasing mobility of the American population and many problems related to the organization of medical care services often make it difficult to maintain this standard.

The principle of family-centered medical care is somewhat less widely accepted than the others. It places emphasis on providing medical care to the family as a whole rather than to each family member as an isolated individual. Disease in one family member is thus seen as having aspects which affect and are affected by the family group; in addition, the family is seen as a major source of community strength in attempts to promote treatment and rehabilitation, especially in cases of chronic disease. In addition, many preventive measures have more chance of success if the whole family is involved. The classic example frequently cited by Dr. James is that parents who do not smoke enhance the possibility of preventing this habit in their children.

Emphasis on preventive services is a very important but much neglected principle in good medical care. Such an emphasis supports the concept that medical care should be applied at the earliest possible stage in the natural history of any disease. Today, efforts are focused primarily on the strictly clinical aspect, i.e., the point at which symptomatic disease presents itself for treatment. The basic assumption underlying emphasis on tertiary prevention is that the earlier medical care intervenes to modify, cure, or arrest the process of disease development, the greater the chances of more permanent and effective results and often the less costly the care.

The fifth principle of good medical care is an insistence on the highest quality. Although the four previously mentioned criteria can be conceived as integral to quality, this additionally means the establishment and maintenance of professional qualifications, the accreditation of facilities, licensure laws, and education requirements for paramedical personnel. Of course, there are already well-established standards which govern the practice of medicine. For example, hospitals that are accredited by the Joint Commission on Accreditation require that certain surgical procedures be performed only by qualified and competent surgeons. In turn, the professional boards which certify specialists require that such practitioners complete certain training and reach a specified level of competence and experience before certification is granted.

The qualitative aspects of medical care cannot be dissociated from the quantitative. Quantitative adequacy implies that good medical care services be available in sufficient amounts and that they be effectively timed and balanced. There must be *enough* qualified personnel, *enough* facilities, and *enough* supplies. In addition, organized arrangements must exist whereby facilities and personnel working in the medical care system coordinate activities to cover the medical needs of the population and the community being served, and there must be ways of financing both the delivery and the receipt of the services.

The Organization and Financing of Medical Care Services

Organization simply refers to the arrangements made for the distribution of a product or products to prospective consumers. In terms of our discussion, there has been much concern about the gap which exists between the potentially available product (medical care services) and its dispensation to prospective consumers (the American public). The Trustees and Council of the New York Academy of Medicine reflected this concern when they stated that "in the United States today, a serious gap exists between the state of health of significant numbers of people and that state of health which would be attainable if the best of present day medical knowledge were more universally available and more fully utilized by the people of this country."

Organization of medical services is both a cause and effect of specialization. Some of the advances in modern medical care have occurred as a result of improved organization methods and skills which have made possible a division of labor and the coordination of specialized tasks. At the same time, technologic advances have generated increasing specialization, and this creates a need for organization which integrates services, helps focus on the total needs of the patient, and reduces the difficulties encountered by patients in their attempts to find and use medical care from numerous independent, specialized sources.

There are literally hundreds of different organized programs for the provision of health services. "Organization" may imply simply the scheme of financing a health service through some collective means, or it may involve the patterns of providing the service. Frequently, both the economic and technologic forms of organization are involved in the program. The organization may be undertaken by government or nongovernment agencies. It may be for profit or it may be on a nonprofit basis. It may function at various geographic or political levels: city, county, state, region, national, or international. In addition, the goal of the service or program may vary within a wide range—from a limited, specific interest in a categorical disease to a comprehensive health service covering preventive, curative, rehabilitative, and restorative aspects of health care. Let us first review some generic elements to be considerd in organizing medical care services and then explore some specific ways in which more rational, more appropriate, and more responsive organization of these services can be achieved.

Essential elements in any organized program of medical care include the following:

1. *There must be an administrative structure.* This refers to the agency or source responsible for the program. It may be a source exclusively designed to provide medical care, such as a health clinic or hospital, or it may be part of an administrative setting responsible for a broader function, such as a unit of government. The administrative structure defines lines of authority, accountability, and relationship with other health

service agencies. It sets the functional basis for the operation of the program.

2. *There must be an adequate funding source or sources for the program.* Funding may come from government sources (federal, state, or local), from insurance contributions of beneficiaries, from private payments, from philanthropic donations, or from a combination of these and other sources. The total funding base must be sufficient to meet the demands of the program; at the same time, the problems associated with each source of funding (either in terms of allocation or collection) must be recognized and handled within the administrative structure.

3. *The benefits of the program must be clearly identified.* Very few medical care programs or arrangements offer the total gamut of available services. In the broadest sense, comprehensive medical services might include the services of physicians (generalists and specialists) in the office, home, and hospital; nursing care in the home and elsewhere; hospitalization, including all of the hospital's specialty services; complete dental care; drugs; prosthesis; laboratory and x-ray services; eyeglasses and appliances; physical therapy; and all the other speciality modalities.

Since such comprehensive benefits are rarely offered (except by military medical programs), it is essential to clarify what benefits are provided and where there are limits. For example, hospitalization may be covered only for a specified number of days, or nursing care visits may be available but restricted to a certain number.

4. *Eligibility for a program's services must be defined.* In the United States at the present time there are not only restrictions on the number and nature of services offered by organized programs but on which persons and how many will be covered and on conditions for which services are provided. Until or unless such restrictions are removed, those concerned with the organization of services must define the many aspects of eligibility. Sometimes the method of financing precircumscribes the eligible population; or there might be geographic boundaries. There are situations where some members of a family are eligible for care while other family members are excluded. The success of any organized plan for delivering medical care services depends heavily on the rational development of a system for eligibility determination. Otherwise, needed funds cannot be accurately calculated or adequately allocated.

5. *The participatory roles of the providers of medical services must be considered, planned, and coordinated.* The delivery of services is dependent on the availability of health professionals. In any attempt to organize medical care services, one has to deal with physicians, dentists, nurses, pharmacists, and many other health workers as well as with the local health organizations which these personnel represent. The relation-

ships, responsibilities, and obligations of the health professionals to the program and its supporting health agencies must be clearly defined. In addition, any working agreements must be in harmony with the licensure laws governing the particular professionals and meet the approval of the official agency responsible for public health in any given community.

6. *Quality of care must be a primary concern.* All of the above elements have an impact on quality. High quality of care depends on access to a wide spectrum of technical resources. The administrative structure, method of payment, level of professional staff, and so on are also equally important forces which affect quality of care. There are many organization arrangements and opportunities for continuing professional education which can be made to help raise the quality of care. Moreover, audit and evaluation systems to review services rendered can be useful tools in measuring and maintaining quality of care. It should be emphasized that critically important and intimately related to high quality is the provision of services which are relevant and responsive to the needs of the target population.

7. *There must be a mechanism for establishing and enforcing control.* A medical care program, like any other organized arrangement, must have rules and regulations governing the provision and use of its services. One of the most effective tools for guaranteeing control is a continuous and planned educational effort which makes the providers and consumers aware of the program, its goals, its objectives, and its attempts to service the community at large. Relationships between consumers and the program may vary between a highly bureaucratic setting and an extremely democratic one. As more consumer participation in the organization and delivery of medical care services becomes the rule rather than the exception, there will be increasing opportunity for consumers and providers to influence and direct the type of services offered in their own communities.

These, then, are some of the most important and basic considerations involved in any attempt to order or organize medical care resources and services. As was indicated in Chapter 11, there is indeed an urgent need for reordering and reorganizing; this reorganization must be grounded on a comprehensive approach which engages all components of the health care system. Professor John Thompson of the Yale University School of Medicine has suggested that such a system must be conceived as regional, rational, responsible, and responsive so that it can then, perhaps, be legally instituted as a "social utility." As such, the social aspects of the health care system's role in society are emphasized. Unlike the more familiar public-utility model, the social utility does not have a primary concern with financial control and public safety; instead, its commitment must be to the development of new services and new systems for delivering those services. In addition, the social utility must have much more citizen and community participation in its planning and management.

The concept of a regionalized system of care, for example, wherein a network of hospitals service the needs of a specific geographic area, is not new. It developed in Sweden during the latter part of the 1800s and began in Great Britain in the 1920s. In the United States this concept was implemented on a voluntary basis in the mid 1930s. Since that time, three federal programs have provided further impetus for the development of this idea. One of the objectives of the Hill-Burton Act, passed by Congress immediately following World War II, was the construction of hospital facilities based on regional hospital plans from various states. Later, chronic disease hospitals, nursing homes, and other types of health institutions were included; but the original limitation to hospitals minimized the Act's impact on the development of a comprehensive health care system.

In 1965 Congress enacted Public Law 79-239 (Regional Medical Programs) in an attempt to direct the resources of medical schools, the medical profession, voluntary and government health agencies, and paramedical and technical groups toward regionalization of activities concerning heart disease, cancer, and stroke. This program had varying success throughout the nation and, as we have already mentioned, is currently enlarging its scope to include an overall consideration of regionalization in the delivery of medical care.

The Comprehensive Health Planning Act of 1965 (Public Law 79-749) is a program concerned with planning rather than providing institutional medical services. Although it may be too early to assess the impact of this program, it is an important one to watch because of its mandate to develop state, regional, and local comprehensive health planning directed, in the words of the public law, at activities "to insure comprehensive health services of high quality for every person. . . ."

Other programs, such as Medicare and Medicaid, by increasing the financial availability of health care services to selected segments of the population (the aged, indigent, and medically indigent) without changing either the amount or the organization of those services, have compounded the problems of rising costs, fragmented care, quality control, and so on. They have underscored even further the need for a more rational, more effective, and more efficient organization of health resources and services. The process of regionalization is seen by many as an important first step toward a solution of the problems.

As has been mentioned previously, new organizational approaches must be responsive to patient needs, which are multiple, of varying complexity, and which require different levels of service at different times. One encouraging scheme designed to meet these needs is that of **progressive patient care.** Three principles are germane to this plan: (1) The patient will be admitted to that facility which can most appropriately meet his immediate medical needs. (2) He will be transferred to another type of facility as his condition changes. (3) Each facility will be designed, equipped, and staffed for patients with similar needs.

The original idea of this organizational arrangement was to contain progressive patient care within the hospital. There were to be three "zones of care" available: **intensive care** for the very ill, **intermediate care** (closely resembling the usual hospital inpatient unit), and **self-care** for the ambulatory patient at the beginning or the end of his hospital stay. This basic concept has been expanded considerably. First, there has been the development of a number of "care elements," or patient activities, and these now include (in addition to intensive care, intermediate care, and self-care) **long-term care, home care,** and **outpatient care.** Secondly,

---

PROGRESSIVE PATIENT CARE: a system designed to enhance efficiency of hospital care by furnishing personal health services tailored to the particular needs of the patient's condition; patients who require constant and intensive medical, nursing, and supportive care are grouped in one location; when their condition permits, they are moved to an area where only routine care is provided; patients who are capable of a measure of self-care are located in still another portion of the hospital where staff and services are appropriately reduced

INTENSIVE CARE: services rendered to seriously ill and critical patients who are unable to communicate their needs or who require extensive nursing care and observation; all necessary lifesaving emergency equipment, drugs, and supplies are immediately available

INTERMEDIATE CARE: services for hospital patients who require a moderate amount of nursing care; some patients may be ambulatory for short periods of time, and emergency care and frequent observation are rarely needed; this category includes patients who are beginning to participate in caring for themselves; further, the terminally ill may be cared for under these circumstances

SELF-CARE: for ambulatory and physically self-sufficient patients who require therapeutic or diagnostic services or who may be convalescing; this is a homelike atmosphere, and patients are instructed in self-care within the limits of their physical capacity

LONG-TERM CARE: for patients requiring skilled prolonged medical and nursing care; rehabilitation, occupational therapy, and physical therapy services are usually available; emphasis is placed on instructing those patients who must learn to adjust to a chronic illness and/or disability

a change in thinking has developed, and the concept of a progressive patient-care *hospital* has evolved into one of a progressive patient-care facilities *system* (including hospitals and other health care institutions, resources, and programs).

Within this system, the hospital outpatient department, while not ideally suited to provide high-quality primary care, can nevertheless function as a referral center for ambulatory patients. As such, it can provide complicated diagnostic and treatment procedures or consultations by highly specialized physicians (super-specialists). This type of function helps to maximize use of the hospital's expensive ancillary services—such as x-ray, radiotherapy, and laboratory—since utilization is not controlled by the number of beds filled at a given time. The development of formal cooperative arrangements or affiliations between hospitals and primary-care organizations would make it unnecessary for the latter to duplicate these expensive facilities or to add medical super-specialists to their own staffs.

Long-term care activities within the progressive patient-care scheme appear to be expanding into hospital-related care. Nursing home care is a familiar example of this. Less well known is the "social care institution," a foster home with nursing supervision; this form of delivering care within a total system is new to the United States but not to Europe. Patients who are for the most part ambulatory and require only limited medical or supervisory care can be supported in these institutions at considerably less cost than in nursing homes.

Implicit in the regional concept of organizing services is that health care institutions must be so operated as to maximize their responsiveness to the specific needs of their communities. This must be fortified by the added dimension of increased community participation even though attempts to augment community involvement are complicated by many problems—including the fact that various health care facilities are under different kinds of ownership (proprietary hospitals, for example, do not have any community boards). Techniques must be found to include representatives of various community groups on the policy-making boards

---

HOME CARE: for patients who can be cared for adequately in the home through the extension of certain services from the hospital and other sources; in this case, hospitals usually assume responsibility for coordinating services; such a home-care program provides personnel and equipment from the hospital or through community agencies such as the local health department, Visiting Nurse Association, and so on

OUTPATIENT CARE: as an element of progressive patient care, outpatient care is for ambulatory patients requiring diagnostic, curative, preventive, and rehabilitative services

of health care institutions, and ways must be developed to increase community involvement in both the planning and operation of these institutions. This is another crucial step in working toward a more effective organization of health care services.

The Role of Government

Government is assuming an ever-increasing responsibility in the medical care industry—not only in the financing of health care services but in influencing the organization and distribution of those services. We have previously mentioned some legislation which reflects this, but it is important at this point to review and to describe briefly the roles of federal, state, and local governments in medical care organization, financing, and delivery.

FEDERAL GOVERNMENT

It will be remembered from Chapter 10 that, early in its development, the federal government became involved in the direct provision of medical care services when it formed the merchant seamen's sick fund. This program evolved into the United States Public Health Service, which has had massive involvement in the health care field. At present, the federal government owns and operates medical services to the military under the Department of Defense. The budget for this is close to $2 billion annually, and medical care is provided for military personnel (and their families) in federal hospitals and clinics staffed by federal employees. Through the Veteran's Administration, another $1.5 billion is spent annually to provide direct medical care services to veterans. In addition, many other direct health services (such as the Indian Health Service) are provided through the United States Public Health Service, and, in recent years, there has been some federally controlled and supported health care under the program of the Office of Economic Opportunity. Health units have been established in urban and some rural poverty areas to provide primary health care in these areas of medical care scarcity.

In addition to providing direct services, the federal government functions in the regulation of personal health services and indirectly supports other health services in the country. Although the federal government does not grant licenses, federal legislation providing health benefits *does* set standards, such as those for the care of crippled children. Federal standards must be met in the construction of health facilities (under the

DISTRIBUTION OF PUBLIC AND PRIVATE HEALTH CARE
EXPENDITURES FOR AGED* (U.S.A. 1966, 1970)

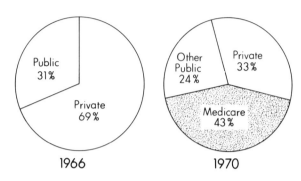

* AGE 65+

FIG. 12-1.   *After four years of medicare, much of the burden of financing health care for the aged has been shifted to the government. In fiscal 1966, 69 cents of every dollar spent on health care for an aged person came primarily out of the individual's pocket. In fiscal 1970, 67 cents of every health dollar for the aged was paid for by all levels of government with medicare contributing nearly three-fifths of this spending. (From* Basic Facts on The Health Industry, *prepared for the use of The Committee on Ways and Means, June 28, 1971, U.S. Government Printing Office, Washington, D.C.)*

Hill-Burton Act), and standards for the control of drugs to be used in practice are set by the Food and Drug Administration. Further regulating activities have been associated with the allocation of funds for various health activities where federal guidelines governing participation are specified. With the passage of the Social Security Act in 1935 and the many amendments which have followed since, there has been steadily more federal involvement in health care financing. As we have indicated at other points in this book, the 1965 amendments establishing Medicare and Title XIX were particularly important. A precedent was set for use of government funds to provide health care for a larger segment of the population (all those over 65) (Fig. 12-1). This was based on the insurance principle, and there was no means test included. Through the mechanism of grants-in-aid to the states, Title XIX (for the indigent and medically indigent) was an attempt to equalize the financial access to medical care services in this country.

STATE GOVERNMENT

In the evolution of medical care services, state government has tended to take on large-scale problems that are beyond the resources of local communities. The largest responsibility assumed by the states has been in the area of services to care for the mentally ill. States operate mental health hospitals and are now expanding their role to include provision for outpatient services. States have also been involved in the development and operation of special hospitals (such as tuberculosis facilities), most of which are now being used as chronic-disease, long-term care facilities.

LOCAL GOVERNMENT

In most communities in the United States, local government assumes responsibility for those who cannot afford private medical care by maintaining hospitals (in larger centers) and/or contracting to pay for services in voluntary hospitals. Most often these services are provided through county or municipal facilities in the form of hospital care and various outpatient clinic services. Examples of such facilities are Cook County Hospital in Chicago and Bellevue Municipal Hospital in New York City.

The above sketch of government's role in medical care organization highlights the fact that there are multiple inputs from different sources. This means that it is possible to visit certain areas of the country and find federal, state, and municipally operated health facilities offering identical services—and sometimes these facilities are directly adjacent to each other! There are few other countries in the world that can afford the luxury of such extensive duplication in such expensive areas as the provision of medical services.

The Private Role

There is a tradition of voluntarism in health matters which has influenced the patterns and configuration of health organizations in the United States. The voluntary health agency, an institution which emerged in the United States in the early part of the twentieth century, grew out of the health concerns of interested citizens. Voluntary health agencies focus public attention on health in general and stimulate action with respect to specific health problems, such as cancer, heart disease, tuberculosis, cerebral palsy, and muscular dystrophy, or health problems of a particular group, such as mothers and children or the poor. These agencies play an important role in identifying health problems and in devising approaches to solve them. They have also been concerned with the education of health professionals, and so have been involved in developing medical schools, i.e., voluntary teaching hospitals. They have also been supportive of and engaged in research pertaining to the causes, prevention, and cure of specific diseases; the direct provision of health care to specific groups and individuals with certain diseases; and the provision of institutional care for the aged, infirm, and so on.

Voluntary agencies are generally more flexible in their operation than government agencies, and are often able to attract the services of health professionals more readily than government. On the other hand, they tend to concentrate on specific areas within the health field and thus reflect the vested interests of their leaders or donors rather than the importance or magnitude of the total health need.

Within the private domain, another strong influence on the organization of medical care has been that of the health professionals and their organizations, notably physicians and the American Medical Association. Traditionally, medical care for the majority of individuals in this country is provided by private practitioners, usually on a *fee-for-service* basis. Fee for service means that the patient is billed each time he receives treatment from the physician. The patient decides when he is in need of a doctor's services and seeks his help at that time. The physician, after seeing the patient, submits his bill either to the patient or to a third party (government or insurance program). Fee-for-service practitioners can either practice alone (solo practitioners) or in group-practice settings (see Chap. 11). There is also a specialty group of physicians who generally develop hospital-based practices. These physicians are in the fields of radiology, pathology, and anesthesiology, and generally provide services for the patients at the request of the patient's personal physician.

Besides fee-for-service practice, another major category of private practice is *prepaid* group practice. In this arrangement, groups of physicians contract with subscribers or groups of subscribers to provide all their required medical care over a period of time and for a preestablished charge. This charge is the same whether the patient is never seen or is treated quite frequently during the particular period. Groups involved in prepaid practice are generally multispecialty in nature, and their services include hospital care. In such groups, it is to the fiscal advantage of the physicians to keep the patients as well as possible and to avoid hospitalizations—the costliest part of medical care services. Prepaid group practice is probably best known as it has evolved in the Kaiser Permanentee group on the west coast. The current national concern over escalating costs of medical care has been responsible for a strong federal effort to introduce prepayment on a national scale. Such a plan would hopefully lower the rate of increase in the cost of health care generally. The Nixon Administration has proposed the development of Health Maintenance Organizations—prepaid group practice which places emphasis on preventive medicine. Unfortunately, this controversial proposal was made not in response to demands for better medical care but rather in response to political pressure to moderate health costs; to date it has failed to receive financial backing from the Congress.

The Role of Insurance

The primary purpose of insurance is to protect people against the risks of large and unusual costs or losses. The concept of insurance dates back to the European guilds and their establishment of sick funds paid for by small weekly contributions from the members. Catastrophic financial losses during periods of illness were thus minimized. Almost 80 percent of the population have some kind of hospital insurance coverage (Fig. 12-2). In the nonprofit group of insurance organizations, Blue Cross and Blue Shield dominate the field and offer insurance coverage for hospital and physician services. There is also a large group of consumer-controlled insurance plans, such as Group Health Cooperative of Puget Sound and Health Insurance Plan of Greater New York, which contract for or provide medical services. Other insurance plans in existence are controlled by labor groups in various health and welfare funds and by management. As originally designed, the Kaiser Health Plan is an example of the management-owned group. While selling other kinds of insurance as well, the commercial companies have also provided insurance coverage for sickness. All of these forms of private health insurance received their biggest push at the end of the 1940s when, under government wage-stabilization programs, collective bargaining agreements began to shift emphasis from pay to fringe benefits. Over the last 30 years, labor has continued to support increasing health insurance coverage; this is currently demonstrated by its support for a form of national health insurance.

Most commercial insurance carriers serve only as fiscal agents and play no role in relation to the problems of health care delivery. These

Hospital Insurance Coverage Percentages by Specified Population Characteristics*(U.S.A.,1968).

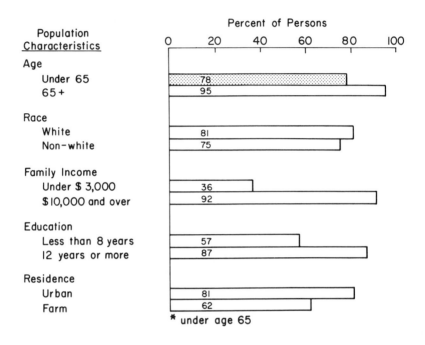

Fig. 12-2. *The shaded bar shows that 78 percent of all persons under age 65 have hospital insurance coverage. Note that the importance of having health insurance and the ability to pay for it (see income bars) are two determining factors in the extent of coverage. (From statistics prepared by U.S. National Center for Health Statistics, Hospital and Surgical Insurance Coverage, 1968, Public Health Service Publication No. 1000, Series 21, No. 15, Washington, D.C., 1972.)*

companies typically provide indemnity health insurance, i.e., the insurance company reimburses the client in accordance with preestablished scales; and this reimbursement is usually far less than the charges for medical services. It is theorized that because the client has to pay some of the bill himself, he will not over-utilize these services.

Blue Cross uses the service approach to insurance. It guarantees its members certain stipulated units of service—a certain number of hospital days, coverage of specified procedures, and so on. These insured services are provided through contracts between the insured and the providers of care. Thus, Blue Cross writes contracts for hospital services with various institutions. Under this plan the client does not have to pay the entire bill. He applies to the insurance company for the allowable payment and he pays the provider the difference between the amount covered by the particular policy and the total amount due.

Under the prepaid group insurance contract such as Kaiser, the same organization which insures also is responsible for providing the medical care services. The proponents of prepaid group insurance claim that by combining the insurance and service functions in the same organization it is not only easier to control cost but there is a built-in incentive to work towards keeping patients well.

In summary, it would seem clear that a genuinely effective and orderly organization of health services would require a plan that includes coverage of all health needs from prevention to rehabilitation, the elimination of gaps in services, the assurance of continuity of care, the avoidance of duplication, and the dissemination of information about what is available and where it can be obtained. In the United States no legislation has yet been passed to make such a plan feasible (even the so-called "comprehensive benefits" plans rarely cover dental care, psychiatric service, drugs, social services, and so on). However, as we have seen in this chapter, there are trends which hold real promise for improvement in the organization and financing of medical care services. The expansion of the health insurance concept and the special governmental health programs of the past few decades have demonstrated the advantages to be gained in group rather than individual financing for health care. To cover that portion of the population that currently has no prepayment protection, the trend is clearly toward community-wide, state, and national financing, with increasing dependence upon public funds and social insurance to cover the special risk groups.

The trends toward regionalization and increased cooperation and affiliation between health care institutions, as well as the development of such programs as progressive patient care, will immensely improve the efficiency and quality of health care delivery. As was pointed out in Chapter 11, there is also increasing coordination and cooperative effort among health care personnel. As health personnel function more in a team fashion and various physical facilities establish more rational inter-relationships, the value of and need for specially organized health services will become increasingly clear. In addition to some of the more hopeful developments already discussed, the concept of the community "health service center" or "multiservice center" is also evolving. Within these centers, local health and welfare activities are coordinated and services are dispensed from a central base of operation which serves a geographically defined area. Finally, it should be reemphasized that the lay public is becoming much more knowledgeable about health and disease and more interested in assuming an active role in organizational planning of health care services. It can be predicted that this trend will increase until the delivery of health care services reaches the level of adequacy that is needed and demanded.

Utilization of Medical Care Services

Whether, how, when, or to what extent medical care services are utilized is of course influenced by their adequacy, how they are organized, and what financial resources are required and available. In addition, utilization reflects functional aspects of need and effective demand, and is directly related to such prime determinants as socioeconomic level, age, demographic factors, and so on.

Some of the factors which affect the ability to perceive or identify a need for medical care were discussed in Chapter 2. Such studies as Koos reported in The Health of Regionville (1954) demonstrate the divergent attitudes toward illness, health, and medical care among different socioeconomic classes. The lower socioeconomic groups tend to have less information and knowledge about illness and medical care and therefore differ from higher socioeconomic classes in their perceived needs for medical services. Cultural factors also influence perceived need. Even in persons from similar socioeconomic and cultural circumstances, differences in personality, in threshold levels for pain, and in concepts of how the body functions affect attitudes and the perception of need. For example, if two individuals have nosebleeds, one might perceive his condition as requiring hospitalization, while the other might dismiss the episode as insignificant and merely apply ice until the bleeding stopped.

Needs, particularly as perceived by the consumer of medical services, may be real in the psychologic sense but may or may not be real in purely medical terms. Although the importance of psychologic and social variables in health and disease has been clearly documented, the medical care system does not have endless resources; therefore, in terms of both the individual and the community, some limits must be placed on what is defined as real need for medical care services. Such definitions are generally made by the persons or agencies representing professional expertise —the physician, the voluntary health agency, government, universities, and so on. However, the successful use of any medical care is ultimately dependent on the extent to which it is favorably accepted by the consumer. In providing services, the medical care system therefore must not only deal with what it defines as real need but must also bring into balance perceived medical needs.

Demand for a medical service can be defined as action taken by individuals, groups, or politically motivated organizations to secure some desired health goal. Although demand and need are related, we have already seen that demand does not always represent a real need. Many patients demand that their physicians prescribe penicillin to cure a common cold although there is no real need for this drug without some associated infection. On the other hand, the presence of a real need (even when it is perceived as such) does not always get mobilized into a demand. There is a real need for people to maintain immunization against tetanus—a serious disease which potentially can affect most people in the population—but there is no sustained demand for this service.

Many factors are involved in the translation of a perceived need into an effective demand for medical service. Rosenstock has grouped these factors into five categories: (1) perceived susceptibility, (2) perceived seriousness, (3) perceived benefits, (4) perceived barriers, and (5) cues to action. As an example of how these factors come into play, let us hypothesize that a potential consumer of medical care starts throwing up blood as the result of an ulcer as diagnosed at a previous visit to a physician. At that contact the patient learned enough about his disease to know that he might need an operation to cure his symptoms. His perceived need for medical care is a real need. However, before he mobilizes effective demand for service, he contemplates some of the following questions: What is the risk involved if he does not seek medical care and the surgical procedure? Is less risk involved in having the surgery than in not seeking medical care? What will surgery and medical care cost him, and can he afford it? Is there a qualified surgeon and adequate facilities in the area to treat him, and will the surgeon accept his case?

The economist defines effective demand in terms of the amount of goods and services that the consumer is willing and able to purchase at a given price level. Within this context, such factors as consumer preference, the size of the market, the price level of the goods or service, the income level of the consumer, and the price level of substitute and alternate goods must be considered. Medical services have to compete in the market place with a wide variety of other consumer goods and services—a family's decision to purchase a color television set might represent a financial postponement of needed medical services. Third-party systems of financing (e.g., Blue Cross) *do* provide an alternative in the open competition between certain medical services and consumer goods. There is also a growing feeling that personal health services should not compete with other goods and services for consumer dollars, but rather should be included in the list of services (such as public education, public health, disaster relief, and a standing army) which society provides for its constituents.

In Chapter 10 we reviewed major socioeconomic and demographic trends and factors and indicated that they significantly affect the utilization of medical care services. Although their complex interrelationship makes it impossible to identify the exact impact of any one of these factors, some broad conclusions have been established. There has been a definite increase in the utilization of personal health services over the years of this century. Along with the increased rates in hospitalization and use of physicians' services, there has been a marked movement toward the hospital as the center for the medical care system. In addition, as shown in Figure 12-3, there has been a decided trend toward more office and clinic visits and toward a corresponding decrease in the much-lamented "house call." Almost three-fourths of all visits now take place in physicians' offices; visit to clinics represent about 9 percent, and home visits have

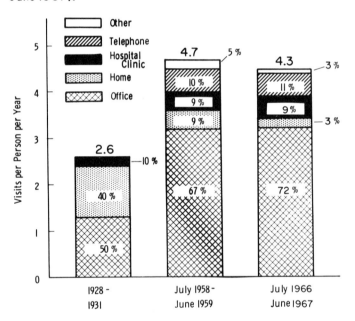

Physician Visits* per Person per Year, by Place of Visit (U.S.A.,1928-1931,** July 1958-June1959, and July 1966 – June 1967).

* Excludes visits to patients in hospital. Number in bar indicates percent of all visits.

**White families only.

Fig. 12-3. *(Adapted from* Medical Chart Book, *University of Michigan, School of Public Health, Third Edition, Revised 1968.)*

Utilization of General Hospitals (U.S.A., 1928–1970).

Year	Admissions per 1000 persons per Year	Hospital Days per 1000 Persons per Year
1928–31*	58.6	746
1946**	98.3	896
1950**	110.5	900
1956**	121.1	934
1960**	128.9	977
1963**	135.4	1036
1965**	137.9	1071
1970**	145	1198

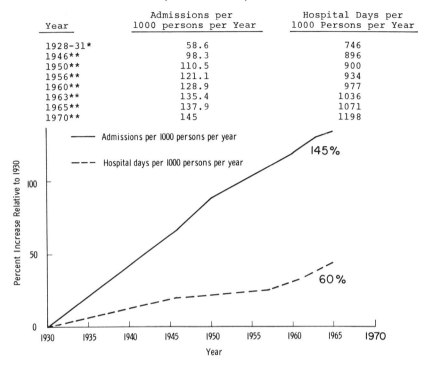

* Pertain to all hospitals except tuberculosis and psychiatric.
** Pertain to all non-federal short-term, long-term, and special hospitals
listed by the American Hospital Association.

Fig. 12-4.   (*Adapted from* Medical Chart Book, *University of Michigan, School of Public Health, Third Edition, Revised 1968.*)

dropped dramatically from 40 percent in 1928–31 to the present figure of about 3 percent. The rapid increase in the utilization of general hospitals is shown (for the years 1930 through 1970) in Figure 12-4. In the United States, utilization rates in terms of physician visits have shown some changes over the years. Figure 12-3 also shows an increase in average number of visits per year from 2.6 in the early 1930s to about 4.3 visits per year in the late 1960s. Since that time there has been very little change in the average number of annual visits to the physician.

In general, the poor, the nonwhite, and the poorly educated have lower utilization rates in terms of both hospitalization and visits to a physician. Studies indicate that there is also a marked difference between these groups and the more affluent, the white, and the educated population in the use of specialists (i.e., psychiatrists, dermatologists, orthopedics, and so on). The former groups receive far less care from these medical experts. The barriers related to economic and discriminatory disadvantages can partially account for the lower utilization rates in population groups whose members are generally more ill and in greater need of medical care services. With reference to visits to physicians, the fact that lower income families generally receive less medical care than families with moderate or high incomes is demonstrated in Figure 12-5.

Females have a higher rate (114 persons per 1,000 population) of hospitalization than males (70 per 1,000) and, similarly, tend to have more physician visits than males. One must immediately take into consideration that, for most women, childbirth is a hospital admission, although not related to an episode of illness.

The distribution of hospitalization based on geographical region shows that persons living in the North Central area of the nation are admitted to hospitals more than others (96 per 1,000 population); the West follows with 93, the South with 92, and the Northeast with 89. Persons living in the West use physicians more than those in other

Number of Physician Visits per Person per Year, by Family Income and Age (U.S.A. July '66 – June '67).

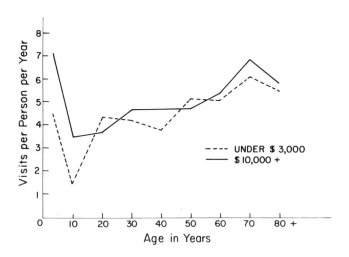

FIG. 12-5. *(Adapted from statistics prepared by U.S. National Center for Health Statistics, Volume of Physician Visits, U.S. 1966–1967, Public Health Service Publication No. 1000, Series 10, No. 49, Washington, D.C., 1968.)*

areas, while persons in the South have the lowest rate of physician utilization. In general, residents of rural communities receive less medical care
than residents of urban areas. This is partly due to lower incomes and
also to less availability of facilities and health personnel to provide
medical care services.

Age is an important variable in the utilization of medical care services.
Young persons (under age 15) are hospitalized less frequently than
those in other age groups, and individuals between ages 15 and 44 have
the highest rate of hospital use. Aged persons—65 years and over—have
the second highest rate, with 112 individuals being hospitalized per
1,000 persons; for those between the ages of 45 and 64, the rate per
1,000 is 95. More physician visits are made by the young and the old than
by other age groups. Between persons under 5, who average about five
visits per year, and those aged 65 or older, who have about six physician
visits annually, there is a steady increase in utilization. Overall, the aged
need and generally use more medical services than the general population.
In addition, as was indicated in Chapter 10, the percentage of aged persons
in this country continues to increase. These factors are particularly im-

Number of Physician Visits in Each Age Group,
by Education of Family Head (U.S.A. July '66-'67).

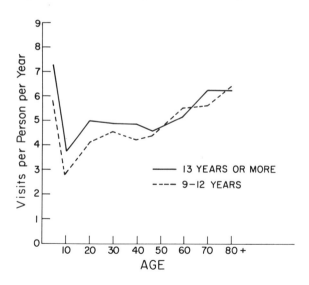

FIG. 12-6.   *(Adapted from statistics prepared by U.S. National Center for Health
Statistics,* Volume of Physician Visits, U.S. 1966–1967, *Public Health
Service Publication No. 1000, Series 10, No. 49, Washington, D.C., 1968.)*

portant in terms of their impact on the demand for medical care. With an increasingly aged population, marked changes in the nature of illness can also be observed. There is more chronic disease, more mental illness, and longer periods of disability among the aged than among other groups. Chronic disease demands more and longer periods of medical services and is accompanied by an increasing need for long-term rehabilitative health services.

It has been demonstrated that education level is related to the utilization of medical care services. The more educated members of the population tend to use most health services more frequently; this is reflected in Figure 12-6. The increase in education at all levels has had a significant effect on planning health services. A more informed, aware, and articulate public makes a greater demand for adequate medical care services.

It must be emphasized that rising rates in utilization of medical and hospital services do not necessarily indicate that community needs are being met more effectively. A real determination of needs and utilization depends on the eradication of economic, social, and cultural barriers, and on the adequacy, availability, and accessibility of all medical care services.

References

Closing the Gap in the Availability and Accessibility of Health Services. Bull. N.Y. Acad. Med. 41:(12) (1965).

Council of Social Work Education and Public Health Service. Effective Community Health Services. Public Health Concepts in Social Work Education, Proceedings of Seminar held at Princeton Universty, 1962.

Dimensions and Detriments of Health Policy. The Milbank Memorial Fund Quarterly **XLVI**:(1) Part 2 (1968).

Garfield, S. R. The delivery of medical care. Sci. Amer. **222**:(4) (1970).

A Guide to Medical Care Administration, Vol. I: Concepts and Principles. Washington, D. C., American Public Health Association, 1969.

Jones, L. W., and Lee, R. I. The Fundamentals of Good Medical Care. Publication No. 22 of the Committee on the Cost of Medical Care. Chicago, University of Chicago Press, 1933.

Katz, A., and Felton, J. S., eds. Health and the Community. Readings in the Philosophy and Sciences of Public Health. New York, The Free Press, 1965.

Kilbourne, E., and Smillie, W. G. Human Ecology and Public Health, 4th ed. London, The MacMillan Co., Collier-MacMillan Ltd., 1969.

Lenner, M. The Extent to Which Patients Use Hospital and Physician Services. Proceedings, The First National Conference on Utilization, Joint Commission for Prevention of Voluntary Nonprofit Prepayment Health Plans, Chicago, March, 1962.

National Center for Health Statistics. Family Use of Health Services, U.S., July, 1963–June, 1964. Vital and Health Statistics, Ser. 10, No. 55, Washington, D.C., U.S. Department of Health, Education, and Welfare, 1969.

Roemer, M. I. Medical Care Administration: Content, Positions, and Training in the United States. Western Branch, American Public Health Association (San Francisco) and the U.C.L.A. School of Public Health (Los Angeles), January, 1963.

Schorow, M., ed. Hearings on Issues and Trends in Medical Care. Intermountain Regional Medical Program, Colloquium of the Air Series, 1969.

Somers, H. M., and Somers, A. R. Doctors, Patients, and Health Insurance. Washington, D.C., The Brookings Institution, 1961.

Straus, A. L. Where Medicare Fails. Transaction Books, 1970.

The University of Michigan School of Public Health Medical Care Chart Book, Bureau of Public Health Economics, 1968.

Concluding Note

The most fundamental value in the American dream is equal opportunity for all—regardless of race, color, socioeconomic status, or cultural differences. Two centuries ago the American system was founded by men whose philosophy was formalized in the Bill of Rights and the Constitution. By virtue of the former, all Americans are entitled to "life, liberty, and the pursuit of happiness"; and according to the Constitution, Congress is charged with the responsibility "to promote the general welfare." The belief in universal entitlement to equal rights and equal opportunity is thus expressed formally in the essential law of the land. However, it was not until 1966, when the Partnership for Health Act (Public Law 89-749) was passed, that universal entitlement to health care services was officially linked with our national purpose and specifically mandated in legislation. In this Act's *Findings and Declaration of Purpose,* it was stated that

the Congress declares that fulfillment of our national purpose depends on promoting and assuring the highest level of health attainable for every person . . . and . . . marshaling of all health resources to assure comprehensive health services of high quality for every person. . . .

This formal resolution of entitlement has three direct implications:

1. Entitlement should be universal; that is, all barriers to adequate health care—barriers deriving from limited financial resources, health manpower shortages, geographic maldistribution, and so on—should be removed for *everyone.*

414

2. Entitlement should be comprehensive and functionally translated into action; that is, all aspects of the health care services spectrum—from prevention to rehabilitation, emergency care to chronic care, inpatient to outpatient treatment—should be of high quality and available to all in the appropriate quantity, 7 days a week, 24 hours a day.

3. Health care should be delivered to every man, woman, and child in a dignified and humane manner.

It is clear that our current health care system must be significantly altered if we are to move towards a society where all Americans receive the health care to which they are entitled in the manner to which they are entitled. We have reviewed many aspects and problems of the traditional health care system and many areas in which new and promising developments can be seen. However, the most fundamental and crucial step still has not been taken: *The United States has not yet formulated a health care policy for the whole nation.* This may seem rather incredible when we pause to think that most developed nations have a formal health policy and that we are pouring over $60 billion into health enterprises with exceedingly little cost control, quality control, or forethought. There are many ideas which have been and continue to be advanced about what constitutes an optimum national health policy. Decisions must be made. Most important, there must ultimately emerge a *National Health Act* which will be a responsive, encompassing, responsible, and genuinely effective base for practically implementing a national health policy.

In summary, the efforts of all committed and concerned persons must be dedicated to the establishment of a national health policy and a system for implementing that policy which incorporate the following:

1. the principle of universal entitlement
2. economic efficiency
3. cohesive and coordinated operation
4. systematically high-quality care
5. an emphasis on comprehensive health rather than sickness
6. the rapid and widespread application of advances in biomedical knowledge
7. social commitment to the common good rather than to the narrow economic advantage of any particular group
8. enlightened organization and planning of health resources for all people and areas of the United States.

Five Leading Causes of Death by Age Groups in the United States, 1967

Rank	Cause of Death	Rate per 100,000 Population
1.	25–34 Years (Overall Death Rate 150)	
1.	Accidents	52.0
2.	Cancer	17.5
3.	Homicide	14.6
4.	Heart disease	12.4
5.	Suicide	12.4
	35–44 Years (Overall Death Rate 310)	
1.	Heart disease	71.7
2.	Cancer	60.3
3.	Accidents	47.8
4.	Cirrhosis of liver	17.2
	45–54 Years (Overall Death Rate 730)	
1.	Heart disease	252.1
2.	Cancer	179.4
3.	Accidents	54.1
4.	Strokes	53.5
5.	Cirrhosis of liver	34.8
	55–64 Years (Overall Death Rate 1,670)	
1.	Heart disease	687.4
2.	Cancer	412.4
3.	Stroke	120.9
4.	Accidents	66.0
5.	Cirrhosis of liver	45.7

[a]*Statistics for other age groups appear in Table 6-3 (ages 1-24) and Table 6-4 (age 65 and over.*
Source: Facts of Life and Death, National Center for Health Statistics, Pub. No. 600 (1970).

APPENDIX
II

Examples of Energy Expenditures by Reference Man and Woman[a]

Activity	Time (hr)	Man		Woman	
		Rate (kcal[b]/min)	Total	Rate (kcal/min)	Total
Sleeping[c] and reclining	8	1.1	530	1.0	480
Sitting[d]	7	1.5	630	1.1	460
Standing[e]	5	2.5	750	1.5	450
Walking[f]	2	3.0	360	2.5	300
Other[g]	2	4.5	540	3.0	360

[a]Reference man is 22 years old and weighs 154 lb. Reference woman is 22 years old and weighs 128 lb.
[b]The amount of heat necessary to raise 1 kg of water $1°C$.
[c]Essentially resting metabolic rate.
[d]Includes normal activity carried on while sitting, e.g., reading, driving automobile, eating, and desk or bench work.
[e]Includes normal indoor activities while standing and walking intermittently in limited area, e.g., cooking and washing and moving from room to room.
[f]Includes purposeful walking, largely outdoors, e.g., home to commuting station to work site, and other comparable activities.
[g]Includes intermittent activities in occasional sports, exercises, limited stair-climbing, or occupational activities involving light physical work. This category may include weekend swimming, golf, tennis, etc. using 5 to 20 kcal/min for a limited time.

Source: Adapted from Recommended Dietary Allowances, 7th ed. Pub. No. 1694, Washington, D.C., National Academy of Sciences–National Research Council, 1968.

APPENDIX

III

Calorie Values of Common Foods and Beverages

Dairy Products and Eggs	Serving	Calories
Cheese, cream	1 oz	100
Cream, heavy	1 tbsp	50
Egg, boiled	1	80
Egg, scrambled, fried	1	100
Yogurt, plain	½ cup	60

Desserts	Serving	Calories
Brownies	1	150
Chocolate cake, icing	2-in. slice	450
Ice cream, vanilla	½ cup	200
Pie, apple, cherry	1 slice	350
Sponge cake, plain	2-in. slice	100

Fruits and Fruit Juices	Serving	Calories
Apple	1 large	100
Applesauce, unsweetened	½ cup	50
Banana	1 medium	100
Cantaloupe, honeydew	½	50
Grapefruit	½	70
Orange, grapefruit juice	8 oz	100
Tomato juice	8 oz	50
Watermelon	1 slice	100
	(4 in. by 6 in.)	

Meats and Poultry	Serving	Calories
Bacon, broiled	2 strips	100
Beef, hamburger	3 oz	200
Boiled ham (sliced)	3 oz	200
Bologna	1 slice	70
Chicken or turkey, roast	3 oz	150
Frankfurter on roll	1	300
Hamburger on roll	4 oz	350
Porkchop	1	300
Steak, broiled	3 oz	250
Veal cutlet	3 oz	250

Sandwiches (White Bread)	Serving	Calories
Bacon, lettuce, tomato	1	300
Cheese, American, Swiss	1	250
Club (bacon, chicken, tomato)	1	600
Peanut butter	1	300
Roast beef	1	300

Vegetables (Cooked)	Serving	Calories
Beans, canned, baked	1 cup	300
Beets	½ cup	35
Carrots, tomatoes	1 cup	45
Corn	2/3 cup	100
Macaroni and cheese	1 cup	350
Peas	½ cup	50
Potato, white	1	100
Rice	½ cup	100

Vegetables (Raw and Salads)	Serving	Calories
Carrot	1 medium	20
Lettuce	¼ head	10
Mixed green salad	1 cup	15
Onions	1 medium	50

Beverages (Non-alcoholic)	Serving	Calories
Carbonated beverages	6 oz	80
Carbonated beverages (artificially sweetened)	6 oz	1
Cocoa, milk	1 cup	150
Coffee, black	1 cup	0
Coffee, milk, sugar (1 tsp)	1 cup	35
Milk, skim	8 oz	80
Milk, whole	8 oz	150
Tea, plain	1 cup	0
Tea, milk, sugar (1 tsp)	1 cup	35

Alcoholic Beverages	Serving	Calories
Beer	8 oz	100
Martini, dry	3½ oz	150
Whiskey, gin, vodka, rum	1½ oz	100
Wine, dry	3½ oz	80
Wine, sweet	3½ oz	150

Courtesy of Standard Brands Incorporated.

APPENDIX

IV

Desirable Weights for Men and Women of Ages 25 and Over [a]

Height (shoes on 1-in. heel)	Men Small Frame	Men Medium Frame	Men Large Frame
5'2"	112–120	118–129	126–141
5'3"	115–123	121–133	129–144
5'4"	118–126	124–136	132–148
5'5"	121–129	127–139	135–152
5'6"	124–133	130–143	138–156
5'7"	128–137	134–147	142–161
5'8"	132–141	138–152	147–166
5'9"	136–145	142–156	151–170
5'10"	140–150	146–160	155–174
5'11"	144–154	150–165	159–179
6'0"	148–158	154–170	164–184
6'1"	152–162	158–175	168–189
6'2"	156–167	162–180	173–194
6'3"	160–171	167–185	178–199
6'4"	164–175	172–190	182–204

Height (shoes on 2-in. heel)	Women Small Frame	Women Medium Frame	Women Large Frame
4'10"	92–98	96–107	104–119
4'11"	94–101	98–110	106–122
5'0"	96–104	101–113	109–125
5'1"	99–107	104–116	112–128
5'2"	102–110	107–119	115–131
5'3"	105–113	110–122	118–134
5'4"	108–116	113–126	121–138
5'5"	111–119	116–130	125–142
5'6"	114–123	120–135	129–146
5'7"	118–127	124–139	133–150
5'8"	122–131	128–143	137–154
5'9"	126–135	132–147	141–158
5'10"	130–140	136–151	145–163
5'11"	134–144	140–155	149–168
6'0"	138–148	144–159	153–173

[a] Weight in pounds according to frame (in indoor clothing).
Courtesy of Standard Brands Incorporated.

Calorie Intake to Lose Weight for Men and Women Ages 25 and Over

CALORIE ALLOWANCES FOR MEN

Weight (lb)	Daily Intake to Maintain Weight	Daily Calorie Intake to Lose 1 lb per Week	Daily Calorie Intake to Lose 2 lb per Week
130	2300	1800	1300
140	2400	1950	1450
150	2500	2100	1600
160	2700	2200	1700
170	2800	2300	1800
180	2900	2450	1950
190	3100	2600	2100
200	3200	2700	2200
210	3300	2800	2300
220	3400	2950	2450

CALORIE ALLOWANCES FOR WOMEN

110	1700	1200	700
120	1800	1300	800
130	1900	1400	900
140	2000	1550	1050
150	2100	1650	1150
160	2300	1750	1250
170	2400	1900	1400
180	2500	2000	1500
190	2600	2100	1600
200	2700	2200	1700

Courtesy of Standard Brands Incorporated.

APPENDIX VI

Recommended Daily Dietary Allowances (Abridged)^a

[Designed for the maintenance of good nutrition of practically all healthy persons in the U.S.A.]

Persons	Age in Years^b From up to	Weight in Pounds	Height in Inches	Food Energy Calories	Protein Grams	Calcium Grams	Iron Milligrams	Vitamin A International Units	Thiamin Milligrams	Riboflavin Milligrams	Niacin Equivalent Milligrams	Ascorbic Acid Milligrams
Infants	0-1/6	9	22	lb. X 264	lb. X 4.8	0.4	6	1,500	0.2	0.4	5	35
	1/6-1/2	15	25	lb. X 242	lb. X 4.4	0.5	10	1,500	0.4	0.5	7	35
	1/2-1	20	28	lb. X 220	lb. X 4.0	0.6	15	1,500	0.5	0.6	8	35
Children	1-2	26	32	1,100	25	0.7	15	2,000	0.6	0.6	8	40
	2-3	31	36	1,250	25	0.8	15	2,000	0.6	0.7	8	40
	3-4	35	39	1,400	30	0.8	10	2,500	0.7	0.8	9	40
	4-6	42	43	1,600	30	0.8	10	2,500	0.8	0.9	11	40
	6-8	51	48	2,000	35	0.9	10	3,500	1.0	1.1	13	40
	8-10	62	52	2,200	40	1.0	10	3,500	1.1	1.2	15	40
Boys	10-12	77	55	2,500	45	1.2	10	4,500	1.3	1.3	17	40
	12-14	95	59	2,700	50	1.4	18	5,000	1.4	1.4	18	45
	14-18	130	67	3,000	60	1.4	18	5,000	1.5	1.5	20	55
Men	18-22	147	69	2,800	60	0.8	10	5,000	1.4	1.6	18	60
	22-35	154	69	2,800	65	0.8	10	5,000	1.4	1.7	18	60
	35-55	154	68	2,600	65	0.8	10	5,000	1.3	1.7	17	60
	55-75+	154	67	2,400	65	0.8	10	5,000	1.2	1.7	14	60

Girls											
10-12	77	56	2,250	50	1.2	18	4,500	1.1	1.3	15	40
12-14	97	61	2,300	50	1.3	18	5,000	1.2	1.4	15	45
14-16	114	62	2,400	55	1.3	18	5,000	1.2	1.4	16	50
16-18	119	63	2,300	55	1.3	18	5,000	1.2	1.5	15	50
Women											
18-22	128	64	2,000	55	0.8	18	5,000	1.0	1.5	13	55
22-35	128	64	2,000	55	0.8	18	5,000	1.0	1.5	13	55
35-55	128	63	1,850	55	0.8	10	5,000	1.0	1.5	13	55
55-75+	128	62	1,700	55	0.8	18	5,000	1.0	1.5	13	55
Pregnant			+200	65	+0.4	18	6,000	+0.1	1.8	15	60
Lactating			+1,000	75	+0.5	18	8,000	+0.5	2.0	20	60

Source: Adapted from Recommended Dietary Allowances, Seventh edition 1968, Publication 1694, 169 pages. Published by National Academy of Sciences—National Research Council, Washington, D. C. 20418. Also available in libraries. This publication includes discussion of allowances, eight additional nutrients, and adjustments needed for age, body size, and physical activity.

aNiacin equivalents include dietary sources of the vitamin itself plus 1 milligram equivalent for each 60 milligrams of dietary tryptophan.

bEntries for age range 22 to 35 years represent the reference man and woman at age 22. All other entries represent allowances for the midpoint of the specified age group.

NOTE.—The Recommended Daily Dietary Allowances should not be confused with Minimum Daily Requirements. The Recommended Dietary Allowances are amounts of nutrients recommended by the Food and Nutrition Board of National Research Council, and are considered adequate for maintenance of good nutrition in healthy persons in the United States. The allowances are revised from time to time in accordance with newer knowledge of nutritional needs.

The Minimum Daily Requirements are the amounts of selected nutrients that have been established by the Food and Drug Administration as standards for labeling purposes of foods and pharmaceutical preparations for special dietary uses. These are the amounts regarded as necessary in the diet for the prevention of deficiency diseases and generally are less than the Recommended Dietary Allowances. The Minimum Daily Requirements for the adult man are: Vitamin A, 4000 I.U.; thiamin, 1 milligram; riboflavin, 1.2 milligram; niacin, 10 milligrams; ascorbic acid, 30 milligrams; calcium, 750 milligrams; iron, 10 milligrams. For additional information on Minimum Daily Requirements see the Federal Register, vol. 6, No. 227 (Nov. 22, 1941), beginning on p. 5921, and amended as stated in the Federal Register (June 1, 1957), vol. 22, No. 106, p. 3841 (effective July 1, 1958).

VII

Major Categories of American Abortion Laws: United States—January 1, 1971

Major Categories of State Abortion Laws	States Having Similar Abortion Laws
I. Abortion allowed only when necessary to preserve the life of the pregnant woman.	Arizona, Connecticut, Florida, Idaho, Illinois, Indiana, Iowa[a], Kentucky, Louisiana[b], Maine, Michigan, Minnesota, Missouri, Montana, Nebraska, Nevada, New Hampshire, North Dakota, Ohio, Oklahoma, Rhode Island, South Dakota, Tennessee, Utah, Vermont, West Virginia, Wyoming.
II. Indications for legal abortion include threats to the pregnant woman's life and forcible rape:	Mississippi.
III. "Unlawful" or "unjustifiable" abortions are prohibited:	Massachusetts, New Jersey, Pennsylvania.
IV. Abortions allowed when continuation of the pregnancy threatens the woman's life or health:	Alabama.
V. American Law Institute Model Abortion Law; "A licensed physician is justified in terminating a pregnancy if he believes that there is substantial risk that continuance of the pregnancy would gravely impair the physical or mental health of the mother or that the child would be born with grave physical or mental defect, or that the pregnancy resulted from rape, incest or other felonious intercourse":	Arkansas, California (does not include fetal deformity), Colorado, Delaware, Kansas, Maryland (does not include incest), New Mexico, North Carolina, South Carolina, Virginia.
VI. Abortion law based on the May 1968 recommendations of the American College of Obstetricians and Gynecologists. Allows abortion when the pregnancy resulted from felonious intercourse, and when there is risk that continuance of the pregnancy would impair the physical or mental health of the mother. "In determining whether or not there is substantial risk (to the woman's physical or mental health), account may be taken of the mother's total environment, actual or reasonably foreseeable":	Oregon.

Major Categories of State Abortion Laws	States Having Similar Abortion Laws
VII. No legal restriction on reasons for which an abortion may be obtained prior to viability of the fetus:	Alaska, Hawaii, New York, Washington.
VIII. Legal restrictions on reasons for which an abortion may be obtained were invalidated by court decision:	District of Columbia, Georgia, Texas, Wisconsin.[c]

From Abortion Surveillance Report—Legal Abortions, United States Annual Summary, 1970 Center for Disease Control, Public Health Service, U. S. Department of Health, Education, and Welfare.

[a]*In State vs Dunklebarger, the Iowa statute which is couched in terms of saving the life of the woman, has been interpreted to suggested that preservation of health is sufficient. 221 N.W. 592 (Iowa, 1928).*

[b]*Although the Louisiana abortion statute does not contain an express exception to the "crime of abortion" the Louisiana Medical Practice Act authorizes the Medical Board to suspend or institute court proceedings to revoke a doctor's certificate to practice medicine in the state when the doctor has procured or aided or abetted in the procuring of an abortion "unless done for the relief of a woman whose life appears imperiled after due consultation with another licensed physician." La. Rev. Stat. Ann. 37:1261.*

[c]*The abortion law of several other states has been ruled unconstitutional by lower state trail courts; however, these decisions are binding only in the jurisdiction in which the decision was rendered.*

APPENDIX
VIII

Antidote and First Aid for Poisoning

The following represent substances most frequently ingested by children, and first aid measures that may be employed until medical aid can be summoned.

Substance	Emergency Treatment
MEDICINE (OVERDOSAGE) Aspirin and aspirin-containing medications Cough medicine Hormones (including thyroid preparations)	Give 2-3 glasses of water or milk, then induce vomiting UNLESS patient is unconscious or convulsing.
Vitamins and iron tablets	Induce vomiting. Then give glass of milk.
Sleeping pills	Induce vomiting. Do **not** induce vomiting or force fluids if patient is unconscious.
Tranquilizers	Induce vomiting unless patient is unconscious. Give 2 tablespoons epsom salts in 2 glasses of water.
HOUSEHOLD CLEANING AND POLISHING AGENTS Laundry bleach Automatic dishwasher detergents Household cleaners Furniture polish Cleaning fluid (gasoline, kerosene) Charcoal fire starter	Give 2-3 glasses of milk or water immediately. Do **not** induce vomiting.
Toilet bowl and drain cleaners	Do **not** induce vomiting. Give 2-3 glasses of milk or water at once. **A**void gas-forming carbonates and bicarbonates.
Wax remover	Give milk or water. Do **not** induce vomiting.
Fabric softeners	Give milk. Neutralize with **weak** soap (not detergent) solution. Induce vomiting.
Household ammonia	Give citrus juice or diluted (1 tablespoon per glassful) vinegar. Then give 2 raw egg whites or 2 oz. olive oil. Do **not** induce vomiting.

Substance	Emergency Treatment
INSECTICIDES, POISON SUBSTANCES, PAINTS (Read labels for content)	
Arsenic	Give glass of milk immediately and induce vomiting. Then give activated charcoal (available from pharmacist).
DDT	Induce vomiting. Give 2 tablespoons epsom salts in 2 glasses water.
Lye	Do **not** induce vomiting. Give solution of vinegar (2 tablespoons vinegar in 2 glasses water). Next give 2 raw egg whites or 2 oz. olive oil.
Paint (dry)	Give milk or water. Induce vomiting.
Paint (liquid)	Give 2-3 glasses of milk or water. Do **not** induce vomiting.
COSMETICS Cologne or perfume Hand lotion Liquid makeup Skin lotion After-shave lotion	Give milk. Induce vomiting if large amounts ingested.
Deodorant	Give milk of magnesia. Induce vomiting.
Bubble bath liquid Hair rinse (conditioners) Shampoo	Give milk or water at once. Induce vomiting.
Nail polish and removers Lacquers Bath oil	Give milk. Induce vomiting.
Home permanent neutralizer Permanent wave solution	Give milk or water. Induce vomiting. Then give weak acid such as lemonade, citrus juice, diluted vinegar.
PLANTS Any plant is a potential poison.	Induce vomiting if convulsions not imminent. Give artificial respiration if necessary.

An emergency **always** *exists if someone swallows poison.* **Do not delay contacting hospital or physician to obtain advice concerning first aid materials that are not readily available. If necessary, summon police or rescue squad for assistance.** *Keep telephone numbers immediately available. Even after emergency measures have been taken,* **always** *consult physician. A delayed reaction could be fatal.*

It is important to dilute or remove poisons as soon as possible. Keep Syrup of Ipecac (available from most pharmacies or poison centers) in your home to induce vomiting if recommended by physician or indicated on product label. If Syrup of Ipecac is not available, try to make patient vomit by tickling back of throat with finger, spoon, or similar blunt object after giving water.

HOWEVER. . .

Vomiting is **not** *recommended in all cases.* **Never induce vomiting in a patient who is unconscious or convulsing. Do not induce vomiting if swallowed substance is acidic or corrosive or petroleum distillate products.**

If poison is from a container, take container with intact label to medical facility treating patient. If poisonous substance is a plant or other unlabeled substance, be prepared to identify suspected substance. Save evidence such as portions of ingested materials from vomitus which may help identify plant or object involved.

IX

Expenditures for Health and Medical Care

Introduction

Economic resources play an important part in determining the evolution and development of health services. The United States has vast and increasing economic resources, but this does not mean that funds have always been readily available for all types of health services. In the eyes of many people, financial support of community-wide public health services and for many personal health services has been lacking.

Indexes of our total national economic resources are not enough to measure the nation's capacity for providing health and medical care services because one must take into account (1) decisions (national-governmental and private) to spend money for one purpose or another, and (2) priorities in expenditures which reflect preferences, desires, pressures, public values, etc. One must also consider the social institutions and practices which influence how much of the gross national product (or national income, or spendable wealth) is actually devoted to one purpose or another. Further, one must bear in mind that the nation's total economic resources are not in one overall pool from which expenditures are made by some centralized national authority. Rather, there are myriads of decisions and actions made by the federal government, state and local governments, organized voluntary services (philanthropic, charitable, business groups, etc.), *and by millions of individuals and families.*

In addition, there are special institutions of our society which have a strong influence on expenditure patterns. The medical professions and their practices, the hospitals, and other health facilities provide both pressures and resistances. Finally, if one thinks of just expenditures from the private sector, one might accept the assumption that most of what is spent privately is still spent not on the prevention of illness, but for the treatment of disease. Therefore, personal expenditures for medical care are determined mainly by the impact of illness on individuals and families.

National Expenditures

In fiscal year 1969–70, with a GNP of $956 billion, the United States spent about $143 billion (15 percent) for **social welfare** purposes. In the same year over $60 billion was spent on health and medical care. A review of the data in Table 1 shows a considerable rise in all the totals (*all expenditures, private and public*). To be somewhat dramatic, "socialized medicine" (public expenditures) now represents well over one-third (37.2 percent) of all health and medical care expenditures. Note also the rise of *All expenditures* as a percent of the GNP —from 3.6 percent in 1928–29 to 7.0 percent in 1969–70.

Considering private expenditures, there has been a vast growth in absolute amounts—from over $3 billion to well over $42 billion. However, as a percent of all expenditures, private payments have decreased from about 87 percent in 1928–29 to about 63 percent in 1969–70. For **personal health care,** the percent from private expenditures decreased from 91.4 to 64.7 percent. Insurance expenditures were negligible in 1928–29 (less than 1 percent), but accounted for 22.3 percent of the 64.4 percent in the 1969–70 expenditures for personal health care. It is interesting to note that over 80 percent of the population has some form of voluntary health insurance, but their insurance covered less than one-fourth of their incurred costs; only 23.8 percent of private expenditures for personal health care is derived from insurance benefits.

Public expenditures also show vast growth in absolute amounts to the point that in 1969–70 almost $25 billion was spent on health and medical care by governmental (federal, state, local) agencies and programs. As private expenditures as a percent of all expenditures has been decreasing, public expenditures have been increasing rather steadily from 13.3 percent to over 37 percent in the last two reporting years. The following are offered as reasons for this increase. Public spending has been (1) filling

---

SOCIAL WELFARE EXPENDITURES: these expenditures are limited to those activities that directly concern the economic and social well-being of individuals and families; examples are social insurance, public aid and other welfare services, health and medical programs, veterans' programs and education

PERSONAL HEALTH CARE EXPENDITURES: all expenditures for health services and supplies except expenses for prepayment and administration, government public health activities, and amounts spent by private voluntary agencies for fund-raising and general health services

gaps for those who could not themselves obtain needed services, (2) expanding community services, (3) providing for special groups, and (4) developing new kinds of service.

TABLE 1. Private and Public Expenditures (in Millions) for Health and Medical Care: United States, Selected Fiscal Years 1928-29 through 1969-70

Type of Expenditure	1928-29	1959-60	1965-66	1969-70
I. *All expenditures*	$3,589	$26,367	$42,286	$67,240
percent of GNP	3.6	5.3	5.9	7.0
per capita	$29.16	$144.93	$212.74	$324.32
A. *Private expenditures* (total)	$3,112	$119,971	$31,464	$42,258
per capita	$25.28	$109.78	$158.29	$203.82
percent of all expenditures	86.7	75.7	74.4	62.8
1. services	$3,010	$19,326	$30,136	$39,647
2. facilities	$ 012	$ 524	$ 1,159	$ 2,416
3. research	...	$ 121	$ 169	$ 195
B. *Public expenditures* (total)	$ 477	$ 6,395	$10,822	$24,982
per capita	$3.88	$35.15	$54.45	$120.50
percent of all expenditures	13.3	24.3	25.6	37.2
1. services	$ 372	$ 5,346	$ 8,702	$22,275
2. facilities (construction)	$ 105	$ 578	$ 744	$ 1,013
3. research	...	$ 471	$ 1,376	$ 1,695
II. *Personal health care* (total)	$3,272	$23,236	$36,398	$58,048
A. Percent from:				
1. *private expenditures*	91.4	78.8	78.3	64.7
direct payments	88.6	56.3	51.8	39.5
insurance benefits	...	20.2	24.5	23.8
2. *public expenditures*	8.6	21.2	21.7	35.3
III. *Gross national product* (in billions)	$101	$493	$718	$956

Source: Adapted from A. M. Skolnik and S. R. Dales, Social welfare expenditures, 1968–69, Social Security Bulletin, Dec., 1969, and Social welfare expenditures 1969–70, Social Security Bulletin, Dec., 1970; Dorothy P. Rice and Barbara S. Cooper, National health expenditures, 1929–70, Social Security Bulletin, Jan., 1971.

Table 2 shows the rate of change for health and medical care expenditures. While the average rate of change in medical care expenditures from 1929 to 1968 was only 7.3 percent, there has been an accelerating rate of increase in each successive time period since 1935, with the exception of the period after 1940–50 when the rate dropped from 12.5 to 7.0 percent. A number of influences account for the peak increases in 1940–1950, immediately postwar. Among those which increased accessibility to medical care were (1) the growth of health insurance as an alternative to the wage increases forbidden during the early 1940s as part of the government's wage and practice control program, (2) more employment, and (3) a higher standard of living and general recovery from depression. Other demographic influences which increased demand were a higher level of education, and increased birth rates and a corresponding decrease in death rates with an increase in the percentage of persons over 65 who use a disproportionate amount of medical care.

From 1950 to 1965 the annual rate of change approximated the average for the 40-year period. From 1966 on, however the rate increased on an average of about 12 percent yearly, reflecting the two additional influences of the general inflation of the economy and the further inflation in medical care costs.

TABLE 2. Expenditures for Health and Medical Care: Rate of Change, United States, Selected Periods 1929–1970

Time Period	Annual Rate of Change
1929–68	7.3
1929–35	-3.6
1935–40	6.2
1940–50	12.5
1950–55	7.0
1955–60	8.4
1960–65	8.5
1966–70[a]	12.3

[a]*Average annual rate for this four-year period from D. P. Rice and B. S. Cooper, National health expenditures, 1929–70. Social Security Bulletin, Jan., 1971.*

Source: D. P. Rice and B. S. Cooper, National health expenditures, 1929–68, Social Security Bulletin, Jan., 1970.

The Private Expenditure Sector

Table 3 presents information limited to private expenditures. Since 1950 total private expenditures have increased about four times as much in total dollars. There has been a rise in each of the categories (types of expenditures), but there has been a change in the percentage distribution. In 1969 a greater percentage went for hospital care than for physicians' services; in the earlier time periods the reverse was true.

The upward streak in expenditures comes about primarily because of a larger amount and variety of available medical care coupled with increased unit prices.

TABLE 3. Private Consumer Expenditures (in Millions) for Health and
Medical Care: United States, Selected Years 1929, 1950, 1969

Type of Expenditure	1929		1950		1969	
	Amount	Percent[a]	Amount	Percent	Amount	Percent
Total	$2,937	100.0	$8,501	100.0	$36,567	100.0
Hospital care	403	13.7	1,965	23.1	11,729	32.1
Physicians' services	959	32.6	2,597	30.5	9,458	25.9
Dentists' services	482	16.4	961	11.3	3,813	10.4
Other professional services	250	8.5	370	4.3	1,152	3.2
Drugs and drug sundries	604	20.6	1,716	20.2	6,196	16.9
Eyeglasses and appliances	131	4.5	482	5.7	1,701	4.6
Nursing home care	...	...	110	1.3	911	2.5
Expenses for prepayment	108	3.7	300	3.5	1,607	4.4
Total per capita[b] consumer expenditures	$67.66		$108.82		$177.27	

[a]*May not total due to rounding.*
[b]*Based on total population including Armed Forces and federal civilian employees abroad.*
Source: Adapted from Social Security Bulletin, Jan., 1970, Table 7, p. 15; Research and Statistics Note, No. 25, Social Security Administration, 1970.

The Public Expenditure Sector

Data given in Table 4 show aggregate expenditures of local, state, and federal governments for health and medical care. As with private expenditures, there has been a fantastic increase in absolute amounts. Health and medical *services* are an increasing proportion of total public expenditures as compared with research and construction; note the considerable rise in absolute amounts for services compared to research and construction combined (in 1969–70 *services* were over $22 billion compared to under $3 billion for medical research and facilities construction combined). Therefore, public expenditures are mainly for care of the acute and chronically ill. It is estimated that 20 percent of these expenditures go for preventive services and 80 percent for diagnosis and treatment.

Table 5 portrays where the money comes from in public expenditures. From 1928–29 to 1965–66, state and local governments contributed over one-half of all public health and medical care expenditures; but note the rapid rise of the federal percentage. Now, with programs like Medicare, the federal government contributes about two-thirds of the total public expenditures, and state and local governments make up the remaining one-third.

TABLE 4. Public Expenditures (in Millions and Rounded) for Health and Medical Care: United States, Selected Fiscal Years 1928–29 to 1969–70

Type of Expenditure	1928–29	1959–60	1966–67	1969–70
Total	$477	$6,395	$15,878	$24,982
Health and medical services	372	5,346	13,727	22,275
OASDHI	...	...	3,395	7,149
Temporary disability insurance	...	40	54	60
Workmen's compensation	75	420	695	970
Public assistance[a]	...	493	2,383	5,042
General hospital and medical care	117	1,973	2,822	3,132
Defense Department	29	820	1,323	1,650
Military dependents	5	60	109	250
Maternal and child health	6	141	310	429
School health[b]	9	101	178	263
Other public health activities	89	401	1,040	1,429
Veterans' hospitals and medical care	47	879	1,249	1,599
Medical vocational rehabilitation	0.1	18	67	152
OEO health and medical care	...	...	103	149
Medical research	...	471	1,428	1,695
Medical facilities construction	105	578	722	1,013

[a]*Vendor medical payments.*
[b]*Educational agencies only.*

Source: Adapted from Social Security Bulletin, Dec., 1969 (1928–29 to 1966–67) and Dec., 1970 (1969–70).

TABLE 5. Source of Funds (in Millions) Used in Public Medical Care Programs: United States, Selected Years 1928–29 to 1969–70

Fiscal Year	Total	Percent of Total	
		Federal	State and Local
1928–29	$ 477	20.5	79.5
1939–40	782	22.8	77.2
1959–60	6,395	45.6	54.4
1965–66	10,822	49.8	50.2
1966–67	15,878	61.5	38.5
1969–70[a]	24,985	66.7	33.3

[a]*Preliminary estimates.*

Source: Adapted from Social Security Bulletin, Dec., 1969, Table 7, p. 13, and Social Security Bulletin, Dec., 1970, Table 7, p. 14.

TABLE 6. Consumer Price Indices[a] for Medical Care Items:
United States, 1935-1970 (1957-1959 = 100.00)

Year	All Commodities and Services	Total Medical Care	Hospital Daily Service Charges	Drugs and Prescriptions	Professional Services	
					Physician's Fees	Dentist's Fees
1935	48	49	24	69	54	52
1945	63	58	33	73	63	63
1955	93	89	83	93	90	93
1965	110	122	153	98	121	118
1968	121	145	227	98	145	135
1970	135	165	288	101	167	152

[a]Figures are rounded to nearest whole number.

Source: U. S. Department of Commerce, Statistical Abstract of the United States, 91st ed., Washington, D. C., U. S. Government Printing Office, 1971.

434

Medical Care Prices

Using the time period of 1957–59 as a base, Table 6 shows the rise in medical care prices; these figures can be read as percentages (for example, hospital daily service charges have increased 288 percent over the base period of 1957–59). Of particular importance is that all commodities and services in the consumer price index increased 135 percent by 1970, but the medical care index was higher (165 percent); therefore, medical care prices rose at a higher rate than all commodities and services. As the data indicate, hospital prices have risen higher than the other prices shown in the table, and physicians' fees have increased more than the other professional services. Prices for drugs and prescriptions have remained rather stable.

Private Expenditures and Economic Indicators

Table 7 relates private expenditures to certain economic indicators. Note the fantastic growth in the GNP—from $103 billion to $976 billion—as well as the significant increase in disposable personal income (personal income minus personal taxes, i.e., the amount of money people can spend, save, etc., after taxes) and personal consumption expenditures (what people actually spend). Private health and medical care expenditures in relation to the GNP show an increase of 2.8 to 4.7 percent. The DPI distribution is 3.5 to 6.7 percent and the PCE is 3.7 to 7.5 percent. Personal consumption expenditures for health and medical care used to

TABLE 7. Private Expenditures (in Billions) for Health and Medical Care Related to Economic Indicators: United States, Selected Year 1929–1970

Income or Expenditure; Economic Indicator	1929	1948	1961	1968	1970
Gross national product	$103	$257	$518	$866	$976
Disposable personal income	$ 83	$188	$364	$590	$685
Personal consumption expenditures	$ 79	$177	$337	$537	$617
Private expenditures for health and medical care	$2.9	$7.6	$21.1	$35.9	$42.1
Percent of GNP	2.8	3.0	4.1	4.1	4.7
Percent of DPJ	3.5	4.1	5.8	6.1	6.7
Percent of PCE	3.7	4.3	6.3	6.7	7.5

account for less than 4¢ of the consumer dollar (3.7¢), and now take over 7¢ (7.5¢). Society must determine whether it is justifiable and sound to spend more—in absolute amounts and as a proportion of all consumption—on medical care; as these indicators show, the trend has been to spend more, in both absolute amounts and proportionately, for health and medical care.

Professional Health Organizations [a]

Audiologist and Speech Pathologist

American Speech and Hearing Association
9030 Old Georgetown Road
Washington, D. C. 20014

Biomedical Equipment Technician

Biomedical Engineering Society
P. O. Box 1600
Evanstown, Illinois 60204

Certified Laboratory Assistant

Registry of Medical Technologists
P. O. Box 4872
Chicago, Illinois 60680

Dental Assistant

American Dental Assistants Association
211 East Chicago Avenue
Chicago, Illinois 60611

Dental Hygienist

American Dental Hygienists Association
211 East Chicago Avenue
Chicago, Illinois 60611

Dental Laboratory Technician

National Association of Certified
  Dental Laboratories
3801 Mt. Vernon Avenue
Alexandria, Virginia 22305

Dentist

American Dental Association
211 East Chicago Avenue
Chicago, Illinois 60611

Dietitian and Nutritionist

American Dietetic Association
840 North Lake Shore Drive
Chicago, Illinois 60611

Environmental Health Technician

National Environmental Health Association
1600 Pennsylvania
Denver, Colorado 80203

Health Educator

Society of Public Health Educators
419 Park Avenue South
New York, New York 10016

Hospital Administrator

American College of Hospital Administrators
840 North Lake Shore Drive
Chicago, Illinois 60611

Inhalation Therapist

American Association for Inhalation Therapy
3554 Ninth Street
Riverside, California 92501

Medical Assistant

American Association of Medical Assistants
One East Wacker Drive, Suite 1510
Chicago, Illinois 60601

Medical Illustrator

Association of Medical Illustrators
Medical College of Georgia
Augusta, Georgia 30902

Medical Technologist

Registry of Medical Technologists
P. O. Box 4872
Chicago, Illinois 60680

Nurse Aide and Orderly

American Hospital Association
840 North Lake Shore
Chicago, Illinois 60611

[a]This is only a partial listing of health occupations and organizations. For further information contact: Health Manpower Service, United Hospital Fund of New York, 3 East 54th Street, New York, New York 10022.

Nurse, Licensed Practical

National League for Nursing
10 Columbus Circle
New York, New York 10019

Nurse, Registered Professional

American Nurses Association
2420 Pershing Road
Kansas City, Missouri 64108

Occupational Therapist

American Occupational Therapy Association
251 Park Avenue South
New York, New York 10010

Operating Room Technician

Association of Operating Room Nurses
The Denver Technological Center
8085 East Pretice Avenue
Englewood, Colorado 80110

Optician

Guild of Prescription Opticians of America
1250 Connecticut Avenue, N. W.
Washington, D. C. 20036

Optometrist

American Optometric Association
7000 Chippewa Street
St. Louis, Missouri 63119

Orthoptist

American Orthoptic Council
3400 Massachusetts Avenue, N. W.
Washington, D. C. 20007

Osteopathic Physician

American Osteopathic Association
212 East Ohio Street
Chicago, Illinois 60611

Pharmacist

American Pharmaceutical Association
2215 Constitution Avenue, N. W.
Washington, D. C. 20037

Physical Therapist

American Physical Therapy Association
1156 15th Street, N. W.
Washington, D. C. 20005

Physician

American Medical Association
535 North Dearborn Street
Chicago, Illinois 60610

Physician's Assistant/Associate

American Association of Physician's
  Associates
Duke University Medical Center
P. O. Box 2914 CHS
Durham, North Carolina 27706

Podiatrist

American Podiatry Association
20 Chevy Chase Circle, N. W.
Washington, D. C. 20015

Prosthetist and Orthotist

American Orthotic and Prosthetic
  Association
1440 N Street, N. W.
Washington, D. C. 20005

Psychologist

American Psychological Association
1200 17th Street, N. W.
Washington, D. C. 20036

Recreation Therapist

National Recreation and Park Association
Community Services Department
1700 Pennsylvania Avenue, N. W.
Washington, D. C. 20006

Sanitarian

National Association of Sanitarians
1550 Lincoln Street
Denver, Colorado 80203

Social Worker

National Commission for Social Work Careers
2 Park Avenue
New York, New York 10016

Veterinarian

American Veterinary Medical Association
600 South Michigan Avenue
Chicago, Illinois 60605

X-Ray Technologist

American Society of Radiologic Technologists
537 South Main Street
Fond du Lac, Wisconsin 54935

XI

U.S. Vital Statistics Rates–1920-1970

U.S. VITAL STATISTICS RATES: 1920-1970

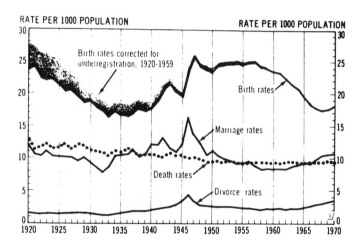

RATE PER 1000 POPULATION

RATE PER 1000 POPULATION

Birth rates corrected for underregistration, 1920-1959

Birth rates

Marriage rates

Death rates

Divorce rates

1/ 1969 and 1970 preliminary.

Index

Boldface numbers indicate that word or term is defined at bottom of specified page.

Abortion, 165-67. *See also* Contraception.
Abruptio placentae, 169
Abscess, **176**
Accidents, 179, 262-70
 alcohol and, 269
 carbon monoxide (CO) and, 265-66
 mortality from, 265
 motor vehicle, 268-70
 occurrence, 266-68
 public attitudes towards, 270
 technologic determinants of, 265
 types of injury in, 265-66
Addiction *see* Drug abuse
Aedes aegypti, 289-90
Affect, **211**
Air pollution
 asbestos and, 313-16
 bronchitis and, 308
 cardiovascular disease and, 310
 chronic respiratory disease and, 308
 emphysema and, 308
 energy consumption and, 322-24
 lead and, 314
 in New York City, 311
 sources of, 309
 sulfur dioxide and, 310
 temperature inversions and, 309
 types of, 309-10
Alcohol *see* Alcoholism

Alcoholics Anonymous, 247, 248-49
Alcoholism, 237-50
 cancer and, 246
 definition of, 244
 "D. T.'s," 243
 effect on body organs, 246
 extent of, 238-39
 factors encouraging alcohol consumption, 239
 familial occurrence, 245
 "hangover," 242-43
 medicolegal definitions of, 242
 motor vehicle accidents and, 269
 nationality and, 244
 schizophrenia and, 244
 sex and ethnicity and, 244
 treatment modalities for, 248-49
Algae, 318
Allele, **16**
Allelomorph *see* Allele
Allergen *see* Allergic disorders
Allergic disorders. *See also* Immunity.
 anamnestic response, 148
 asthma, 149-50
 "auto-immune" diseases, 150
 collagen diseases, 151
 contact dermatitis, 150
 eczema, 150
 hay fever, 149
 hives, 150

Allergic disorders (*Cont.*)
  immediate vs. delayed reactions, 148-49
  organ transplants and, 150
  rheumatoid arthritis, 151
Allied health manpower
  characteristics of, 379-82
  education and training of, 382-87
  preponderance of nurses, 379
  scarcity of, 387-88
Alpha particles *see* Radiation
Ambulatory care, **362**
Amebiasis, 305
American Dental Association, 341
American Hospital Association, 361
American Medical Association, 341, 402
American Public Health Association, 342
American Red Cross, 342
Amino acids, **25**
Amnionic fluid, **167**
Amphetamines, 233-35
Anaerobic, **287**
Analgesic, **224**
Analytic epidemiology, 74-80
Anamnestic response *see* Allergic disorders
Anaphylactic shock, **56**. *See also* Allergic disorders, immediate vs. delayed reactions.
Anemia
  aplastic, **57**
  hemolytic, **58**
  iron-deficiency, 33-34
  pregnancy and, 168
  sickle cell disease, 17-19, 23
Aneurysm, **206**
Angina pectoris *see* Cardiovascular diseases
Anoxia, **168**
Antabuse *see* Alcoholism, treatment modalities for
Anthrax, **123**
Antibiotics, 33, 106-7
  broad spectrum, **40**
  cephalothin, 106
  chloramphenicol, 57, 107
  erythromycin, 106
  isoniazid (INH), 107, 117

Antibiotics (*Cont.*)
  kanamycin, 107
  lincomycin, 106
  para-aminosalicylic acid (PAS), 107, 120
  penicillin, 90, 106, 257, 258
  polymycin, 107
  streptomycin, 107, 120
  sulfonamides, 106
  tetracycline, 58
  radiation sickness and, 329
  use in developing countries, 39-40
Antibody, **4**. *See also* Allergic disorders; Immunity.
Antigen, **4**. *See also* Allergic disorders; Immunity.
Anxiety, **217**
"A. P. C." tablets, **58**
Aphasic, **6**
Aplastic anemia *see* Anemia
Arteriosclerosis *see* Cardiovascular diseases
Artery, **133**
Arthritis, 179. *See also* Rheumatoid arthritis.
Arthropod, **99**, 112
Asbestos, 313-16
  asbestosis, 313-14
Ascariasis, 305
Ascaris lumbricoides, **305**
Ascorbic acid *see* Vitamins, C
Asepsis, **366**
Asphyxia, 171
Asthma *see* Allergic disorders
Astigmatism *see* Visual defects
Atelectasis, 171
Athlete's foot, 111
Atomic Energy Commission, 330
Attenuated, **96**
Attributable risk, 80
Autosomal, **23**

Bacillary dysentery, 305
Bacillus *see* Bacteria
Bacteria, 4, 90, 93. *See also individual bacterial diseases.*
  aerobacter, 90
  Clostridium botulinum, 302
  Clostridium perfringens, 302

Bacteria (*Cont.*)
   Corynebacterium diphtheriae, 102
   Gram's stain and, 90
   Hemophilus ducreyi, 259
   Hemophilus influenza, 102
   Hemophilus pertussis, 102
   identification of, as disease agents,
     41
   klebsiella, 90
   Mycobacterium tuberculosis, 12
   Neisseria gonorrhoeae, 257
   pneumococcus (i), 90
   Salmonella typhimurium, 303
   Salmonella typhosa, 300
   Spirillum minus, 333
   staphylococcus *see* Staphylococcus
   Streptobacillus moniliformis, 333
   Streptococcus *see* Streptococcus
   Treponema pallidum, 253
   tubercle bacillus, 90
Bacteriophage, 93
Barbiturates, 231-32. *See also* Drug
   abuse.
BCG, 120
Beriberi, 32. *See also* Malnutrition;
   Vitamins.
Beta particles *see* Radiation
Bias, **74**
Birth rate, **36**
Births, registration of, 83
Bismarck, Otto von, 341, 342
Bleuler, Paul, 193
Blindness
   cataract and, 156
   corneal injury and, 156
   diabetes mellitus and, 146
   glaucoma and, 156
   legal definition of, 155
   trachoma and, 157
   and vitamin A, 29
Blood
   donations and hepatitis, 113-15
   groups, 142
   transfusion and malaria transmis-
     sion, 291
   type and disease risk, 23
Blue Cross, 403-4
Blue Shield, 403
Botulism, 302-3
Bradycardia, **290**

Brill's disease, 297. *See also* Typhus.
Broad-spectrum antibiotics *see* Anti-
   biotics
Bronchitis *see* Air pollution; Chronic
   respiratory disease
Bronchus, **95**
Brucellosis, **123**, 301
BTUs, **320**

Calorie, **25**, 27
Cancer, 138-43
   alcoholism and, 246
   benign vs. malignant, 139
   breast, 142
   carcinogens, 140
   colon and rectum, 140-41, 176
   early detection of, 140
   international variation and, 67-68,
     140
   leukemia, 143
   lung, 143
   nature of, 138-39
   pernicious anemia and, 32
   prevalence, 138
   prostate, 143, 179
   radiation and, 329
   registries for, 85
   skin, 327
   stomach, 142
   uterus, 142
Candida albicans see Candidiasis
Candidiasis, 111
Capillary, **145**
Carbohydrate, **25**
Carbon monoxide (CO), 322. *See also*
   Accidents.
Carcinogenic, **140**
Carcinoma *see* Cancer
Cardiovascular diseases, 132-38
   air pollution and, 310
   angina pectoris in, 135
   arteriosclerosis and hypertension, re-
     lationship between, 133
   arteriosclerotic, 133-35
   cerebrovascular accident, **6**, 135-37
   congenital cardiac defects, 137
   coronary insufficiency in, 135
   hypertension, 133-34

Cardiovascular diseases (*Cont.*)
  hypertension, hemorrhage, and heart failure, relationship between, 133
  maternal rubella and, 168
  myocardial infarction in, 134
  peripheral vascular disease, 137
  rheumatic heart disease, 122, 137. *See also* Streptococcus.
  affecting vision *see* Visual defects
Caries, **35**
Carrier of infectious disease, **98**
Case history study *see* retrospective study
Cataract *see* Visual defects
Catatonia, 218. *See also* Schizophrenia.
Cause, 12
Central nervous system, **32**
Cephalothin *see* Antibiotics
Cerebral palsy, **159**
Cerebrovascular accident *see* Cardiovascular diseases
Chancroid, 259
Cheilosis, 32. *See also* Malnutrition; Vitamins.
Chiarugi, Vincinzo, 190
Chickenpox, 98, 103
Child health, 168-75
Childhood diseases, 95-96
Childhood poisoning, 173-74
Children's Bureau, 342
Chloramphenicol, 57, 107. *See also* Antibiotics.
Chlorination *see* Water treatment
Chloroquine, 291
Cholelithiasis *see* Gallstones
Cholera, 100-101, 106, 305
Cholesterol, 13
Chordotomy, **198**
Chromosome, **15**
  nondisjunction, **16**
  X and Y, 23-24
Chronic, **13**
Chronic diseases, 126-62
  allergies *see* Allergic disorders
  cancer *see* Cancer
  as causes of disability, 132
  cirrhosis of the liver, 246

Chronic diseases (*Cont.*)
  contrasted with infectious diseases, 126, 128-29
  dental *see* Dental disorders
  diabetes *see* Diabetes mellitus
  effect on infections, 95
  hearing loss *see* Hearing defects
  of heart and vessels *see* Cardiovascular diseases
  interrelationship with infectious diseases, 130, 132
  and a "national health crisis," 130
  prevalence of, 126
  reporting of, 85
  resource allocation and, 159-62
  respiratory *see* Chronic respiratory disease
  rising prevalence of, 123
  vision *see* Visual defects
Chronic respiratory disease, 146-48
Cigarette smoking, 129, 147, 261-62
Circadian rhythm, **321**
Cirrhosis, 246
Clinic *see* Outpatient care
Clinical medicine, 6, 62-63
Clostridium botulinum, 302. *See also* Botulism.
Clostridium perfringens, 302
Cockroaches, 333
Cohort study *see* Prospective study
Coitus, **46**
Coitus interruptus *see* Contraception
Colds, 103
Collagen, **151**. *See also* Allergic disorders.
Collective protection, **340**
Communicable, **4**
Communicable diseases *see* Infectious diseases
Communicable period, **105**
Community Mental Health Centers Act, 196
Comprehensive Health Planning Act, 308, 390
Comprehensive services, **354**
Condom *see* Contraception
Congenital, **137**
Congenital cardiac defects *see* Cardiovascular diseases

Congenital malformations, 170-71. *See also* Congenital cardiac defects.
Congestive heart failure, **121**, 128
Conjunctivitis, **103**
Connective tissue, 33
Constipation, 178
Consumer price index, **346**
Contact dermatitis *see* Allergic disorders
Contraception
    abortion, 46
    coitus interruptus, 46
    condom, 47
    diaphragm, 47
    douche, postcoital, 46
    in family planning, role of, 47-48
    intrauterine device (IUD), 47
    "the pill," 46-47
    rhythm method, 46
    surgical intervention, 46
Contraindication, **169**
Control group, **75**
Cornea, **29**, 156
Coronary insufficiency *see* Cardiovascular diseases
Correlation, **13**
Cortisone, **95**, 119, 145, 179. *See also* Steroids.
Corynebacterium diphtheriae see Diphtheria
"Cross-eyes," *see* Strabismus
Cross-sectional study *see* Prevalence study
Crude death rate *see* Death rate
Culture (laboratory), **104**
Cupping, **186**
CVA (cerebrovascular accident) *see* Cardiovascular diseases
Cytomegalic inclusion disease, 168

DDT (dichloro-diphenyl-trichloroethane), 293-94
Death rate, 29, **36**, 71-72
Deaths, registration of, 83
Decibel, **158**
Delirium tremens ("D.T.'s") *See* Alcoholism
Delusion, **205**

Demand (for medical care), 406-7
Dementia, **32**
Dementia praecox, 214
Demography, **37**. *See also* Population and Population growth.
Dental disorders, 152-54
    fluoridation, 152
    gingivitis, 152
    periodontitis, 154
Deoxyribonucleic acid *see* DNA
Descriptive epidemiology, 65-68
Diabetes mellitus, 19-22, 143-46, 168, 179
    cortisone and, 145
    in the elderly, 179
    genetic inheritance and, 19-22
    hyperthyroidism and, 145
    obesity and, 145
    pregnancy and, 145, 168
    thiazide diuretics and, 145
Diagnosis, **6**
    process of, 7-12
Diaphragm *see* Contraception
Diaphragmatic hernia, 176
Digitalis, 128, 224
Diphtheria, 102, 174
Diploid, **16**
Disease. *See also* Health.
    causality and, 7-14
    chronic *see* Chronic diseases
    coexistence with health, 2
    contrasted with health, 2
    country-by-country variation, 67-68, 140
    definition of, 2
    drugs, relation to, 56
    foodborne, 301-4
    iatrogenic, **56-58**
    infectious *see* Infectious diseases
    milkborne, 299-301
    outbreaks of infectious disease, characteristics of, 65-66
    quarantinable, 106
    rates *see* Rates
    seasonal variations, 66-67
    variations by age, 68
    variations by scx, 68
    vector-borne *see* Vector-borne diseases

Disease (*Cont.*)
  venereal *see* Venereal disease
  waterborne, 304-5
  zoonoses *see* Zoonoses
Disposable personal income, **350**
Diuretic, **145**, 247
Diverticulitis, 176
Dix, Dorothy, 341
DNA (deoxyribonucleic acid), 15
Doctors *see* Physicians
Domiciliary care home, **357**
Dominant (gene), **19**
Donora, Pennsylvania, 309
Donovania granulomatis, 259
DPT (immunization), 174
Drug Abuse, 223-237
  addiction, 225
  alcohol *see* Alcoholism
  amphetamines, 233-35
  barbiturates, 231-32
  costs of, 230
  definition of, 224
  habituation and, 225
  Harrison Act, 227
  hepatitis and, 113
  marihuana, 235-37
  marihuana vs. hashish vs. THC, 235
  mortality and, 230
  narcotic addiction, 225-31
  in New York City, 229-30
  opium vs. morphine vs. heroin, 225
  physical dependence vs. habituation, 225
  reasons for, 224
  tolerance and, 225
  treatment methods, 230-31
  withdrawal symptoms, 225
Drug addiction *see* Drug abuse
Drugs
  abuse of *see* Drug abuse
  antibiotics, 106-7
  chloroquine, 291
  cortisone, 95, 119, 145, 179
  definition of, 224
  epinephrine, **133**
  hemolytic anemia and, **58**
  Librium, 195
  lithium carbonate, 195
  methadone *see* Drug abuse, treatment methods

Drugs (*Cont.*)
  Metrazol, 194
  Miltown, 195
  narcotic *see* Drug abuse
  over-the-counter, **224**
  phenacetin, 57
  place in American society, 222-23
  quinine, 291
  reactions to, 56-58
  steroids, 169
  thiazides, 145
  Thorazine, 195
  tranquilizers, 195
  Valium, 195
"D. T.'s." *see* Alcoholism
Dubos, René, 318
Duodenum, **177**
Dysentery, 100-101

Eclampsia *see* Toxemia
Ecology
  definition of, 311
  pollution and, 311-12
Economies of scale, **372**
Edema, **121**
Education (as a factor in the utilization of medical care services), 349
Elderly, the, 175-80, 208-13
Electroshock treatment, 194-95
Emetic, **186**
Emphysema, 74. *See also* Chronic respiratory disease.
  air pollution and, 308
Endemic, **23**
Endocarditis, **132**
Endogenous, **120**
Entamoeba histolytica, 305
Enteric, **100**
Enterotoxin, **71**
Environmental pollution *see* Pollution
Enzyme, **89**
Epidemic, **95**
Epidemiologic approach to disease *see* Epidemiology
Epidemiology, 62-86
  analytic, 74-80
  definition of, 64
  descriptive, 65-68

Epidemiology (*Cont.*)
  descriptive vs. analytic, 65
  uses of, 64
Epilation, **329**
Epilepsy, **170**
Epinephrine, **133**
Erysipelas, 103, 104
Erythroblastosis fetalis, 171
Erythromycin *see* Antibiotics
Esophagus, **34**
Etiology, **134**
Eutrophication, 318-19
Extended care facilities, **353**
Extrinsic, **149**

Fair Labor Standards Act, 382
Fallopian tubes, **46**
False negatives, **83**
False positives, **83**
Familial, **32**
Familial polyposis, 142
Family health maintenance, **353**
Family planning *see* Contraception
Feces, **34**
Federal Food and Drug Act, 342
Fetal death, 169
Fetal death rate, 73
Fetus, **33**
Flies *see* Housefly
Flora, **33**
Fluoridation *see* Dental disorders
Folic acid, 32. *See also* Vitamins.
Foodborne diseases, 301-4
Food poisoning, 303. *See also* Food-
  borne diseases.
Fungus (i), **58**, 107, 111

Gallstones, 177
Gamete, **16**
Gamma globulin, 95, 96
Gamma rays *see* Radiation
Gangrene, **138**
Gastroenteritis, viral, 101
Gastrointestinal tract, **32**
Genes, 15
  dominant vs. recessive, **19**
  "drift of," 25

Genes (*Cont.*)
  "fixed," 25
  heterozygote, 19
  homozygote, 19
Genetic inheritance, 15-25
  blood type and, 23
  diabetes and, 19-22
  hemophilia and, 23-24
  malaria and, 23
  racial mixing and, 25
  sickle cell disease and, 17-19
Genetics. *See also* Genetic inheritance.
  poverty and, 48
Genotype, **22**
Geriatrics, **175**. See also Elderly, the.
German measles *see* Rubella
Gestation, **169**
Gingivitis *see* Dental disorders
Glaucoma *see* Blindness; Visual de-
  fects
Glomerulonephritis, 103, 121
Glossitis, **32**
Glucose *see* Diabetes mellitus
Goiter, **34**
Gout, **135**
Government. *See also* Health adminis-
  tration.
  role in medical care, 399-406
  role in mental illness, 401
  taxation as a health measure, 129
Gram negative, **58**
Gram positive, 58
Gram's stain *see* Bacteria
Grand Junction, Colorado, 331-32
Granuloma inguinale, 259
Greenfield, Harry I., 379
Group Health Cooperative of Puget
  Sound, 403
Group practice, **373**

Hallucination, **205**
Hangover *see* Alcoholism
Haploid, **16**
Harelip, **171**
Hashish, 235-37
Haverhill fever *see* *Streptobacillus
  moniliformis*
Hay fever *see* Allergic disorders

Health. *See also* Disease.
  causality and, 7-14
  coexistence with disease, 2
  data sources for, 85-86
  definition of, 2
  discussion of, 1-14
  population and, 36
  poverty and, 48-56
Health administration. *See also* Government.
  nature of, 3-4
  objective of, 4
Health care, 339-42. *see also* Medical care.
  in America, eighteenth century, 341
  in America, nineteenth, early twentieth centuries, 342
  in ancient Greece, 339
  ancient Hebrews and, 339
  in ancient Rome, 339-40
  and change in role of the physician, 344
  Code of Hammurabi and, 339
  demographic and socioeconomic determinants of, 346
  in Europe, nineteenth century, 341
  growth of specialization in, 344
  historical development of, 339-42
  the Industrial Revolution and, 340
  in the Middle Ages, 340
  planning and national wealth, 349-50
  rising costs of, 344-46
  shamanism, 339
  trends in, 350-54
Health departments, 4. *See also* Government.
Health education, 2-3
Health insurance, 403-6
  Blue Cross, 403, 404
  Blue Shield, 403
  commercial carriers and, 403-4
  Group Health Cooperative of Puget Sound, 403
  Health Insurance Plan of Greater New York (HIP), 403
  indemnity vs. service benefit, 404
  Kaiser Permanentee, 403, 405
  role of organized labor, 403

Health Insurance Plan of Greater New York (HIP), 403
Health Maintenance Organizations, 403
Hearing defects, 158-59
  in the elderly, 179
  maternal rubella and, 168
"Heart attack," *see* Cardiovascular diseases; Myocardial infarction
Helminthic diseases, 111-12
Hematuria, **121**
Hemiplegia, **179**
Hemoglobin, **17**
Hemolytic anemia *see* Anemia
Hemophilia, **23-24**
Hemophilus ducrey, 259
Hemophilus influenza see Infectious diseases
Hemophilus pertussis see Pertussis
Hemorrhage, 133, 137, 164
Hernia *see* Diaphragmatic hernia
Heroin *see* Drug abuse, narcotic addiction
Hepatitis, 112-14
  blood donations and, 113-15
  drug addiction and, 113
  infections, 93, 101, 305
  infectious vs. serum, 113
  isolation in, 115
  nonmedical solutions and, 115
  pregnancy and, 168
  serum, 99, 105
Herpangina, 101
Herpes zoster *see* Chickenpox
Heterozygous, **19**
Hill-Burton Act, 396
Hippocrates, 185
Hiroshima, 143, 328, 329, 331
Hives *see* Allergic disorders
Home care, **353**, 397, 398
Homozygous, **19**
Hookworm, 33-34, 111
Hormone, **247**
Hospitals, **301-72**
  and causes of increased costs, 371
  changing role of, 361-62
  community, 361
  consumers and, 367
  controlling costs, 371-72
  costs to patients, 370-72

Hospitals (*Cont.*)
definition of, 361
educational programs in, 369
as hazards to health, 56
increasing utilization of, 409
legislation affecting, 368-69
mergers and collaborative agreements among, 372
number of, 361
origins of, 365-66
and planning, agencies of, 369
providers vs. consumers, 370
psychiatric, 197-98, 365
and society, pressures affecting, 366-67
types of, 365
Housefly, 288, 300, 303
Housing, 270-77
code, 271
health and, 271-74
maintenance, importance of, 276-77
Huntington's chorea, 159
Hydrocephaly, 171
Hyperopia *see* Visual defects
Hypertension. *See also* Cardiovascular diseases.
in toxemia, 165
Hypertrophy, 179
Hypothesis, 65
Hypothyroidism, 34

Iatrogenic disease *see* Disease
"Iceberg effect," 63-64
Immunity, 93-98. *See also* Allergic disorders; Infectious diseases.
active vs. passive, 95-97
antigen vs. antibody in, 94-95
gamma globulin and, 95
immunizations and, 96, 287, 290, 300
immunizations in childhood, 174-75
natural vs. acquired, 93
toxins and, 96
Immunization, 4. *See also* Immunity.
Impetigo, 102, 104
Incidence (of disease), 70-71
Incubation period, 66
Index case, 66
India, 43, 48, 305

Indigent, 340
Infant, 4
Infant mortality, 173
Infection, 13
Infectious diseases, 88-125. *See also* Immunity.
due to adenovirus, 103
amebiasis, 305
antibiotics and, 106-7
ascariasis, 305
athlete's foot, 111
bacillary dysentery, 305
bacterial, 90, 93
botulism, 302-3
candidiasis, 111
chancroid, 259
chickenpox, 98
cholera, 100-101, 305
chronic, in course of, 130
due to *Clostridium perfringens,* 302
common, in reporting, 124
conjunctivitis, 103
control of, 98-107
debilitation and, 93
diphtheria, 102
dysentery, 100-101
eclipse of, 123
enteric, 101
enteroviruses, 101
foodborne, 301-4
gonorrhea *see* Venereal disease
granuloma inguinale, 259
due to *Hemophilus influenzae,* 102
hepatitis, 112-14, 305
herpangina, 101
immunity to, 93-98
influenza, 103
insecticides and, 293-94, 296
isolation in, 104-5
latency in, 98
leprosy, 100, 104, 105
leptospirosis, 305, 333-34
lymphogranuloma venereum, 259
malaria, 23, 39, 99, 111, 290-96
measles, 103
meningitis, 102
milkborne, 299-301
mumps, 103
murine typhus, 334
outbreaks, characteristics of, 65-66

Infectious diseases (*Cont.*)
   pertussis, 102
   plague, 99-100, 334
   pleurodynia, 101
   pneumonia, 102
   primary vs. secondary lesions in, 89
   quarantine in, 104-5
   rabies, 287-88
   radiation and, 329
   reporting of, 84
   reservoirs of, 98
   respiratory, 89, 102-4
   due to rhinovirus, 103
   Rickettsial, 107, 111
   ringworm, 111
   rubella, 103-4
   salmonellosis, 303
   schistosomiasis, 67, 111-12, 296-97, 305
   smallpox, 93, 103, 105, 169, 174
   due to *Spirillum minus*, 333
   staphylococcal, 58, 71, 90, 98, 102, 172, 301, 303
   staphylococcal food poisoning, 30
   due to *Streptobacillus moniliformis*, 333
   streptococcal, 7, 90, 103, 121, 122, 132, 137, 152, 164, 299
   syphilis *see* Venereal disease
   tetanus, 174, 287
   toxoplasmosis, 168
   trachoma, 157
   transmission of, 98-107
   trichinosis, 112, 284-86, 334
   tuberculosis, 71, 98, 116-20, 247, 301
   tularemia, 305
   typhoid fever, 98, 99, 100-101, 300-301, 305
   typhus, 98, 107, 111, 297-99
   vector-borne diseases, 288-99
   vector control in, 291
   vehicles vs. vectors in transmission of, 99
   venereal diseases *see* Venereal disease
   viral, 93, 101
   waterborne, 304-5
   yellow fever, 289-90
   zoonoses, 99, 284-88

Infestation, **25**
Influenza, 103
INH (isoniazid), 117
Injury *see* Accidents
Insecticides, 293-94, 296
Insulin *see* Diabetes mellitus
Insulin shock, 194
Insurance *see* Health insurance; Social insurance
Intensive care, **397**
Intercurrent, **174**
Intermediate care, **397**
Intrauterine device *see* IUD
Intrinsic, **149**
Inversions, temperature *see* Temperature inversions
Investment rate *see* Population and Poulation growth, rate of investment and
Iodine deficiency, 34
Ionizing radiation *see* Radiation
Ireland, relationship of nutrition and population in, 43
Iron deficiency, 33-34
Irritable colon, 178
Isolation, 104-5
Isoniazid *see* INH
IUD *see* Contraception

James, George, 391
Jargon, 6-10
"Jet-travel syndrome," 327

Kaiser Permanente, 403, 405
Kanamycin *see* Antibiotics
Kernicterus, **158**
King George III, 187
Klarman, Herbert, 371
Koch, Robert, 116, 117
Koos, Earl, 406
Kraepelin, Emil, 193
Kwashiorkor, 29. *See also* Malnutrition.

Labile, **211**
Lactation, **27**
Laennec, René, 116, 117
Laparotomy, **198**

Lead poisoning, 312. *See also* Housing.
nonmedical solutions to, 54
poverty and, 53, 54
Leopold, Pietro, Grand Duke of Tuscany, 190
Leprosy, 100, 104, 105
Leptospirosis, 305, 333-34
Leucopenia, **290**
Leukemia, **7**, 329
Librium, 195
Lice, 332
Lincomycin *see* Antibiotics
Lind, Joseph, 33
Lloyd George, David, 341
Lobotomy, 194
Long-term care, **397**
Lying-in hospitals, **366**
Lymphogranuloma venereum, 259

Malaise, **256**
Malaria, 111, 290-96
in Ceylon, 39
drug addiction and, 291
eradication of, 39
mosquito vector of, 99
population growth and, 39
sickle cell disease and, 23
Malignant, **138**
Malnutrition, 25-35
adverse effects of, 25-26, 27-28
alcoholism and, 246-47
anemia and, 33-34
beriberi, 32
breast feeding and, 29
cheilosis, 32-33
food distribution and, 35, 43
food supplements and, 34
infection and, 25, 29
iodine deficiency, 34
iron deficiency, 33
marasmus vs. kwashiorkor, 29
obesity, 26
pellagra, 32
population growth and, 43-44
protein-calorie, 27
rickets, 29
scurvy, 33
sufficient causes of, 26-27

Malnutrition (*Cont.*)
vitamins and, 25, 29-33
Manic-depressive psychosis, 192
Manpower *see* Allied health manpower; Personnel
Marasmus, 29. *See also* Malnutrition.
Marihuana, 235-37
Masserman, J. H., 249
Mass screening, 81-83
criteria for, 81-82
multiphasic programs in, 354
precision of tests in, **82**
reliability, repeatability, and reproducibility of tests in, **82**
sensitivity of tests in, **83**
specificity of tests in, **83**
validity of tests in, **83**
Maternal health, 162-68
Measles, 93, 103, 119
immunization against, 174
pregnancy and, 168
tuberculosis and, 119
Median, **349**
Medicaid, 342, 358, 360, 368, 396
Medical care, 39, 391-99, 401-12. *See also* Health care.
adequacy, criteria for, 391-92
factors affecting utilization of, 409-11
government, role of in, 399-406
insurance, role of in, 403-6
legislation and, 396
need vs. demand for, 406-7
organization of, 393-95
population growth and, 397
role of voluntary health agencies in, 401-2
as a "social utility," 395-96
utilization of services, 406-12
worldwide availability of, 39
Medically indigent, **340**
Medicare (Title XIX), 342, 358, 360, 368, 396, 400
Meduna, Joseph von, 194
Meiosis, **16**
Meningitis, **7**, 89, 102
Meningococcus *see* Meningitis
Mental illness, 181-220
acute delirium, 204
alcoholism and, 244, 246

Mental illness (*Cont.*)
  availability of therapists, 203
  catatonia, 218
  community psychiatry, 196-97
  dementia praecox, 214
  in the elderly, 179-80, 208-13
  extent of, 200-201
  historical concepts of, 182-200
  organic brain syndromes, 204
  and role of state mental hospitals,
    197-98
  schizophrenia, 213-20, 244
  senility and, 208
  state hospitals, 201
  thought disorder in, 215
Mercury (in foodborne disease), 304
Metabolism, **27**
Metastasis, 139
Methadone *see* Drug Abuse, treatment
    methods
Methemoglobinemia, 335 n
Metrazol, 194
Migration rate, **36**
Milkborne diseases, 299-301
Miltown, 195
Mineral, **33**
Molecule, **19**
Mongolism, **16**, 137, 171
Moniliasis *see* Candidiasis
Morbidity, **67**, 84
Mortality, **67**, 123, 350-51
Mucous membrane, **100**
Multiparous, **142**
Multiple sclerosis, **68**, 159
Mumps, 103
Murine typhus, 334
Mutation, **329**
Mycobacterium tuberculosis, 12
Myocardial infarction, **63**. *See also*
    Cardiovascular diseases.
Myocarditis, **101**
Myopia *see* Visual defects

Nagasaki, 143, 328, 329, 331
National Health Council, 342
National Health Survey, 86
National wealth, 349-50
Necrosis, **134**
Need (for medical care), 406-7

Neisseria gonorrhea, 257
Nematode(a), **286**
Neonatal mortality, 169, 287
Neonatal period, 169
Neonate, **33**
Neoplastic, **138**
Nephritis. *See also* Glomerulonephritis.
Net reproductive rate, **37**
Neurology, **192**
Neurotic, **192**
New York Academy of Medicine, 393
Niacin, 32. *See also* Vitamins.
Nitrate, 318, 319, 335 n
Noise *see* Pollution
Nondisjunction, **16**
Nonmedical solutions (to medical
    problems), 54, 55, 115
Nunberg, Herman, 193
Nursing homes, 357-61
  growth of, 350
  number of, 358
  location of, 358
  size of, 358-59
  types of, 357
Nursing services, 357
Nutrition *see* Malnutrition

Obesity *see* Malnutrition
Occupancy rate, **365**
Occupational health and safety, 324-
    25
Ombudsman, **369**
Organic, **33**
Organism, **4**
Organ transplants *see* Allergic dis-
    orders
Os, 169
Osteomyelitis, **102**
Osteopathy, **377**
Otitis media, **102**
Outpatient, **361**
  care, 397, 398
Over-the-counter (drugs), **224**

Pain (chest), 134, 135
Palpitation, **145**
Pap smear, 142

Papule, **253**
Para-aminosalicylic acid (PAS) *see* Antibiotics
Parkinson's disease, **159**
Partnership for Health Act *see* Comprehensive Health Planning Act
Parturition, **171**. *See also* Pregnancy.
PAS *see* Para-aminosalicylic acid
Pasteurization, 300, 301
Pathogenic, **4**
Pathogens, definition of, 4
Pathognomonic, **12**
Pediculus humanus, 297
Pellagra, 32. *See also* Malnutrition.
Penicillin, 90, 106. *See also* Antibiotics.
  venereal disease and, 257, 258
Per capita income, 44-46, 350
Pericarditis, **101**
Peridontitis *see* Dental disorders
Perinatal mortality, 73, 169
Peripheral vascular disease *see* Cardiovascular diseases
Peritonitis, **101**
Pernicious anemia, 32
  as an "auto-immune" process, 151
  stomach cancer and, 142
Personal care home, **357**
Personal care home with nursing, **357**
Personal consumption expenditures, **350**
Personnel (in Health), 372-88
  allied health workers, 379-88
  autonomous health professional, 373, 379
  physicians, 344, 373-77
Pertussis, 102, 174
Pests, 332-35
Phagocytes, **89**
Phenacetin, 57. *See also* Drugs.
Phenotype, **22**
Phosphates, 318, 319
Physicians, 39, 40, 344, 373-77
  availability of, in developing countries, 39-40
  growing demand for services of, 377
  home vs. office visits, 408
  number of, 377
  patterns of practice, 373-77
  population growth and, 36, 39, 40

Physicians (*Cont.*)
  as proportion of all health workers, 379
  role in hospitals, 367
"the Pill" *see* Contraception
Pinel, Phillipe, 188-89
Placenta, **164**
Placenta praevia, 169-70
Plague, 99-100, 125 n, 334
Pleurodynia, 101
Pneumococcus *see* Pneumonia
Pneumonia, 102
Pneumothorax, **116**
Poisoning *see* Childhood poisoning; Lead poisoning
Poison ivy, 150
Polio, 93, 101, 168, 174-75
Pollution, 305-26
  air, 308-11
  anticipation of, 325-36
  asbestos and, 313-16
  cost as key to control, 314
  definition of, 311
  developing countries and, 317
  ecology and, 311
  energy consumption and, 320-24
  eutrophication and, 318-19
  lead and, 314
  lead-based paint and, 312
  long-term effects on health, 317
  noise as, 312
  occupational health and, 324-25
  population growth and, 319-20
  public policy vs. individual behavior, 325
  water, 305-8
Polyarthritis, **102**
Polymorphism, **23**
Polymycin *see* Antibiotics
Population explosion *see* Population and population growth
Population and population growth, 35-48, 347
  antibiotics and, 39-40
  birth rate, 36
  change in proportions of different age groups, 347
  contraception and, 46-48
  death rate, 36
  growth by ethnicity, 40-43

Population and population growth (*Cont.*)
  factors influencing growth of, 36-38
  growth, long-term, 40-43, 44
  health and, 36
  health care utilization, effect of, 347
  malaria eradication and, 39
  malnutrition and, 43-44
  medical care and, 36
  migration rate, 36
  net reproductive rate and, 37
  numerical increase and growth rates, 44
  pollution and, 319-20
  poverty and, 44-46
  probability of failure of present approaches to, 47-48
  rate of investment and, 44
  relation to per capita income, rate of investment, and productivity, 44-45
  sanitation and, 40
Population at risk, **69**
Porphyria, 188
Postpartum, **162**. *See also* Pregnancy.
Poverty
  business practices and, 53
  criteria for, 48
  definition of, 49
  education and, 52, 53
  employment and, 52-53
  environmental hazards and, 53-54
  family structure and, 54
  genetics and, 48
  health and, 48-56
  income distribution and, 46
  jobs in health and, 55
  lead poisoning and, 53, 54
  medical vs. nonmedical solutions, 54-55
  medical problems associated with, 49-52, 54-55
  population and, 44-46
  racial discrimination and, 53
  relationship to per capita income, productivity, rate of investment, and population growth, 44
  tuberculosis and, 118
Pregnancy
  anemia and, 168

Pregnancy (*Cont.*)
  cytomegalic inclusion disease and, 168
  diabetes mellitus and, 168
  hepatitis during, 168
  measles during, 168
  polio during, 168
  prevention of *see* Contraception
  radiation and, 169
  rickets and, 168
  rubella during, 168
  smallpox vaccination and, 169
  steroid drugs and, 169
  syphilis and, 168
  toxoplasmosis during, 168
Prematurity, 170
Prevalence, 70-71
Prevalence (or cross-sectional) study, 81-83
Prevention, 4-6
Private consumer expenditures, 345, 346
Prodrome, **329**
Prognosis, **134**
Progressive patient care, **397**
Prophylaxis, **258**
Proprietary, **358**
Prospective study, **75**-76, 79
Proteins, 25
Proteinuria, **165**
Prothrombin, **33**
Protozoa, **290**
Pruritic, **256**
Psychoanalysis, **192**
Psychosis, **188**
Psychotherapy, **198**
Public Health Service, 330, 341, 354
Public Law 89-239. *See also* Regional Medical Programs.
Public Law 89-749. *See also* Comprehensive Health Planning Act.
Puerperal, **164**
Purgative, **185**
Purpura, **329**
Purulent, **258**
Pussin, Jean-Baptiste, 188-89
Pustule, **256**
Pyrethrum, **296**

Q fever, 301
Quarantine, 104, 106
Quinine, 291

Rabies, 287-88
Rad, 328
Radiation, 326-32
  alpha particles, 328
  antibiotics and, 329
  Atomic Energy Commission and, 330
  beta particles, 328
  cancer and, 329, 330
  gamma rays, 328
  in Grand Junction, Colorado, 331-32
  heat, 327
  infection and, 329
  ionizing, 327-32
  leukemia and, 329
  light, 327
  as occupational hazard to radiologists and dentists, 329
  pregnancy and, 329, 330
  during pregnancy, exposure to, 169
  Public Health Service and, 330
  Roentgen vs. Rad vs. Rem, 328
  sickness, 329-30
  state health departments and, 330
  X-rays, 328
Radiation sickness see Radiation
Radioactivity see Radiation, ionizing
Radioisotope, 328
Rat-bite fever see Rats
Rates, 68-74
  nature of, 70
  numerator vs. denominator, 70
  uses of, 69-70, 73-74
Rationalize, 182
Rats, 100, 333-35
Recessive, 19
Regional Medical Programs (Public Law 89-239), 368, 396
Rehabilitation, 6
Relative risk, 79-80
Rem, 328
Remission, 151
Renal disease see Glomerulonephritis

Reservoirs (of infection) see Infectious diseases
Restoration, goal of, 6. See also Prevention.
Retrospective study, 76-79
Rheumatic fever, 7, 103, 121-22
Rheumatic heart disease see Cardiovascular diseases
Rheumatoid arthritis, 179. See also Allergic disorders.
Rh incompatibility, 171
Rhinitis, 149
Rhythm method see Contraception
Riboflavin, 32. See also Vitamins.
Ribonucleic acid see RNA
Rickets, 29, 168. See also Malnutrition; Vitamins.
Rickettsiae, 299
Ringworm, 111
Risk factor, 13
RNA (ribonucleic acid), 16
Roentgen, 328
Rosenstock, Irwin, 407
Rubella, 103-4, 137, 168

Salmonella typhimurium, 303. See also Salmonellosis.
Salmonella typhosa, 300
Salmonellosis, 303
Sample, 74
Sanitation, 40. See also Water treatment.
Scarlet fever, 103
Schistosoma, 296
Schistosomiasis, 67, 111-12, 296-97, 305
Schizophrenia, 213-20, 244
Screening see Mass screening
Scrofula, 119, 188. See also Tuberculosis.
Scurvy, 33. See also Malnutrition; Vitamins.
Self-care, 397
Sepsis, 164
Septicemia, 102
Serologic, 257
Serum, 13
Sewage treatment see Water treatment

Sex, influence on disease occurrence, 68
Sex-linked (chromosome), 23
Shingles, 103
Shock, 100, 101
    anaphylactic, 56, 149
    electric, in mental illness, 194-95
    hypoglycemic, 145
    insulin, in mental illness, 194
Sibling, 16
Sickle cell disease, 17-19, 23
Sign (physical), 2
Skilled nursing care home, 353
Smallpox, 93, 103, 105, 169, 174
Social insurance, 357
Solid wastes, 308
Spasm, 176
Spirillum minus, 333
Spore, 287
Staphylococcal food poisoning, 71, 301, 303
Staphylococcus (i), 58, 71, 90, 98, 102, 172, 301, 303. See also Bacteria.
    carrier state and, 98
    diseases caused by, 102
    neonatal death and, 172
Steroids, 95, 119, 145, 179. See also Cortisone.
Stillbirth, 168
Strabismus see Visual defects
Streptobacillus moniliformis, 333
Streptococcus (i), 7, 90, 103, 120-23, 132, 137, 152, 164, 299
    bacterial endocarditis and, 132
    dental disorders and, 152
    diseases arising from, 120-23
    glomerulonephritis and, 121
    milkborne disease and, 299
    puerperal sepsis and, 164
    rheumatic fever and, 121-22
    rheumatic heart disease and, 122, 137
Streptococcus viridans, 132
Streptomycin see Antibiotics
"Stroke" see Cardiovascular diseases
Sulfonamides see Antibiotics
Sulfur dioxide, 322. See also Air pollution.
Sullivan, Harry Stack, 193

Sunburn, 327
Symbiosis, 88
Symptom, 2
Syndrome, 12
Synergistic, 27
Synthesis, 25
Syphilis, 137, 168, 253-57

Tachycardia, 149
TB see Tuberculosis
Temperature, inversions of, 309
Terminology see Jargon
Tests see Mass screening
Tetanus, 174, 287
Tetanus neonatum, 287
Tetracycline, 58. See also Antibiotics.
Thalidomide, 56, 137
Thiamine, 32. See also Vitamins.
Thiazide, 145
Third-party payers, 345
Thompson, John, 395
Thorazine, 195
Thought disorder, 215
Thromboembolism, 47, 133, 134, 137
Thrombophlebitis see Peripheral vascular disease
Thrush see Candidiasis
Title XIX see Medicare
Toxemia, 165
Toxins, 96, 102, 287
Toxoplasmosis, 168
Trachea, 34
Trachoma, 157
Tranquilizers, 195
Transfer agreements, 368
Transplants see Organ transplants
Treponema pallidum, 12, 253
Trichinosis, 112, 284-86, 334
Trimester, 57
Trisomy, 16. See also Chromosome; Mongolism.
Tubercle bacillus see Mycobacterium tuberculosis; Tuberculosis
Tuberculin skin test see Tuberculosis
Tuberculosis, 71, 98, 116-20, 247, 301
    alcoholism and, 247
    BCG and, 120
    bovine, 119
    INH and, 117

Tuberculosis (*Cont.*)
  measles and, 119
  as a milkborne disease, 301
  mortality, rate in New York City, 116
  poverty and, 118
  recurrence of, 98
  scrofula, 119
  steroids and, 119
  tuberculin skin test and, 119-20
Tuke, William, 190
Tularemia, 305
TV dinners, 301, 302
Typhoid fever, 98, 99, 100-101, 300-301, 305
  carrier state, 98
  transmission of, 99
  water treatment and, 35
Typhus, 98, 107, 111, 297-99

Ulcer, 177
Ulcerative colitis, 68
Unconscious (psychiatric term), 192
United Nations, 48
Urbanization, 123, 301, 347-48
Ureter, 95
Urethra, 95
Utilization (of medical care services) *see* Medical care
Utilization review, 368

Vaccination *see* Immunization; Smallpox
Vaccinia, 150
Valium, 195
Variable, 68
Varicella *see* Chickenpox
Varicose veins *see* Peripheral vascular disease
Vascular, 126
Vas deferens, 46
Vector *see* Infectious diseases
Vector-borne diseases, 288-89
Vehicle *see* Infectious diseases
Venereal, 4
Venereal disease, 100, 250-61
  chancroid, 259
  control of, 259-61

Venereal disease (*Cont.*)
  gonorrhea, 257-59
  granuloma inguinale, 259
  lymphogranuloma venereum, 259
  penicillin and, 257, 258
  screening tests for syphilis, 257
  syphilis, 253-57
Viral diseases *see* Infectious diseases, viral
Virulence, 96
Virus, 13, 93-94
  adenovirus, 103
  coxsackie, 101
  echo, 101
  hepatitis, 101
  influenza, 103
  measles, 93, 103, 119
  mumps, 103
  polio, 93, 101, 168, 174-75
  reovirus, 101
  rhinovirus, 103
  rubella, 103-4
  smallpox, 93, 103, 105, 169, 174
Visual acuity, 155
Visual defects, 154-57
  in the elderly, 179
  maternal rubella and, 168
Vital statistics, 83
Vitamins, 25, 29-33
  A, 29
  B_{12}, 32
  C, 32-33
  D, 29, 299
  folic acid, 32
  K, 33, 88
  niacin, 32
  riboflavin, 32
  thiamine, 32
Voluntary health agencies, 401-2

Waterborne diseases, 304-5
Water pollution, 305-8
  fertilizers and pesticides, 307
  heat and, 306-7
  Lake Erie, 306
  in New York City, 281, 306
  nitrates and phosphates and, 306
  solid wastes and, 308
  sources of, 307-8

Water treatment, 305-6
  biological oxygen demand (BOD), 306
  chlorination, 305
  nitrates and phosphates and, 306
  sand filtration, 305
  sewage and, 306
  sewage vs. sewerage, 305-6
  stages of, 306
Wavelength, **327**
Whooping cough *see* Pertussis
Workmen's Compensation laws, 267, 342

World Health Organization, **1**, 40, 244, 290

X-ray *see* Radiation

Yellow fever, 289-90

Zoonosis, 99, 284-88